**Acute Medicine**

For Esme

# Acute Medicine

A practical guide to the management of medical emergencies

**David Sprigings**

Consultant Physician
Northampton General Hospital
Northampton UK

**John B. Chambers**

Reader and Consultant Cardiologist
Guy's and St Thomas' Hospitals
London UK

FOURTH EDITION

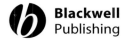
**Blackwell**
Publishing

© 2008 David Sprigings and John B. Chambers
© 1990, 1995, 2001 Blackwell Science Ltd
Published by Blackwell Publishing
Blackwell Publishing, Inc., 350 Main Street, Malden, Massachusetts 02148-5020, USA
Blackwell Publishing Ltd, 9600 Garsington Road, Oxford OX4 2DQ, UK
Blackwell Publishing Asia Pty Ltd, 550 Swanston Street, Carlton, Victoria 3053, Australia

First published 1990
Second edition 1995
Third edition 2001
Fourth edition 2008

1   2008

Library of Congress Cataloging-in-Publication Data

Sprigings, David.
Acute medicine : a practical guide to the management of medical emergencies / David
Sprigings, John B. Chambers. – 4th ed.
p.   ;   cm.
Includes bibliographical references and index.
ISBN 978-1-4051-2962-6
1. Medical emergencies–Handbooks, manuals, etc. I. Chambers, John, MD. II. Title.
[DNLM: 1. Emergency Treatment–methods–Handbooks. 2. Emergencies–
Handbooks. WB 39 S769a 2007]

RC86.8.S68 2007
616.02'5–dc22
2007005512

ISBN: 978-1-4051-2962-6

A catalogue record for this title is available from the British Library

Set in 8 on 11 Frutiger Light by SNP Best-set Typesetter Ltd., Hong Kong
Printed and bound in Singapore by Utopia Press Pte Ltd

Commissioning Editor: Alison Brown
Editorial Assistant: Jennifer Seward
Development Editor: Adam Gilbert
Production Controller: Debbie Wyer

For further information on Blackwell Publishing, visit our website:
http://www.blackwellpublishing.com

# Contents

## Section 2: Specific problems

### Cardiovascular

### Respiratory

### Neurological

## Gastrointestinal/liver/renal

## Endocrine/metabolic

## Dermatology/rheumatology

## Hematology/oncology

## Miscellaneous

# Section 3: Procedures in acute medicine

# Preface

In the 4th edition we have distilled the text to a set of flow diagrams with linked tables. Our aim is to provide the doctor caring for an acutely ill patient with rapid access to key information, including a balanced interpretation of current national and international guidelines.

We have substantially broadened the scope of the book to cover all problems in general medicine likely to be encountered in the emergency department. Integration of the use of echocardiography, which we believe is as important in acute medicine as ECG interpretation, is a particular feature of the text. Our emphasis is on urgent management in the first few hours, but we also give guidance for continuing care.

DCS
JBC
Northampton
January 2007

**ALERT**
Although every effort has been made to ensure that the drug dosages in this book are correct, readers are advised to check the prescribing information in the *British National Formulary* (www.bnf.org) or equivalent.

# Acknowledgments

We are indebted to the following colleagues for expert criticism of sections of the manuscript: Professor John Rees, Professor Tom Treasure, Nicholas Hart, John Klein, Boris Lams, Paul Holmes, Tony Rudd, Mark Wilkinson, David Treacher, Bridget McDonald, Michael Cooklin, Archie Haines, Carole Tallon and Andrew Jeffrey.

We also wish to thank our trainees for their comments on the text, in particular Susie Cary, Richard Haynes and Jim Newton. We are very grateful to Jim Newton for providing the ECGs for illustration.

# Common presentations

# 1 The critically ill patient: assessment and stabilization

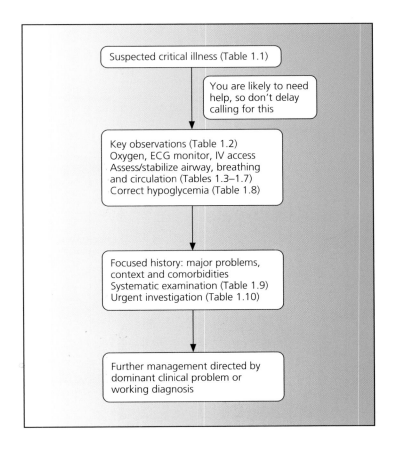

Suspected critical illness (Table 1.1)

You are likely to need help, so don't delay calling for this

Key observations (Table 1.2)
Oxygen, ECG monitor, IV access
Assess/stabilize airway, breathing and circulation (Tables 1.3–1.7)
Correct hypoglycemia (Table 1.8)

Focused history: major problems, context and comorbidities
Systematic examination (Table 1.9)
Urgent investigation (Table 1.10)

Further management directed by dominant clinical problem or working diagnosis

The critically ill patient: assessment and stabilization

MEWS

**TABLE 1.1** Identification of patients with potential critical illness using the Early Warning Score

| Score | 3 | 2 | 1 | 0 | 1 | 2 | 3 |
|---|---|---|---|---|---|---|---|
| Respiratory rate (/min) | | <8 | 8–11 | 12–20 | 21–25 | 26–30 | >30 |
| Arterial oxygen saturation(%) | <85 | 86–89 | 90–94 | >95 | | | |
| Heart rate (/min) | | <40 | 41–50 | 51–100 | 101–110 | 111–130 | >130 |
| Systolic blood pressure (mmHg) | <70 | 71–80 | 81–100 | 101–179 | 180–199 | 200–220 | >220 |
| Temperature (°C) | | <35 | 35.1–36.5 | 36.6–37.4 | >37.5 | | |
| Neurological status | | | New confusion | Alert | Responds to voice | Responds to pain | Unresponsive |

A score of 3 or more suggests potential critical illness and requires immediate assessment. The score is a guide and has not been fully validated.

**TABLE 1.2** Nine key observations in suspected critical illness

| Observation | Signs of critical illness | Action |
| --- | --- | --- |
| **1 Airway** | Evidence of upper airway obstruction | See Table 1.3 and pp. 245–52 for management of the airway |
| **2 Respiratory rate** | Respiratory rate <8 or >30/min | Give oxygen (initially 60–100%) Check arterial oxygen saturation and blood gases (pp. 98–103, 587) See Table 1.5; pp. 104–9 for management of respiratory failure |
| **3 Arterial oxygen saturation** | Arterial oxygen saturation <90% | Give oxygen (initially 60–100% if there are other signs of critical illness) Check arterial blood gases (pp. 587, 98–103) |
| **4 Heart rate** | Heart rate <40 or >130 bpm | Give oxygen 60–100% Connect an ECG monitor and obtain IV access See p. 18 for management of cardiac arrhythmia |
| **5 Blood pressure** | Systolic BP <90 mmHg, or fall in systolic BP by more than 40 mmHg with signs of impaired perfusion | Give oxygen 60–100% Connect an ECG monitor and obtain IV access See p. 53 for management of hypotension/impaired perfusion |

*Continued*

| Observation | Signs of critical illness | Action |
|---|---|---|
| **6 Perfusion** | Signs of reduced organ perfusion: cool/mottled skin with capillary refill time >2 s; agitation/reduced conscious level; oliguria (urine output <30 ml/h) | Give oxygen 60–100% Connect an ECG monitor and obtain IV access See p. 53 for management of hypotension/ impaired perfusion |
| **7 Conscious level** | Reduced conscious level (unresponsive to voice) | Stabilize airway, breathing and circulation Endotracheal intubation if GCS 8 or less Exclude/correct hypoglycemia Give naloxone if opioid poisoning is possible (respiratory rate <12/min, pinpoint pupils) (see Table 11.2) See pp. 118–25 for management of the unconscious patient |
| **8 Temperature** | Core temperature <36 or >38°C, with hypotension, hypoxemia, oliguria or confusional state | See pp. 59–65 for management of sepsis |
| **9 Blood glucose** | Blood glucose <3.5 mmol/l, with signs of hypoglycemia (sweating, tachycardia, abnormal behavior, reduced conscious level or fits) | Give 50 ml of 50% glucose IV via a large vein (or 500 ml of 5% glucose IV over 15–30 min) or glucagon 1 mg IV/IM/SC Recheck blood glucose after 5 min and again after 30 min. See p. 10 |

GCS, Glasgow Coma Scale score (see p. 297).

**TABLE 1.3** Assessment and stabilization of the airway

| | Signs of acute upper airway obstruction | Causes of acute upper airway obstruction | Action if you suspect upper airway obstruction |
|---|---|---|---|
| **Conscious patient** | Respiratory distress* Inspiratory stridor Suprasternal retraction Abnormal voice Coughing/ choking | Foreign body Anaphylaxis Angioedema | Sit the patient up Give high-flow oxygen Call for urgent help from an anesthetist and ENT surgeon |
| **Unconscious patient** | Respiratory arrest Inspiratory stridor Gurgling Grunting/ snoring | Above causes Tongue and soft tissues of oropharynx Inhalation of foreign body, secretions, blood, vomitus | Head-tilt/chin-lift maneuver (p. 249) Remove dentures (if loose) and aspirate the pharynx, larynx and trachea with a suction catheter Call for urgent help from an anesthetist Before intubation, ventilate the patient using a bag-mask device with 100% oxygen |

\* Respiratory distress is shown by dyspnea, tachypnea, ability to speak only in short sentences or single words, agitation and sweating.

**TABLE 1.4** Assessment of breathing

- Conscious level, mental state and speech
- Respiratory rate and pattern
- Arterial oxygen saturation
- Depth and symmetry of chest expansion
- Accessory muscles of respiration active?
- Volume of secretions?
- Tracheal position
- Signs of pleural effusion?
- Signs of pneumothorax?
- Focal/generalized wheeze?
- Focal/generalized crackles?

**ALERT**
Pulse oximetry can give an inaccurate reading of arterial oxygen saturation (see Table 15.3): always check arterial blood gases if in doubt.

**TABLE 1.5** Management of respiratory failure (impaired oxygenation and/or ventilation): general principles

- Maintain patent airway (pp. 245–9)
- Increase inspired oxygen concentration if needed to achieve arterial oxygen saturation >90% (>88% in acute exacerbation of COPD)
- Diagnose and treat underlying cause and contributory factors (see Table 16.3)
- If feasible, sit the patient up to improve diaphragmatic descent and increase tidal volume
- Clear secretions: encourage cough, physiotherapy, aspiration
- Drain large pleural effusion if present
- Drain pneumothorax if present (Table 43.3; p. 619)
- Optimize cardiac output: treat hypotension and heart failure (Table 1.7)
- Consider ventilatory support (p. 108)

COPD, chronic obstructive pulmonary disease.

The critically ill patient: assessment and stabilization

---

**TABLE 1.6** Assessment of the circulation

- Conscious level and mental state
- Heart rate
- Cardiac rhythm by ECG monitor
- Blood pressure
- Skin color, temperature and sweating
- Capillary refill time: squeeze the finger pulp, held at the level of the heart, for 5 s and then release: a capillary refill time of >2 s is abnormal
- Jugular venous pressure
- Auscultation: added heart sounds, murmurs or pericardial rub?
- Major pulses: present and symmetrical?
- Signs of pulmonary and/or peripheral edema?

---

**TABLE 1.7** Management of circulatory failure: general principles

- Stabilize airway and breathing: maintain arterial oxygen saturation >90%
- Correct major arrhythmia (p. 18)
- Fluid resuscitation to correct hypovolemia (e.g. from acute blood loss (pp. 367–9) or severe sepsis (p. 63))
- Consider/exclude tension pneumothorax (p. 282) and cardiac tamponade (p. 216)
- Use inotropic vasopressor agent if there is pulmonary edema, or refractory hypotension despite fluid resuscitation (see Table 9.5)
- Diagnose and treat underlying cause (pp. 53–4, 178–9)
- Correct major metabolic abnormalities (e.g. derangements of electrolytes or blood glucose) (see Table 1.8)

---

**TABLE 1.8** Management of hypoglycemia

**1** If the patient is drowsy or fitting (this may sometimes occur with mild hypoglycemia, especially in young diabetic patients):
- Give 50 ml of 50% glucose IV via a large vein (if not available give 250 ml of 10% glucose over 15–30 min) or glucagon 1 mg IV/IM/SC
- Recheck blood glucose after 5 min and again after 30 min
- In patients with chronic alcohol abuse, there is a remote risk of precipitating Wernicke's encephalopathy by a glucose load; prevent this by giving thiamine 100 mg IV before or shortly after glucose administration

**2** Identify and treat the cause (pp. 423–4)

**3** If hypoglycemia recurs or is likely to recur (e.g. liver disease, sepsis, excess sulfonylurea):
- Start an IV infusion of glucose 10% at 1 litre 12-hourly via a central or large peripheral vein
- Adjust the rate to keep the blood glucose level at 5–10 mmol/L
- After excess sulfonylurea therapy, maintain the glucose infusion for 24 h

**4** If hypoglycemia is only partially responsive to glucose 10% infusion:
- Give glucose 20% IV via a central vein
- If the cause is intentional insulin overdose, consider local excision of the injection site

**TABLE 1.9** Systematic examination of the critically ill patient

| Site | Check list |
|---|---|
| **Central nervous system (pp. 293–302)** | Conscious level and mental state<br>Pupils: size, symmetry, response to light (p. 121)<br>Fundi<br>Lateralized weakness?<br>Tendon reflexes and plantar responses |
| **Head and neck** | Neck stiffness?<br>Jaundice/pallor?<br>Jugular venous pressure<br>Central venous cannula?<br>Mouth, teeth and sinuses<br>Lymphadenopathy? |
| **Chest** | Focal lung crackles/bronchial breathing?<br>Pleural/pericardial rub?<br>Heart murmur?<br>Prosthetic heart valve?<br>Pacemaker/ICD? |
| **Abdomen and pelvis** | Vomiting/diarrhea?<br>Distension?<br>Ascites?<br>Tenderness/guarding?<br>Bladder catheter?<br>Perineal/perianal abscess? |
| **Limbs** | Acute arthritis?<br>Prosthetic joint?<br>Abscess? |
| **Skin** | Cold/flushed/sweating?<br>Rash/purpura?<br>Pressure ulcer/cellulitis?<br>IV cannula/tunneled line? |

ICD, implantable cardioverter-fibrillator.

---

**TABLE 1.10** Investigation of the critically ill patient

**Immediate**
- Arterial blood gases and pH
- ECG
- Blood glucose
- Sodium, potassium and creatinine
- Full blood count

**Urgent**
- Chest X-ray
- Cranial CT if reduced conscious level or focal signs
- Coagulation screen if low platelet count, suspected coagulation disorder, jaundice or purpura
- Biochemical profile
- Amylase if abdominal pain or tenderness
- C-reactive protein
- Blood culture if suspected sepsis
- Urine stick test
- Toxicology screen (serum 10 ml and urine 50 ml) if suspected poisoning

---

## Further reading

Andrews FJ, Nolan JP. Critical care in the emergency department: monitoring the critically ill patient. *Emerg Med J* 2006; 23: 561–4.

Bion JF, Heffner JE. Challenges in the care of the acutely ill. *Lancet* 2004; 363: 970–77.

Reilly B. Physical examination in the care of medical inpatients: an observational study. *Lancet* 2003; 362: 100–5.

# 2 Cardiac arrest

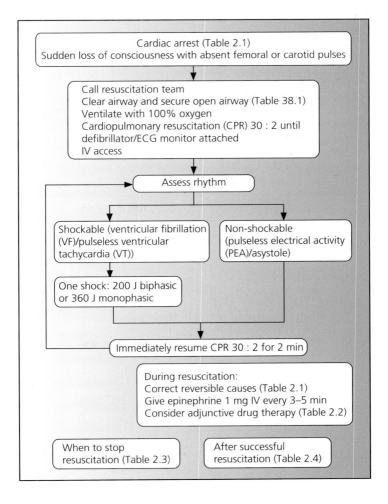

Cardiac arrest (Table 2.1)
Sudden loss of consciousness with absent femoral or carotid pulses

Call resuscitation team
Clear airway and secure open airway (Table 38.1)
Ventilate with 100% oxygen
Cardiopulmonary resuscitation (CPR) 30 : 2 until
defibrillator/ECG monitor attached
IV access

Assess rhythm

Shockable (ventricular fibrillation (VF)/pulseless ventricular tachycardia (VT))

Non-shockable (pulseless electrical activity (PEA)/asystole)

One shock: 200 J biphasic or 360 J monophasic

Immediately resume CPR 30 : 2 for 2 min

During resuscitation:
Correct reversible causes (Table 2.1)
Give epinephrine 1 mg IV every 3–5 min
Consider adjunctive drug therapy (Table 2.2)

When to stop resuscitation (Table 2.3)

After successful resuscitation (Table 2.4)

---

**TABLE 2.1** Causes of cardiac arrest

**With ventricular fibrillation/pulseless ventricular tachycardia**
- Acute coronary syndrome
- Ischemic heart disease with previous myocardial infarction
- Other structural heart disease (e.g. dilated or hypertrophic cardiomyopathy)
- Wolff–Parkinson–White syndrome

**With pulseless electrical activity (PEA) or asystole**
- Hypovolemia
- Hypoxemia
- Hypokalemia/hyperkalemia/hypocalcemia
- Hypothermia
- Toxins (poisoning)
- Tamponade: cardiac
- Tension pneumothorax
- Thromboembolism: pulmonary

---

**ALERT**
Remember the four Hs and four Ts which can cause PEA/asystole.

**ALERT**
Effective basic life support and early defibrillation are the key elements in successful resuscitation.

**TABLE 2.2** Adjunctive drug therapy in cardiopulmonary resuscitation (CPR)

| Drug | Indications | Dose (IV) |
|---|---|---|
| Amiodarone | Shock-refractory VF/VT (persisting after third shock) | 300 mg, diluted in 5% glucose to a volume of 20 ml, or from a prefilled syringe, via a central vein or large peripheral vein, followed by saline flush |
| | Hemodynamically stable VT | See Table 4.2 |
| Atropine | PEA with a rate <60/min Sinus or junctional bradycardia with unstable hemodynamic state | 3 mg bolus |
| Bicarbonate | PEA caused by hyperkalemia, tricyclic poisoning or severe metabolic acidosis | 50 ml of 8.4% sodium bicarbonate (50 mmol) |
| Calcium | PEA caused by hyperkalemia, hypocalcemia, poisoning with calcium-channel blocker | 10 ml of 10% calcium chloride (p. 450, 456) |
| Epinephrine | To augment myocardial and cerebral perfusion during CPR Treatment of anaphylactic shock | 1 mg, repeated every 3–5 min until spontaneous circulation restored See p. 519 |
| Thrombolytic | Proven or suspected pulmonary embolism | Alteplase 100 mg over 2 h (p. 230) |

PEA, pulseless electrical activity; VF, ventricular fibrillation; VT, ventricular tachycardia.

Cardiac arrest

---

**TABLE 2.3** When to stop cardiopulmonary resuscitation

- Resuscitation *should be stopped* if a 'Do not attempt resuscitation' (DNAR) order has been written, or the circumstances of the patient indicate that one should have been
- Resuscitation *should be stopped* if there is refractory asystole for more than 20 min (except when cardiac arrest is due to hypothermia)
- Resuscitation *should not be stopped* while the rhythm is ventricular fibrillation

---

**TABLE 2.4** What to do after successful resuscitation

| Aim | Action |
|---|---|
| **Stabilize airway and breathing** | Maintain clear airway, with placement of endotracheal tube if indicated (pp. 245–52)<br>Give oxygen 100%<br>Check arterial blood gases and pH<br>Consider mechanical ventilation if there is coma (GCS 8 or below) or pulmonary edema<br>Insert a nasogastric tube to decompress the stomach (gastric distension causes splinting of diaphragm) if there is coma<br>Obtain a chest X-ray to check position of endotracheal tube and central venous cannula, and exclude pneumothorax |
| **Stabilize the circulation** | Continuous ECG monitoring and 12-lead ECG<br>If there is evidence of ST elevation acute coronary syndrome, consider revascularization by thrombolysis or PCI (Table 25.2)<br>If cardiac arrest was due to primary brady-asystole, put in a temporary pacing lead (p. 600)<br>Postresuscitation myocardial dysfunction (lasting 24–48 h) may result in hypotension and low cardiac output, requiring inotropic vasopressor support (p. 58) |

*Continued*

| Aim | Action |
|---|---|
| **Protect the brain** | Control seizures (p. 350)<br>Treat hyperthermia by fanning, tepid sponging or paracetamol (Rectal/iv)<br>Control blood glucose (p. 10; Table 67.5)<br>If there is coma, consider induced hypothermia (32–34°C for at least 12–24h, using chilled saline infusion) |
| **Establish cause of arrest** | Establish cause of arrest by clinical assessment, ECG, echocardiography, blood tests<br>Seek expert advice on management to prevent recurrence |
| **Maintain normal plasma potassium** | Correct hypokalemia and hyperkalemia (aim for plasma potassium 4–4.5 mmol/L) (pp. 447, 450) |
| **Prevent sepsis** | IV lines inserted without sterile technique during the resuscitation should be changed |

GCS, Glasgow Coma Scale; PCI, percutaneous coronary intervention.

## Further reading

American Heart Association. Guidelines for cardiopulmonary resuscitation and emergency cardiovascular care (2005). *Circulation* website (http://circ.ahajournals.org/content/vol112/24_suppl/).

European Resuscitation Council. Guidelines for resuscitation (2005). European Resuscitation Council website (http://www.erc.edu/index.php/mainpage/en/).

Weisfeldt ML, Becker LB. Resuscitation after cardiac arrest: a 3-phase time-sensitive model. *JAMA* 2002; 288: 3035–38.

# 3 Cardiac arrhythmias: general approach

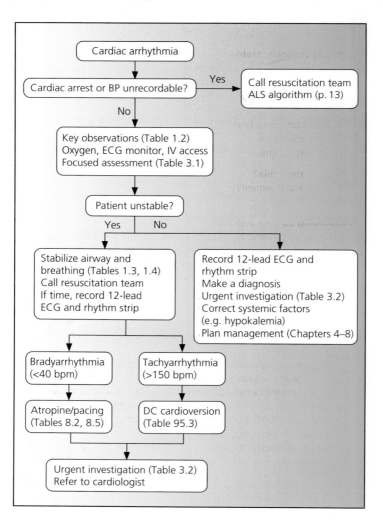

**TABLE 3.1** Focused assessment of the patient with an arrhythmia

**Symptoms?**
- Of arrhythmia (palpitation, presyncope, syncope)
- Of underlying cardiac disease (chest pain, breathlessness)

**Hemodynamically stable?** Signs of instability are:
- Heart rate <40/min or >200/min
- Pauses >3 s
- Systolic BP <90 mmHg
- Syncope
- Reduced conscious level
- Anginal chest pain
- Pulmonary edema

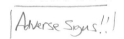
Adverse Signs!!

**Known arrhythmia?**
- Previous management?
- Current therapy?

**Underlying cardiac disease?**
- Evidence of ischemic heart disease (e.g. history, Q waves on ECG)?
  - This makes ventricular tachycardia almost certainly the diagnosis if there is a regular broad complex tachycardia
  - Flecainide should be avoided for cardioversion or prevention of atrial fibrillation because of the risk of precipitating ventricular arrhythmias
- Could LV systolic function be significantly impaired (e.g. exertional breathlessness, large cardiac shadow on chest X-ray, previous echocardiography)?
  - If so, avoid high-dose beta-blockers and flecainide
- Is there Wolff–Parkinson–White syndrome? This may cause:
  - AV re-entrant tachycardia (narrow complex, regular) (conduction forward through the AV node and back via the accessory pathway)
  - Fast conduction of atrial fibrillation down the accessory pathway (broad complex, irregular)
  - Rarely, antidromic tachycardia (broad complex, regular) (conduction forward down the accessory pathway and back via the AV node)

*Continued*

**Associated acute or chronic illness?**
- Atrial fibrillation commonly complicates pneumonia and other infection
- Electrolyte disorders (especially of potassium) should be excluded/corrected

AV, atrioventricular; LV, left ventricular.

**TABLE 3.2** Urgent investigation of the patient with an arrhythmia

- 12-lead ECG and rhythm strip during the arrhythmia and after resolution (Q waves, QT interval, delta wave, evidence of LV hypertrophy?)
- Electrolytes (especially potassium and, if on diuretic, magnesium) and creatinine
- Blood glucose
- Thyroid function (for later analysis)
- Plasma digoxin level (if taking digoxin)
- Plasma troponin
- Chest X-ray (heart size, evidence of raised left atrial pressure, coexistent pathology, e.g. pneumonia?)
- Echocardiogram (for LV function, RV function, valve disease)

LV, left ventricular; RV, right ventricular.

## Further reading
See the Resuscitation Council (UK) website on management of periarrest arrhythmias (http://www.resus.org.uk/pages/periarst.pdf).

# 4 Broad complex regular tachycardia

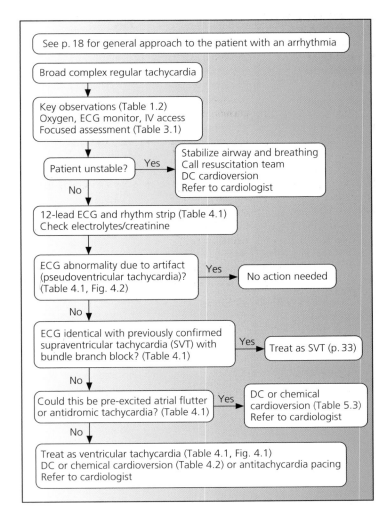

See p. 18 for general approach to the patient with an arrhythmia

Broad complex regular tachycardia

↓

Key observations (Table 1.2)
Oxygen, ECG monitor, IV access
Focused assessment (Table 3.1)

↓

Patient unstable? —Yes→ Stabilize airway and breathing
Call resuscitation team
DC cardioversion
Refer to cardiologist

No ↓

12-lead ECG and rhythm strip (Table 4.1)
Check electrolytes/creatinine

↓

ECG abnormality due to artifact
(pseudoventricular tachycardia)?
(Table 4.1, Fig. 4.2) —Yes→ No action needed

No ↓

ECG identical with previously confirmed
supraventricular tachycardia (SVT) with
bundle branch block? (Table 4.1) —Yes→ Treat as SVT (p. 33)

No ↓

Could this be pre-excited atrial flutter
or antidromic tachycardia? (Table 4.1) —Yes→ DC or chemical
cardioversion (Table 5.3)
Refer to cardiologist

No ↓

Treat as ventricular tachycardia (Table 4.1, Fig. 4.1)
DC or chemical cardioversion (Table 4.2) or antitachycardia pacing
Refer to cardiologist

**TABLE 4.1** Broad complex regular tachycardia: differential diagnosis and management

| Arrhythmia | Comment | Management |
|---|---|---|
| **Monomorphic ventricular tachycardia (Fig. 4.1)** | Commonest cause and should be the default diagnosis (especially if there is a history of previous myocardial infarction or other structural heart disease) Restore sinus rhythm as soon as possible, even in hemodynamically stable patients, as sudden deterioration may occur | DC cardioversion (p. 617) if there is hemodynamic instability or other measures are ineffective In stable patient, DC cardioversion, IV antiarrhythmic therapy (Table 4.2), or antitachycardia pacing Refer to a cardiologist |
| **Supraventricular tachycardia (SVT) with bundle branch block** | Confirm with adenosine test (Table 6.3) | DC cardioversion (p. 617) if there is hemodynamic instability or other measures are ineffective In stable patient, IV adenosine, verapamil or beta-blocker (Table 6.3) Record 12-lead ECG after sinus rhythm restored to check for pre-excitation (WPW syndrome) |

*Continued*

| Arrhythmia | Comment | Management |
|---|---|---|
| | | Refer to a cardiologist if episodes are frequent or severe or if pre-excitation is found |
| **Antidromic tachycardia or atrial flutter WPW syndrome** | These are rarely seen but should be considered in a young patient with known WPW syndrome who does not have structural heart disease | DC cardioversion Refer to a cardiologist |
| **Pseudoventricular tachycardia (Fig. 4.2)** | Caused by body movement and intermittent skin–electrode contact ('toothbrush tachycardia') No hemodynamic change during apparent ventricular arrhythmia | No action needed The importance of recognition is to prevent misdiagnosis as ventricular tachycardia |

WPW, Wolff–Parkinson–White.

*Broad complex regular tachycardia*

## Further reading

American College of Cardiology, American Heart Association and European Society of Cardiology. Guidelines for the management of patients with ventricular arrhythmias and the prevention of sudden cardiac death (2006). American College of Cardiology website (http://www.acc.org/qualityandscience/clinical/topic/topic.htm).

concordance !!

**Broad complex regular tachycardia**

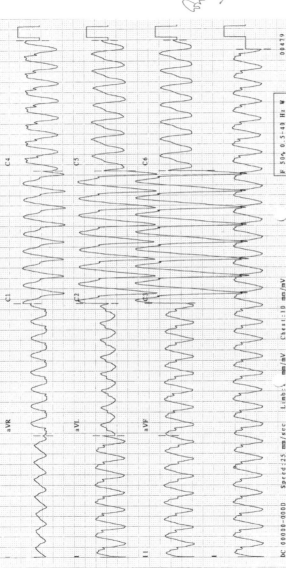

**FIGURE 4.1** Monomorphic ventricular tachycardia (VT). VT is almost certain if there is a broad complex tachycardia with structural heart disease (e.g. myocardial infarction). ECG features of VT (e.g. ventriculo-atrial dissociation, capture or fusion beats and QRS concordance) are specific but not often seen.

**Broad complex regular tachycardia**

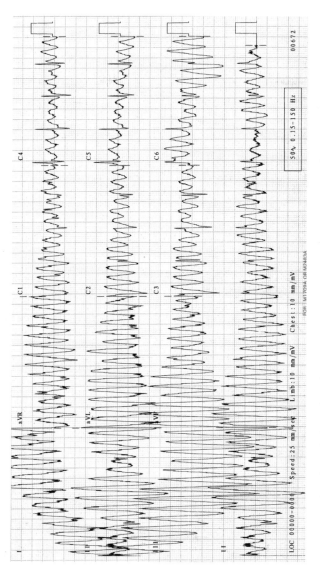

FIGURE 4.2 Pseudoventricular tachycardia. There are native QRS complexes at the cycle length of the baseline rhythm within the artifact, best seen in C4 and C5.

**TABLE 4.2** Drug therapy of hemodynamically stable monomorphic ventricular tachycardia

| Drug | Comment | Dose (IV) |
|------|---------|-----------|
| **Amiodarone** | Efficacy in converting VT uncertain<br>Major role is in suppression of recurrent episodes<br>Needs to be given via central vein to avoid thrombophlebitis | Loading: 300 mg, diluted in 5% glucose to a volume of 20–50 ml, infused over 20 min via a central vein<br>Maintenance: 900–1200 mg over 24 h<br>Supplementary doses of 150 mg can be given as necessary every 10 min for recurrent or resistant VT to a maximum total daily dose of 2.2 g |
| **Procainamide** | Converts ~70%<br>May cause hypotension | Loading: 10 mg/kg at 100 mg/min<br>Maintenance: 1–4 mg/min, diluted in 5% glucose or normal saline (reduce dose in renal failure) |
| **Sotalol** | Converts ~70%<br>May cause hypotension and bradycardia<br>Contraindicated in severe asthma | Loading: 1 mg/kg over 10 min<br>Maintenance: 10 mg/min |
| **Lidocaine** | Converts ~30%<br>Appropriate when VT is due to myocardial ischemia or infarction<br>May cause hypotension and neurological side effects | Loading: 1.5 mg/kg over 2 min<br>Maintenance: 1–4 mg/min |

VT, ventricular tachycardia.

# 5 Broad complex irregular tachycardia

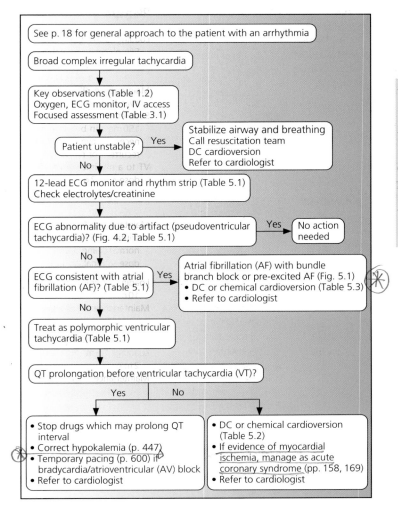

See p. 18 for general approach to the patient with an arrhythmia

Broad complex irregular tachycardia

Key observations (Table 1.2)
Oxygen, ECG monitor, IV access
Focused assessment (Table 3.1)

Patient unstable? — Yes → Stabilize airway and breathing
Call resuscitation team
DC cardioversion
Refer to cardiologist

No

12-lead ECG monitor and rhythm strip (Table 5.1)
Check electrolytes/creatinine

ECG abnormality due to artifact (pseudoventricular tachycardia)? (Fig. 4.2, Table 5.1) — Yes → No action needed

No

ECG consistent with atrial fibrillation (AF)? (Table 5.1) — Yes → Atrial fibrillation (AF) with bundle branch block or pre-excited AF (Fig. 5.1)
• DC or chemical cardioversion (Table 5.3)
• Refer to cardiologist

No

Treat as polymorphic ventricular tachycardia (Table 5.1)

QT prolongation before ventricular tachycardia (VT)?

Yes / No

• Stop drugs which may prolong QT interval
• Correct hypokalemia (p. 447)
• Temporary pacing (p. 600) if bradycardia/atrioventricular (AV) block
• Refer to cardiologist

• DC or chemical cardioversion (Table 5.2)
• If evidence of myocardial ischemia, manage as acute coronary syndrome (pp. 158, 169)
• Refer to cardiologist

**TABLE 5.1** Broad complex irregular tachycardia: differential diagnosis and management

| Arrhythmia | Comment | Management |
|---|---|---|
| **Atrial fibrillation with bundle branch block (Fig. 5.1)** | Difference between maximum and minimum instantaneous heart rates, calculated from the shortest and longest RR intervals is usually >30 bpm, with QRS showing typical LBBB or RBBB morphology | DC cardioversion (p. 617) if there is hemodynamic instability or other measures are ineffective In stable patient, DC cardioversion or antiarrhythmic therapy (see Chapter 7) |
| **Polymorphic ventricular tachycardia (Fig. 5.2)** | | |
| With preceding QT prolongation ('torsade de pointes') | Usually due to therapy with antiarrhythmic and other drugs which prolong the QT interval (e.g. amiodarone, sotalol, erythromycin, psychotropic drugs), especially in patients with hypokalemia and/or bradycardia | DC cardioversion (p. 617) if there is hemodynamic instability or other measures are ineffective Stop drugs which may prolong QT interval Correct hypokalemia (target potassium 4.5–5 mmol/l) If there is bradycardia/AV block, use temporary pacing at 90/min (p. 600) |

*Continued*

| Arrhythmia | Comment | Management |
|---|---|---|
| | Other causes are advanced conduction system disease with AV block and the congenital long QT syndromes | If due to long QT syndrome, give magnesium sulfate 2 g IV bolus over 2–3 min, repeated if necessary, and followed by an infusion of 2–8 mg/min Refer to a cardiologist |
| Without preceding QT prolongation | Usually due to myocardial ischemia in the setting of acute coronary syndrome Other causes include acute myocarditis, cardiomyopathies (e.g. arrhythmogenic right ventricular cardiomyopathy) and Brugada syndrome (VT/VF with RBBB and precordial ST elevation) | DC cardioversion (p. 617) if there is hemodynamic instability or other measures are ineffective In stable patient, DC cardioversion or antiarrhythmic therapy with IV amiodarone or beta-blocker (Table 5.2) Manage as acute coronary syndrome (p. 169) with urgent coronary angiography and revascularization if ischemia is suspected or cannot be excluded Refer to a cardiologist *Continued* |

Broad complex irregular tachycardia

| Arrhythmia | Comment | Management |
|---|---|---|
| **Pre-excited atrial fibrillation (AF) in WPW syndrome (Fig. 5.1)** | AF conducted predominantly over accessory pathway<br>Ventricular rate typically 200–300/min<br>QRS morphology similar to delta wave during sinus rhythm | DC cardioversion (p. 617) if there is hemodynamic instability or other measures are ineffective<br>In stable patient, DC cardioversion or antiarrhythmic therapy with sotalol, flecainide or amiodarone (Tables 5.2 and 5.3)<br>Refer to a cardiologist |
| **Pseudoventricular tachycardia (Fig. 4.2)** | Caused by body movement and intermittent skin–electrode contact ('toothbrush tachycardia')<br>No hemodynamic change during apparent ventricular arrhythmia | No action needed<br>The importance of recognition is to prevent misdiagnosis as VT |

AV, atrioventricular; LBBB, left bundle branch block; RBBB, right bundle branch block; VF, ventricular fibrillation; VT, ventricular tachycardia; WPW, Wolff–Parkinson–White.

**TABLE 5.2** Drug therapy of hemodynamically stable polymorphic ventricular tachycardia (VT) without preceding QT prolongation

| Drug | Comment | Dose (IV) |
|------|---------|-----------|
| **Amiodarone** | Needs to be given via central vein to avoid thrombophlebitis | Loading: 300 mg, diluted in 5% glucose to a volume of 20–50 ml, infused over 20 min via a central vein<br>Maintenance: 900–1200 mg over 24 h<br>Supplementary doses of 150 mg can be given as necessary every 10 min for recurrent or resistant VT to a maximum total daily dose of 2.2 g |
| **Sotalol** | May cause hypotension and bradycardia | Loading: 1 mg/kg over 10 min<br>Maintenance: 10 mg/min |

**TABLE 5.3** Drug therapy of hemodynamically stable pre-excited atrial fibrillation

| Drug | Comment | Dose (IV) |
|------|---------|-----------|
| **Flecainide** | May cause hypotension<br>Avoid if known structural heart disease | 2 mg/kg (to a maximum of 150 mg) over 20 min |
| **Amiodarone** | Needs to be given via central vein to avoid thrombophlebitis | 300 mg, diluted in 5% glucose to a volume of 50 ml, infused over 20 min via a central vein |

Broad complex irregular tachycardia

## Further reading

Knight BP, et al. Clinical consequences of electrocardiographic artefact mimicking ventricular tachycardia. *N Engl J Med* 1999; 341: 1270–4.

Roden DM. Drug-induced prolongation of the QT interval. *N Engl J Med* 2004; 350: 1013–22.

Yap YG, Camm AJ. Drug induced QT prolongation and torsades de pointes. *Heart* 2003; 1363–72.

Broad complex irregular tachycardia

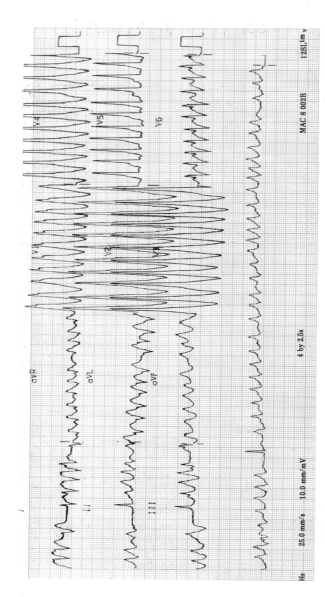

**FIGURE 5.1** Pre-excited atrial fibrillation in Wolff–Parkinson–White syndrome. Despite irregularity of the RR interval over the whole trace, some sections (e.g. $V_{1-6}$) look regular. By contrast, in atrial flutter the tachycardia is usually regular and in antidromic tachycardia, it is reproducibly regular.

# 6 Narrow complex tachycardia

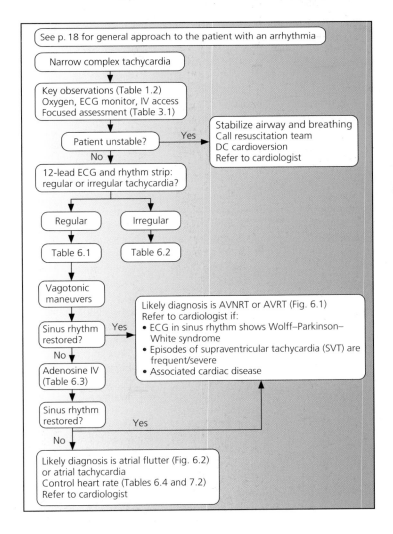

See p. 18 for general approach to the patient with an arrhythmia

Narrow complex tachycardia

Key observations (Table 1.2)
Oxygen, ECG monitor, IV access
Focused assessment (Table 3.1)

Patient unstable? — Yes → Stabilize airway and breathing
Call resuscitation team
DC cardioversion
Refer to cardiologist

No ↓

12-lead ECG and rhythm strip:
regular or irregular tachycardia?

Regular | Irregular

Table 6.1 | Table 6.2

Vagotonic maneuvers

Sinus rhythm restored? — Yes →

Likely diagnosis is AVNRT or AVRT (Fig. 6.1)
Refer to cardiologist if:
• ECG in sinus rhythm shows Wolff–Parkinson–White syndrome
• Episodes of supraventricular tachycardia (SVT) are frequent/severe
• Associated cardiac disease

No ↓

Adenosine IV (Table 6.3)

Sinus rhythm restored? — Yes →

No ↓

Likely diagnosis is atrial flutter (Fig. 6.2)
or atrial tachycardia
Control heart rate (Tables 6.4 and 7.2)
Refer to cardiologist

Narrow complex tachycardia

**TABLE 6.1** Differential diagnosis of narrow complex regular tachycardia

| Arrhythmia | Comment | Management |
|---|---|---|
| Sinus tachycardia | May sometimes be difficult to distinguish from other causes of tachycardia<br>Adenosine causes gradual deceleration of sinus rate followed by acceleration, with or without AV block | Identify and treat the underlying cause<br>Adenosine test (Table 6.3) may be appropriate to exclude other causes of narrow-complex regular tachycardia if in doubt |
| AV nodal re-entrant tachycardia (AVNRT) | The commonest cause of paroxysmal SVT<br>Typically presents in teenagers or young adults with no underlying cardiac disease<br>Retrograde P wave usually hidden within or inscribed at the end of the QRS complex (simulating S wave in inferior leads, partial RBBB in V1)<br>Heart rate usually 140–200 bpm | DC cardioversion (p. 617) if there is hemodynamic instability or other measures are ineffective<br>In stable patient try vagotonic maneuvers. If these fail, use IV adenosine, or verapamil if adenosine is not tolerated or is contraindicated (Table 6.3) Record 12-lead ECG after sinus rhythm restored to check for pre-excitation (WPW syndrome) |

*Continued*

| Arrhythmia | Comment | Management |
|---|---|---|
| | | Refer to cardiologist if episodes are frequent or severe or if pre-excitation is found |
| **AV re-entrant tachycardia involving accessory pathway (AVRT) (Fig. 6.1)** | Typically presents in teenagers or young adults with no underlying cardiac disease<br>Retrograde P wave may be seen between QRS complex in inferior leads, inscribed on T wave<br>Heart rate usually 140–230 bpm | DC cardioversion (p. 617) if there is hemodynamic instability or other measures are ineffective<br>In stable patient try vagotonic maneuvers. If these fail, use IV adenosine, or verapamil if adenosine is not tolerated or is contraindicated (Table 6.3)<br>Record 12-lead ECG after sinus rhythm restored to check for pre-excitation (WPW syndrome)<br>Refer to cardiologist if episodes are frequent or severe or if pre-excitation is found |

*Continued*

Narrow complex tachycardia

**ALERT**
AVRT and AVNRT may be impossible to distinguish from the surface ECG.

| Arrhythmia | Comment | Management |
|---|---|---|
| **Atrial flutter (Fig. 6.2)** | Suspect atrial flutter with 2 : 1 block when the rate is 150 bpm<br>Often associated with structural heart disease<br>Vagotonic maneuvers and adenosine slow the ventricular rate to reveal flutter waves | See Chapter 7<br>DC cardioversion (p. 617) if there is hemodynamic instability or other measures are ineffective<br>In stable patient, aim for rate control with AV node-blocking drugs (Table 6.4)<br>Discuss further management with a cardiologist |
| **Atrial tachycardia** | Caused by discrete focus of electrical activity<br>P wave usually of abnormal morphology, at a rate 130-300/min, conducted with varying degree of AV block<br>May be associated with structural heart disease in older patients | DC cardioversion (p. 617) if there is hemodynamic instability or other measures are ineffective<br>In stable patient, aim for rate control with AV node-blocking drugs (Table 6.4)<br>Discuss further management with a cardiologist |

AV, atrioventricular; RBBB, right bundle branch block; SVT, supraventricular tachycardia; WPW, Wolff–Parkinson–White

**ALERT**
Artial flutter and atrial tachycardia may be irregular if there is variable AV conduction.

**TABLE 6.2** Differential diagnosis of narrow complex irregular tachycardia

| Arrhythmia | Comment | Management |
|---|---|---|
| **Atrial fibrillation** | Difference between maximum and minimum instantaneous heart rates, calculated from the shortest and longest RR intervals is usually >30 bpm<br>No organized atrial activity evident: fibrillation waves of varying amplitude may be seen | See Chapter 7 |
| **Atrial flutter with variable AV conduction** | Often associated with structural heart disease<br>Vagotonic maneuvers and adenosine slow the ventricular rate to reveal flutter waves ('saw-tooth' flutter waves in inferior limb leads and V1) | See Chapter 7<br>DC cardioversion (p. 617) if there is hemodynamic instability or other measures are ineffective<br>In stable patient, aim for rate control with AV node-blocking drugs (Table 6.4) Discuss further management with a cardiologist |
| **Multifocal atrial tachycardia** | Irregular tachycardia, typically 100–130 bpm, with P waves of three or more morphologies and irregular PP interval<br>Most commonly seen in COPD | Treatment is directed at the underlying disorder and correction of hypoxia/hypercapnia<br>Consider verapamil if the heart rate is consistently over 110 bpm<br>DC cardioversion is ineffective |

AV, arterioventricular; COPD, chronic obstructive pulmonary disease.

Narrow complex tachycardia

**TABLE 6.3** Intravenous therapy to terminate supraventricular tachycardia (AV nodal re-entrant tachycardia and AV re-entrant tachycardia)

| Drug | Comment | Dose |
|---|---|---|
| **Adenosine** | May cause facial flushing, chest pain, hypotension, bronchospasm<br>May cause brief asystole, atrial fibrillation and non-sustained ventricular tachycardia<br>Use with caution in patients with severe airways disease<br>Contraindicated in patients with heart transplant | 6 mg IV bolus, followed by saline flush. Repeat as necessary, if no response within 2 min, with 12, 18 and 24 mg boluses |
| **Verapamil** | May cause hypotension<br>Contraindicated in patients taking beta-blockers or in heart failure | 5 mg IV over 5 min, to maximum dose of 15 mg |
| **Esmolol** | Short-acting (half-life 8 min) beta-1 selective beta-blocker | 500 µg/kg over 1 min, followed by 200 µg/kg over 4 min |
| **Metoprolol** | May cause hypotension | 5 mg IV over 5 min, to maximum dose of 15 mg |

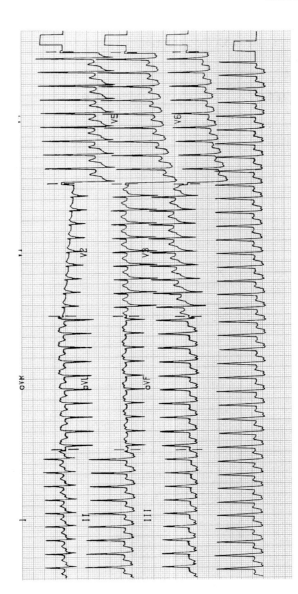

**FIGURE 6.1** Paroxysmal supraventricular tachycardia, in this case due to AV re-entrant tachycardia.

Narrow complex tachycardia

Narrow complex tachycardia

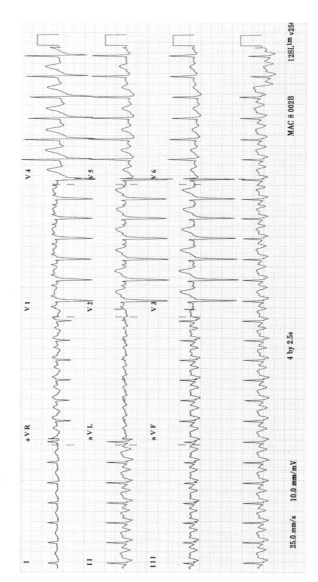

**FIGURE 6.2** Atrial flutter with 2:1 block.

**TABLE 6.4** Intravenous therapy for rate control in atrial fibrillation, atrial flutter and atrial tachycardia

| Drug | Comment | Dose (IV) |
| --- | --- | --- |
| **Esmolol** | Short-acting (half-life 8 min) beta-1 selective beta-blocker | 500 µg/kg over 1 min, followed by 200 µg/kg over 4 min |
| **Metoprolol** | May cause hypotension | 5 mg over 5 min, to maximum dose of 15 mg |
| **Solatol** | May cause hypotension | 1 mg/kg over 10 min |
| **Verapamil** | May cause hypotension Contraindicated in patients taking beta-blockers or in heart failure | 5 mg over 5 min, to maximum dose of 15 mg |
| **Digoxin** | Use if there is heart failure | 500–1000 µg in 50 ml saline over 1 h |
| **Amiodarone** | May be combined with digoxin for rate control in hemodynamically unstable patients | Loading: 300 mg, diluted in 5% glucose to a volume of 20–50 ml, infused over 20 min via a central vein Maintenance: 900–1200 mg over 24 h |

Narrow complex tachycardia

## Further reading

American College of Cardiology, American Heart Association and European Society of Cardiology. Guidelines for the management of patients with supraventricular arrhythmias (2003). American College of Cardiology website (http://www.acc.org/qualityandscience/clinical/topic/topic.htm).

Delacretaz E. Supraventricular tachycardia. *N Engl J Med* 2006; 354: 1039–51.

# 7 Atrial fibrillation and flutter

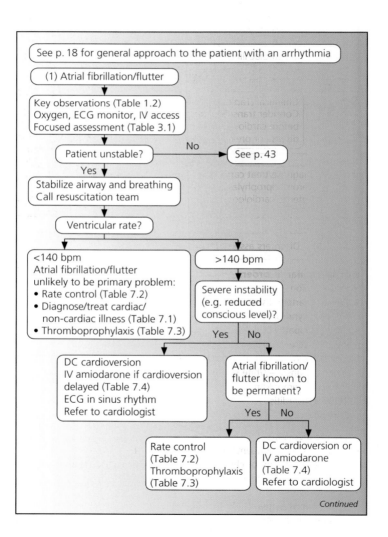

See p. 18 for general approach to the patient with an arrhythmia

(1) Atrial fibrillation/flutter

Key observations (Table 1.2)
Oxygen, ECG monitor, IV access
Focused assessment (Table 3.1)

Patient unstable? — No → See p. 43

Yes ↓

Stabilize airway and breathing
Call resuscitation team

Ventricular rate?

**<140 bpm**
Atrial fibrillation/flutter
unlikely to be primary problem:
• Rate control (Table 7.2)
• Diagnose/treat cardiac/
  non-cardiac illness (Table 7.1)
• Thromboprophylaxis (Table 7.3)

**>140 bpm**

Severe instability
(e.g. reduced
conscious level)?

Yes | No

DC cardioversion
IV amiodarone if cardioversion
delayed (Table 7.4)
ECG in sinus rhythm
Refer to cardiologist

Atrial fibrillation/
flutter known to
be permanent?

Yes | No

Rate control
(Table 7.2)
Thromboprophylaxis
(Table 7.3)

DC cardioversion or
IV amiodarone
(Table 7.4)
Refer to cardiologist

*Continued*

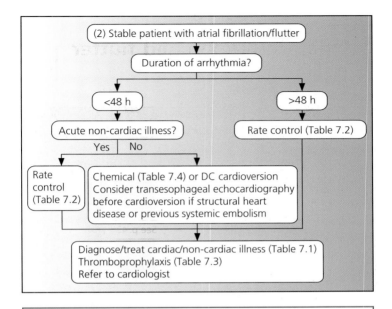

**TABLE 7.1** Disorders associated with atrial fibrillation

**Cardiovascular disorders**
- Hypertension
- Coronary artery disease: previous myocardial infarction or acute coronary syndrome
- Cardiomyopathy
- Valve disease
- Any cause of congestive heart failure
- Wolff–Parkinson–White syndrome
- Pulmonary embolism
- Acute pericarditis
- Cardiac surgery

**Systemic disorders**
- Sepsis, especially pneumonia
- Acute exacerbation of chronic obstructive pulmonary disease
- Excessive alcohol intake
- Thyrotoxicosis
- Severe hypokalemia
- Non-cardiac surgery

**Atrial fibrillation and flutter**

**TABLE 7.2** Rate control in atrial fibrillation and flutter

| Drug | Comment | Dose (IV) | Dose (oral) |
|------|---------|-----------|-------------|
| Esmolol | Short-acting (half-life 2–9 min) beta-1 selective beta-blocker | 500 µg/kg over 1 min, followed by 200 µg/kg over 4 min | Not available |
| Metoprolol | May cause hypotension | 5 mg over 5 min, to maximum dose of 15 mg | 25–100 mg 12-hourly |
| Verapamil | May cause hypotension. Contraindicated in patients taking beta-blockers or in heart failure | 5 mg over 5 min, to maximum dose of 15 mg | 40–80 mg 8-hourly |
| Digoxin | Use if there is heart failure. Verapamil and amiodarone increase plasma digoxin level | 500–1000 µg in 50 ml saline over 1 h | Maintenance dose 62.5–250 µg daily, according to renal function/age |
| Amiodarone | May be combined with digoxin for rate control in hemodynamically unstable patients | Loading: 300 mg, diluted in 5% glucose to a volume of 20–50 ml, infused over 20 min via a central vein. Maintenance: 900–1200 mg over 24 h | 200 mg 8-hourly for one week, then 200 mg 12-hourly for one week, then 200 mg daily |

**TABLE 7.3** Thromboprophylaxis in atrial fibrillation

| | Thromboembolic risk | | |
| --- | --- | --- | --- |
| | **Low** | **Moderate** | **High** |
| **Defining features** | Age <65 years with no moderate or high risk factors | Age >65 years with no high risk factors<br>or<br>Age <75 years with hypertension, diabetes, coronary artery disease or peripheral artery disease | Previous ischemic stroke, TIA or thromboembolic event<br>or,<br>Age >75 years with hypertension diabetes, coronary artery disease or peripheral artery disease<br>or<br>Clinical evidence of valve disease or heart failure, or impaired LV systolic function on echocardiography |
| **Thromboprophylaxis** | Aspirin 75–300 mg daily if no contraindications | Warfarin or aspirin | Warfarin, target INR 2.5 (range 2.0–3.0)<br>Aspirin if warfarin contraindicated |

INR, international normalized ratio; LV, left ventricular; TIA, transient ischemic attack.

**Atrial fibrillation and flutter**

**TABLE 7.4** Drug therapy of atrial fibrillation or flutter: medication to restore sinus rhythm (chemical cardioversion)

| Drug | Comment | Dose |
|------|---------|------|
| **Flecainide** | May cause hypotension Avoid if known/possible structural or coronary heart disease | IV 2 mg/kg (to a maximum of 150 mg) over 10–30 min *or* PO 200–300 mg stat |
| **Amiodarone** | Needs to be given via central vein to avoid thrombophlebitis | IV 300 mg, diluted in 5% glucose to a volume of 20–50 ml, infused over 20 min via a central vein |
| **Sotalol** | May cause hypotension and bradycardia Contraindicated in severe asthma | IV 1 mg/kg over 10 min |

## Further reading

American College of Cardiology, American Heart Association and European Society of Cardiology. Guidelines for the management of patients with atrial fibrillation (2006). American College of Cardiology website (http://www.acc.org/qualityandscience/clinical/topic/topic.htm).

National Institute for Health and Clinical Excellence (NICE). Guidelines for the management of atrial fibrillation (2006). NICE website (http://www.nice.org.uk/guidance).

Peters NS, et al. Atrial fibrillation: strategies to control, combat, and cure. *Lancet* 2002; 359: 593–603.

Wellens HHJ. Contemporary management of atrial flutter. *Circulation* 2002; 106: 649–52.

# 8 Bradycardia and atrioventricular block

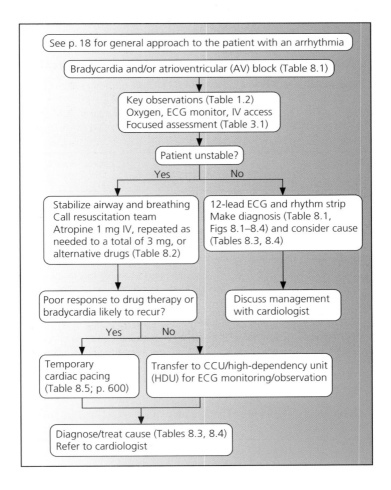

See p. 18 for general approach to the patient with an arrhythmia

Bradycardia and/or atrioventricular (AV) block (Table 8.1)

Key observations (Table 1.2)
Oxygen, ECG monitor, IV access
Focused assessment (Table 3.1)

Patient unstable?

Yes      No

**Yes:**
Stabilize airway and breathing
Call resuscitation team
Atropine 1 mg IV, repeated as
needed to a total of 3 mg, or
alternative drugs (Table 8.2)

**No:**
12-lead ECG and rhythm strip
Make diagnosis (Table 8.1,
Figs 8.1–8.4) and consider cause
(Tables 8.3, 8.4)

Poor response to drug therapy or
bradycardia likely to recur?

Yes      No

Discuss management
with cardiologist

Temporary
cardiac pacing
(Table 8.5; p. 600)

Transfer to CCU/high-dependency unit
(HDU) for ECG monitoring/observation

Diagnose/treat cause (Tables 8.3, 8.4)
Refer to cardiologist

Bradycardia and atrioventricular block

**TABLE 8.1** Classification of bradycardia and atrioventricular (AV) block

**Bradycardia**
- Sinus bradycardia (see Table 8.3 for causes)
- Junctional bradycardia (Fig. 8.1)
- Slow atrial fibrillation (distinguished from atrial fibrillation with complete AV block by variability in RR interval)
- Atrial flutter/atrial tachycardia with 4:1 AV block
- Complete AV block with junctional or ventricular escape rhythm (Fig. 8.4)

**Atrioventricular block** (see Table 8.4 for causes)
- First degree AV block (constant PR interval >200 ms)
- Second degree AV block, Mobitz type 1 (Wenckebach) (Fig. 8.2)
- Second degree AV block, Mobitz type 2 (Fig. 8.3)
- Third degree/complete AV block (Fig. 8.4)

**TABLE 8.2** Drug therapy of bradycardia

| Drug | Comment | Dose (IV) |
|------|---------|-----------|
| **Atropine** | Inhibition of vagal tone | Bolus of 500–1000 μg, with further doses at 5 min intervals up to a total dose of 3 mg to achieve target heart rate |
| **Dobutamine** | Cardiac beta-1 receptor stimulation<br>High doses may provoke ventricular arrhythmias | Start infusion at 10 μg/kg/min<br>Adjust rate of infusion to achieve target heart rate |
| **Glucagon** | To reverse beta-blockade | Bolus of 2–10 mg followed by infusion of 50 μg/kg/h |

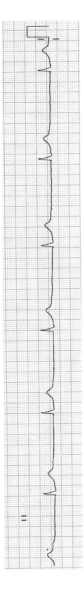

**FIGURE 8.1** Junctional bradycardia. Heart rate 30–60bpm with P wave absent or position constant either after, immediately before or hidden in QRS complex. Occurs when junctional pacemaker overtakes slow sinus node pacemaker.

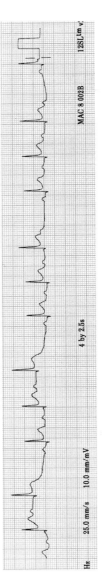

**FIGURE 8.2** Second degree atrioventricular block, Mobitz type 1 (Wenckebach). Progressively lengthening PR interval followed by dropped beat.

**Bradycardia and atrioventricular block**

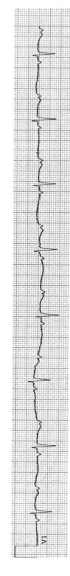

**FIGURE 8.3** Second degree atrioventricular (AV) block, Mobitz type 2. Constant PR interval with dropped beats. Usually due to disorder of His–Purkinje system and often progresses to complete AV block.

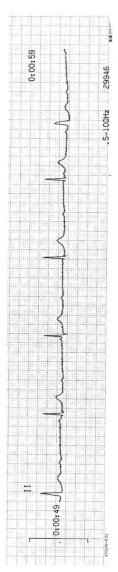

**FIGURE 8.4** Complete atrioventricular block. Relationship of P wave to QRS varies randomly, and P waves are absent if there is atrial fibrillation. Escape rhythm may be junctional (narrow complex) or ventricular (broad complex). Even in asymptomatic patients, this carries a risk of sudden death due to ventricular standstill or polymorphic ventricular tachycardia/ventricular fibrillation.

---

**TABLE 8.3** Causes of sinus bradycardia

**Cardiovascular**
- Chronic sinus node dysfunction (due to idiopathic degenerative/fibrotic change in sinus node)
- Acute sinus node dysfunction due to ischemia (typically in inferior myocardial infarction; sinus node artery arises from right coronary artery in ~90%)
- Maneuvers triggering high vagal tone, e.g. suctioning of airway
- Vasovagal syncope
- Carotid sinus hypersensitivity

**Systemic**
- Drugs (beta-blockers, digoxin, diltiazem, verapamil, other antiarrhythmic drugs)
- Hypothermia
- Hypothyroidism
- Hypokalemia, hyperkalemia
- Raised intracranial pressure

---

**TABLE 8.4** Causes of atrioventricular (AV) block

**Acute**
- High vagal tone (may cause Mobitz type 1 second-degree AV block, but not Mobitz type 2 or complete AV block)
- Myocardial ischemia/infarction
- Drugs (beta-blockers, digoxin, diltiazem, verapamil, other antiarrhythmic drugs)
- Hyperkalemia
- Infections: Lyme disease
- Myocarditis
- Endocarditis with abscess formation

**Chronic**
- Idiopathic conducting system fibrosis
- Congenital complete AV block
- Cardiomyopathy

Bradycardia and atrioventricular block

**TABLE 8.5** Temporary cardiac pacing: indications, contraindications and potential complications (for technique, see p. 600)

**Indications**
- Bradycardia/asystole (sinus or junctional bradycardia or second/third degree AV block) associated with hemodynamic compromise and unresponsive to atropine (p. 48)
- After cardiac arrest due to bradycardia/asystole
- To prevent perioperative bradycardia. Temporary pacing is indicated in:
  - Second degree Mobitz type 2 AV block or complete heart block; *or*
  - Sinus/junctional bradycardia or second degree Mobitz type I (Wenckebach) AV block or bundle branch block (including bifascicular and trifascicular block) only if history of syncope or presyncope
- Atrial or ventricular overdrive pacing to prevent recurrent monomorphic ventricular tachycardia or polymorphic ventricular tachycardia with preceding QT prolongation (torsade de pointes)

**Contraindications**
- Risks of temporary pacing outweigh benefits, e.g. rare symptomatic sinus pauses, or complete heart block with a stable escape rhythm and no hemodynamic compromise
- Discuss management with a cardiologist. Consider using standby external pacing system instead of transvenous pacing
- Prosthetic tricuspid valve

**Complications**
- Complications of central vein cannulation (p. 590), especially bleeding in patients with acute coronary syndromes treated with thrombolytic therapy (reduced with ultrasound-guided approach, p. 591)
- Cardiac perforation by pacing lead (may rarely result in cardiac tamponade)
- Arrhythmias (including ventricular fibrillation) during placement of pacing lead
- Infection of pacing lead

AV, atrioventricular.

## Further reading

Mangrum JM, DiMarco JP. The evaluation and management of bradycardia. *N Engl J Med* 2000; 342: 703–9.

# 9 Hypotension

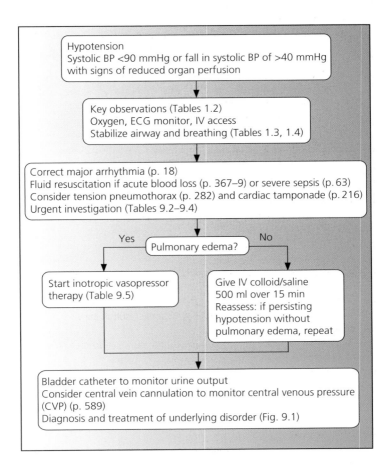

Hypotension
Systolic BP <90 mmHg or fall in systolic BP of >40 mmHg
with signs of reduced organ perfusion

Key observations (Tables 1.2)
Oxygen, ECG monitor, IV access
Stabilize airway and breathing (Tables 1.3, 1.4)

Correct major arrhythmia (p. 18)
Fluid resuscitation if acute blood loss (p. 367–9) or severe sepsis (p. 63)
Consider tension pneumothorax (p. 282) and cardiac tamponade (p. 216)
Urgent investigation (Tables 9.2–9.4)

Pulmonary edema?

Yes

No

Start inotropic vasopressor
therapy (Table 9.5)

Give IV colloid/saline
500 ml over 15 min
Reassess: if persisting
hypotension without
pulmonary edema, repeat

Bladder catheter to monitor urine output
Consider central vein cannulation to monitor central venous pressure
(CVP) (p. 589)
Diagnosis and treatment of underlying disorder (Fig. 9.1)

Hypotension

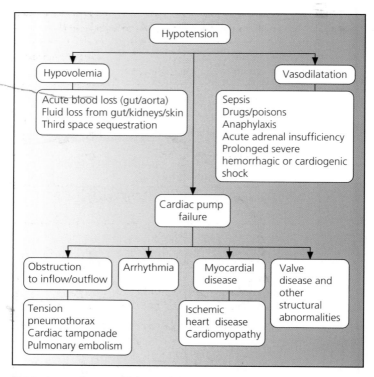

**FIGURE 9.1** Causes of hypotension.

## Further reading

Beaulieu Y, Marik PE. Bedside ultrasonography in the ICU. *Chest* 2005; 128: 881–95 (part 1) and 1766–81 (part 2).

Graham CA, Parke TRJ. Critical care in the emergency department: shock and circulatory support. *Emerg Med J* 2005; 22: 17–21.

Landry DW, Oliver JA. The pathogenesis of vasodilatory shock. *N Engl J Med* 2001; 345: 588–95.

Vincent J-L, Weil MH. Fluid challenge revisited. *Crit Care Med* 2006; 34: 1333–7.

**TABLE 9.1** Clinical signs pointing to the cause of hypotension*

| Cause of hypotension | Pulse volume | Skin temperature | Jugular venous pressure |
|---|---|---|---|
| **Hypovolemia** | Low | Cool | Low |
| **Cardiac pump failure** | Low | Cool | Normal or raised |
| **Vasodilatation** | Normal or increased | Warm | Low |

* Disorders which result in hypovolemia, cardiac pump failure and vasodilatation are given in Fig. 9.1.

**ALERT**
If the jugular venous pressure is raised in a hypotensive patient not known to have cardiac disease, consider acute major pulmonary embolism and cardiac tamponade: arrange urgent echocardiography.

**ALERT**
Hypotension needs urgent correction if systolic BP is <90 mmHg and there are signs of low cardiac output.

**ALERT**
All inotropic vasopressor agents (with the exception of dobutamine) must be given via a central vein, as tissue necrosis due to vasoconstriction may occur if there is extravasation from a peripheral vein.

Hypotension

---

**TABLE 9.2** Urgent investigation in hypotension

- ECG
- Chest X-ray
- Echocardiography if indicated (see Tables 9.3, 9.4)
- Arterial blood gases and pH
- Blood glucose
- Sodium, potassium and creatinine
- Full blood count
- Group and save (cross-match 6 units if acute hemorrhage suspected)
- Coagulation screen if low platelet count, suspected coagulation disorder, jaundice or purpura
- Blood culture
- Urine stick test

---

**Hypotension**

---

**TABLE 9.3** Indications for urgent or emergency echocardiography in hypotension

- Suspected cardiac tamponade (p. 216)
  - Hypotension and breathlessness following placement of central venous cannula or pacing lead, or in a patient with known cancer
  - Raised jugular venous pressure
  - Pulsus paradoxus >10 mmHg
- Suspected acute major acute pulmonary embolism (p. 231)
  - Risk factors for venous thromboembolism
  - Raised jugular venous pressure
- Hypotension with pulmonary edema (cardiogenic shock; p. 174)
- Unexplained severe hypotension

**TABLE 9.4** Echocardiographic findings in hypotension

| Cause of hypotension | IVC | LV size | LV contraction | RV size | RV contraction |
|---|---|---|---|---|---|
| **Hypovolemia** | Flat | Small | Increased | Small | Increased |
| **Sepsis** | Flat | Normal or large | Normal or reduced | Normal or large | Normal or reduced |
| **LV dysfunction due to ischemia** | Normal or dilated | Large | Reduced regionally or globally | Normal | Normal (unless associated RV infarction) |
| **Acute major pulmonary embolism** | Dilated | Normal or small | Normal or increased | Large | Reduced |
| **Cardiac tamponade** | Dilated | Normal | Normal or increased | Normal | Diastolic free wall collapse |
| **RV infarction** | Dilated | Normal or large if associated LV inferior infarction | Normal or reduced if associated inferior infarction | Large | Reduced |

IVC, inferior vena cava; LV, left ventricular; RV, right ventricular.

**Hypotension**

**Hypotension**

**TABLE 9.5** Inotropic vasopressor therapy

| Cause of hypotension/clinical setting | Choice of therapy |
|---|---|
| Left ventricular failure | Systolic BP >90 mmHg: dobutamine |
| Right ventricular infarction | Systolic BP 80–90 mmHg: dopamine |
| Pulmonary embolism | Systolic BP <80 mmHg: norepinephrine |
| Bradycardia and hypotension | Epinephrine |
| Cardiac tamponade while awaiting pericardiocentesis | Norepinephrine |
| Septic shock (after fluid resuscitation) | Norepinephrine as first-line agent Dobutamine should be added if cardiac output is low |
| Anaphylactic shock | Epinephrine |

| Drug | Dosage (μg/kg/min) | Effect |
|---|---|---|
| Dobutamine | 5–40 | Beta-1 inotropism and beta-2 vasodilatation |
| Dopamine | 5–10 | Beta-1 inotropism |
|  | 10–40 | Alfa-1 vasoconstriction |
| Epinephrine | 0.05 | Beta-1 inotropism and beta-2 vasodilatation |
|  | 0.05–5 | Beta-1 inotropism and alfa-1 vasoconstriction |
| Norepinephrine | 0.05–5 | Alfa-1 vasoconstriction and beta-1 inotropism |

# 10 Sepsis and septic shock

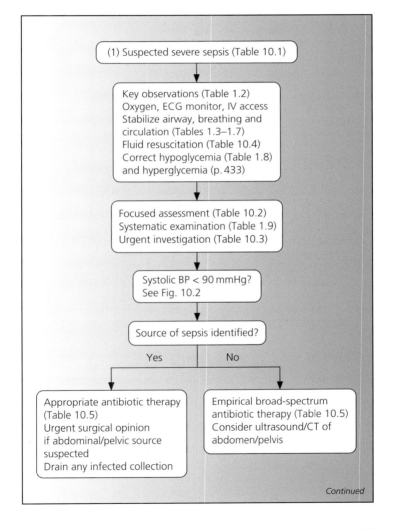

(1) Suspected severe sepsis (Table 10.1)

Key observations (Table 1.2)
Oxygen, ECG monitor, IV access
Stabilize airway, breathing and
circulation (Tables 1.3–1.7)
Fluid resuscitation (Table 10.4)
Correct hypoglycemia (Table 1.8)
and hyperglycemia (p. 433)

Focused assessment (Table 10.2)
Systematic examination (Table 1.9)
Urgent investigation (Table 10.3)

Systolic BP < 90 mmHg?
See Fig. 10.2

Source of sepsis identified?

Yes

No

Appropriate antibiotic therapy
(Table 10.5)
Urgent surgical opinion
if abdominal/pelvic source
suspected
Drain any infected collection

Empirical broad-spectrum
antibiotic therapy (Table 10.5)
Consider ultrasound/CT of
abdomen/pelvis

*Continued*

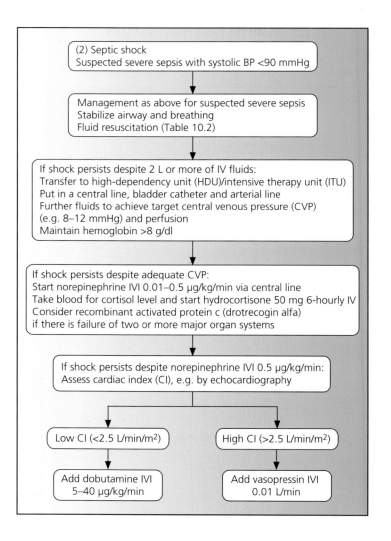

(2) Septic shock
Suspected severe sepsis with systolic BP <90 mmHg

Management as above for suspected severe sepsis
Stabilize airway and breathing
Fluid resuscitation (Table 10.2)

If shock persists despite 2 L or more of IV fluids:
Transfer to high-dependency unit (HDU)/intensive therapy unit (ITU)
Put in a central line, bladder catheter and arterial line
Further fluids to achieve target central venous pressure (CVP)
(e.g. 8–12 mmHg) and perfusion
Maintain hemoglobin >8 g/dl

If shock persists despite adequate CVP:
Start norepinephrine IVI 0.01–0.5 µg/kg/min via central line
Take blood for cortisol level and start hydrocortisone 50 mg 6-hourly IV
Consider recombinant activated protein c (drotrecogin alfa)
if there is failure of two or more major organ systems

If shock persists despite norepinephrine IVI 0.5 µg/kg/min:
Assess cardiac index (CI), e.g. by echocardiography

Low CI (<2.5 L/min/m²)

High CI (>2.5 L/min/m²)

Add dobutamine IVI
5–40 µg/kg/min

Add vasopressin IVI
0.01 L/min

**TABLE 10.1** Definitions of sepsis and septic shock

| Disorder | Definition |
|---|---|
| **Systemic inflammatory response syndrome** | Two or more of the following:<br>• Body temperature >38.5 or <35.0°C<br>• Heart rate >90 bpm<br>• Respiratory rate >20/min or $PaCO_2$ <32 mmHg or need for mechanical ventilation<br>• White blood cell count >12 or <4 × $10^9$/L or immature forms >10% |
| **Sepsis** | Systemic inflammatory response syndrome<br>*and*<br>Documented infection (culture or Gram stain of blood, sputum, urine or normally sterile body fluid positive for pathogenic microorganism; or focus of infection identified by visual inspection) |
| **Severe sepsis** | Sepsis and at least one sign of organ hypoperfusion or organ dysfunction:<br>• Areas of mottled skin<br>• Capillary refull time >3 s<br>• Urine output <0.5 ml/kg for at least 1 h or renal replacement therapy<br>• Arterial lactate level >2 mmol/L<br>• Abrupt change in mental status or abnormal EEG<br>• Platelet count <100 × $10^9$/L or disseminated intravascular coagulation<br>• Acute lung injury – acute respiratory distress syndrome (p. 192)<br>• Cardiac dysfunction on echocardiography |
| **Septic shock** | Severe sepsis and one of:<br>• Mean blood pressure <60 mmHg (<80 mmHg if previous hypertension) after 20–30 ml/kg colloid or 40–60 ml/kg crystalloid<br>• Need for dopamine >5 µg/kg/min or norepinephrine or epinephrine <0.25 µg/kg/min to maintain mean blood pressure >60 mmHg (>80 mmHg if previous hypertension) |
| **Refractory septic shock** | Need for dopamine >15 µg/kg/min or norepinephrine or epinephrine >0.25 µg/kg/min to maintain mean blood pressure >60 mmHg (>80 mmHg if previous hypertension) |

**TABLE 10.2** Focused assessment of the patient with suspected severe sepsis

- Context: age, sex, comorbidities, medications, hospital or community acquired
- Current major symptoms and their time course
- Risk factors for sepsis? Consider immunosuppressive therapy, AIDS, cancer, renal failure, liver failure, diabetes, malnutrition, splenectomy, IV drug use, prosthetic heart valve, other prosthetic material, peripheral IV cannula, central venous cannula, bladder catheter
- Recent culture results?
- Recent surgery or invasive procedures?
- Recent foreign travel?
- Contact with infectious disease?

**ALERT**

A good outcome in sepsis depends on prompt diagnosis, vigorous fluid resuscitation, appropriate initial antibiotic therapy and drainage of any infected collection.

**TABLE 10.3** Urgent investigation in suspected severe sepsis

- Full blood count
- Coagulation screen if there is purpura or jaundice, prolonged oozing from puncture sites, bleeding from surgical wounds or low platelet count (see Table 78.2)
- Blood glucose
- Sodium, potassium and creatinine
- C-reactive protein
- Blood culture
- Urinalysis and urine microscopy/culture
- Chest X-ray
- Arterial blood gases and pH
- Additional investigation directed by the clinical picture (e.g. lumbar puncture, aspiration of pleural effusion or ascites, joint aspiration)

---

**TABLE 10.4** Fluid resuscitation in severe sepsis and septic shock

- 1 L of normal saline over 30 min
- 1 L of sodium lactate (Hartmann solution; Ringer lactate solution) over 30 min
- 1 L of sodium lactate (Hartmann solution; Ringer lactate solution) over 30 min
- Start norepinephrine infusion if shock persists despite 2 L or more of IV fluid
- Give further maintenance/bolus fluid guided by clinical condition and hemodynamic monitoring (e.g. maintenance 200 ml/h Ringer lactate solution)

---

**TABLE 10.5** Initial antibiotic therapy in severe sepsis

| Suspected source of sepsis | Initial antibiotic therapy (IV, high dose) | |
|---|---|---|
| | **Not allergic to penicillin** | **Penicillin allergy (Table 10.6)** |
| **Bacterial meningitis (p. 327)** | See Table 50.3 | |
| **Community-acquired pneumonia (p. 268)** | See Table 41.5 | |
| **Hospital-acquired pneumonia (p. 277)** | See Table 42.1 | |
| **Infective endocarditis (p. 203)** | See Table 31.5 | |
| **Intra-abdominal sepsis** | Piperacillin/tazobactam + gentamicin + metronidazole | Meropenem + gentamicin + metronidazole |

*Continued*

| Suspected source of sepsis | Initial antibiotic therapy (IV, high dose) | |
| | **Not allergic to penicillin** | **Penicillin allergy (Table 10.6)** |
| --- | --- | --- |
| **Urinary tract infection** | Ciprofloxacin | |
| **IV line related** | Vancomycin or teicoplanin (+ gentamicin if Gram-negative sepsis possible) | |
| **Septic arthritis (p. 473)** | See Table 75.4 | |
| **Cellulitis (p. 469)** | See Table 74.3 | |
| **No localizing signs: neutropenic** | Piperacillin/tazobactam + gentamicin (+ teicoplanin if suspected tunneled line sepsis) (+ metronidazole if oral or perianal infection) | Ciprofloxacin + gentamicin (+ teicoplanin if suspected tunneled line sepsis) (+ metronidazole if oral or perianal infection) |
| **No localizing signs: not neutropenic** | Ceftazidime + gentamicin + metronidazole (omit if anaerobic infection unlikely) | Meropenem + gentamicin + metronidazole (omit if anaerobic infection unlikely) |

---

**TABLE 10.6** Penicillin allergy

- Patients with previous anaphylactic reaction to a penicillin should not receive penicillins or other beta-lactam antibiotics (penicillins, cephalosporins, carbapenems (e.g. meropenem) and monobactams (e.g. aztreonam))
- Up to 85% of patients allergic to a penicillin can tolerate the drug when given it again, as sensitization may only be temporary. Late reactions can occur up to several weeks after exposure and account for 80–90% of all reactions, most commonly rash
- Penicillin-allergic patients without a history of anaphylaxis are no more likely to have an allergic reaction to a cephalosporin than patients without a history of penicillin allergy

---

## Further reading

Annane D, et al. Corticosteroids for severe sepsis and septic shock: a systematic review and meta-analysis. *BMJ* 2004; 329; 480–4.

Annane D, et al. Septic shock. *Lancet* 2005; 365: 63–78.

Dellinger RP, et al. Surviving Sepsis. Campaign guidelines for management of severe sepsis and septic shock. *Crit Care Med* 2004; 32: 858–73.

Gordon RJ, Lowy FD. Bacterial infections in drug users. *N Engl J Med* 2005; 353: 1945–54.

Gruchalla RS, Pirmohamed M. Antibiotic allergy. *N Engl J Med* 2006; 354: 601–9.

Hollenberg SM, et al. Practice parameters for hemodynamic support of sepsis in adult patients: 2004 update. *Crit Care Med* 2004; 32: 1928–48.

Johns Hopkins Hospital. Antibiotics guide. Johns Hopkins Hospital website (http://hopkins-abxguide.org/show_pages.cfm?content=s_faq_content.html).

Russell JA. Management of sepsis. *N Engl J Med* 2006; 355: 1699–713.

Safdar N, et al. Meta-analysis: methods for diagnosing intravascular device-associated bloodstream infection. *Ann Intern Med* 2005; 142: 451–66.

Sepsis and septic shock

# 11 Poisoning: general approach

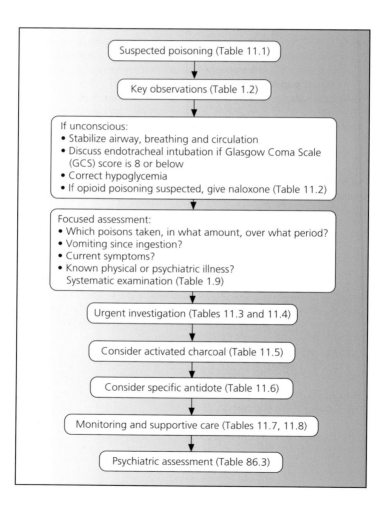

Suspected poisoning (Table 11.1)

↓

Key observations (Table 1.2)

↓

If unconscious:
- Stabilize airway, breathing and circulation
- Discuss endotracheal intubation if Glasgow Coma Scale (GCS) score is 8 or below
- Correct hypoglycemia
- If opioid poisoning suspected, give naloxone (Table 11.2)

↓

Focused assessment:
- Which poisons taken, in what amount, over what period?
- Vomiting since ingestion?
- Current symptoms?
- Known physical or psychiatric illness?
  Systematic examination (Table 1.9)

↓

Urgent investigation (Tables 11.3 and 11.4)

↓

Consider activated charcoal (Table 11.5)

↓

Consider specific antidote (Table 11.6)

↓

Monitoring and supportive care (Tables 11.7, 11.8)

↓

Psychiatric assessment (Table 86.3)

| TABLE 11.1 Clues to the poison taken | |
|---|---|
| **Feature** | **Poisons to consider** |
| **Coma** | Barbiturates, benzodiazepines, ethanol, MDMA, opioids, trichloroethanol, tricyclics |
| **Fits** | Amphetamines, cocaine, dextropropoxyphene, insulin, oral hypoglycemics, phenothiazines, theophylline, tricyclics, lead |
| **Constricted pupils** | Opioids, organophosphates, trichloroethanol |
| **Dilated pupils** | Amphetamines, cocaine, phenothiazines, quinine, sympathomimetics, tricyclics |
| **Arrhythmias** | Antiarrhythmics, anticholinergics, MDMA, phenothiazines, quinine, sympathomimetics, tricyclics |
| **Hypertension** | Amphetamines, cocaine |
| **Pulmonary edema** | Carbon monoxide, ethylene glycol, irritant gases, MDMA, opioids, organophosphates, paraquat, salicylates, tricyclics |
| **Ketones on breath** | Ethanol, isopropyl alcohol |
| **Hypothermia** | Barbiturates, ethanol, opioids, tricyclics |
| **Hyperthermia** | Amphetamines and MDMA, anticholinergics, cocaine, monamine oxidase inhibitors |
| **Hypoglycemia** | Insulin, oral hypoglycemics, ethanol, salicylates |
| **Hyperglycemia** | Theophylline, organophosphates, salbutamol |
| **Renal failure** | *Amanita phalloides*, ethylene glycol, MDMA, paracetamol, salicylates, prolonged hypotension, rhabdomyolysis |
| **Hypokalemia** | Salbutamol, salicylates, theophylline |
| **Metabolic acidosis** | Carbon monoxide, ethanol, ethylene glycol, methanol, paracetamol, salicylates, tricyclics |
| **Raised plasma osmolality** | Ethanol, ethylene glycol, isopropyl alcohol, methanol |

MDMA, methylene dioxymethamfetamine ('ecstasy').

**TABLE 11.2** Naloxone in suspected opioid poisoning

If the respiratory rate is <12/min, or the pupils are pinpoint or there is other reason to suspect opioid poisoning:
- Give 0.4–2 mg IV every 2–3 min, to a maximum of 10 mg, until the respiratory rate is around 15/min.
- If there is a response, start an IV infusion: add 4 mg to 500 ml glucose 5% or saline (8 μg/ml) and titrate against the respiratory rate and conscious level. The plasma half-life of naloxone is 1 h, shorter than that of most opioids
- If there is no response to naloxone, opioid poisoning is excluded

**TABLE 11.3** Urgent investigation in poisoning

- Blood glucose
- Sodium, potassium and creatinine
- Plasma osmolality* if the ingested substance is not known
- Paracetamol and salicylate levels (as mixed poisoning is common), and plasma levels of other drugs/poisons if indicated (Table 11.4)
- Full blood count
- Urinalysis (myoglobinuria due to rhabdomyolysis gives a positive stick test for blood; see Table 65.3)
- Arterial blood gases and pH in the following circumstances:
  - If the patient is unconscious, hypotensive, has respiratory symptoms or a reduced arterial oxygen saturation on oximetry
  - If the poison can cause metabolic acidosis (Table 11.1)
  - After inhalation injury
- Chest X-ray if the patient is unconscious, hypotensive, has respiratory symptoms or a reduced arterial oxygen saturation on oximetry
- ECG if there is hypotension, heart disease, suspected ingestion of cardiotoxic drugs (antiarrhythmics, tricyclics) or age >60 years
- If the substance ingested is not known, save serum (10 ml), urine (50 ml) and vomitus (50 ml) at 4°C in case later analysis is needed

* The normal range of plasma osmolality is 280–300 mosmol/kg. If the measured plasma osmolality (by freezing point depression method) exceeds calculated osmolality (from the formula [2(Na + K) + urea + glucose]) by 10 mosmol/kg or more, consider poisoning with ethanol, ethylene glycol, isopropyl alcohol or methanol.

**TABLE 11.4** Poisoning in which plasma levels* should be measured

| Drug/poison | Plasma level at which specific treatment is indicated | Treatment |
| --- | --- | --- |
| **Aspirin and other salicylates** | See Table 12.2 | Fluids, HD, PD |
| **Barbiturates** | Discuss with Poisons Information Center | RAC, HP |
| **Digoxin** | >4 ng/ml (>5 mmol/L) | Digoxin-specific antibody fragments |
| **Ethylene glycol** | >500 mg/L | Ethanol/fomepizole, HD, PD |
| **Iron** | >3.5 mg/L[†] | Desferrioxamine |
| **Lithium (plain tube)** | >5 mmol/L | HD, PD |
| **Methanol** | >500 mg/L | Ethanol/fomepizole, HD, PD |
| **Paracetamol** | See Figure 12.1 | Acetylcysteine |
| **Theophylline** | >50 mg/L | RAC, HP, HD |

HD, hemodialysis; HP, hemoperfusion; PD, peritoneal dialysis; RAC, repeated oral activated charcoal.

* Always check the units of measurement used by your laboratory.

[†] Also measure plasma iron level if clinical evidence of severe iron toxicity (hypotension, nausea, vomiting, diarrhea) or after massive ingestion (>200 mg elemental iron/kg body weight; one 200 mg tablet of ferrous sulphate contains 60 mg elemental iron).

**TABLE 11.5** Activated charcoal: indications* and contraindications[†]

| Multiple-dose activated charcoal may be indicated | Single-dose activated charcoal may be indicated | Activated charcoal contraindicated |
|---|---|---|
| Barbiturates | Antihistamines | Acids |
| Carbamazepine | Paracetamol | Alkalis |
| Dapsone | Salicylates | Carbamate |
| Paraquat | Tricyclics | Cyanide |
| Quinine | | Ethanol |
| Theophylline | | Ethylene glycol |
| | | Hydrocarbons |
| | | Iron |
| | | Lithium |
| | | Methanol |
| | | Organophosphates |

* Administration of activated charcoal (50 g mixed with 200 ml of water) should be considered if a potentially toxic amount of a poison known to be adsorbed to charcoal has been ingested within 1 h, and an oral antidote is not indicated.
[†] Because of the risk of inhalation, and the absence of evidence that administration improves clinical outcomes, activated charcoal should not be given to a patient with a reduced conscious level unless the airway is protected by a cuffed endotracheal tube.

**TABLE 11.6** Specific antidotes*

| Poison | Antidote |
|---|---|
| **Anticholinergic agents** | Physostigmine |
| **Arsenic** | Dimercaprol, penicillamine |
| **Benzodiazepines** | Flumazenil |
| **Beta-blockers** | Glucagon |
| **Calcium antagonists** | Calcium gluconate |
| **Cyanide** | Dicobalt Edentate *or* Sodium nitrite + sodium thiosulfate |
| **Digoxin** | Digoxin-specific antibody fragments |
| **Ethylene glycol** | Ethanol, fomepizole |
| **Fluoride** | Calcium gluconate |
| **Iron** | Desferrioxamine |
| **Lead** | Dimercaprol, penicillamine, sodium calcium edetate |
| **Mercury** | Dimercaprol, penicillamine, sodium calcium edetate |
| **Methanol** | Ethanol, fomepizole |
| **Opioids** | Naloxone |
| **Organophosphates** | Atropine, pralidoxime mesylate |
| **Paracetamol** | Acetylcysteine |
| **Warfarin** | Vitamin K, fresh frozen plasma, prothrombin complex concentrate (see Table 79.7, p. 512) |

* Discuss the case with a Poisons Information Center first, unless you are familiar with the poison and its antidote, as some antidotes may be harmful if given inappropriately.

---

**TABLE 11.7** Monitoring and supportive care after poisoning

---

**1 Criteria for admission to ITU after poisoning:**\*
- Endotracheal tube placed
- Glasgow Coma Scale score of 8 or below
- Hypoventilation ($PaCO_2 > 6\,kPa$)
- $PaO_2 < 7\,kPa$ breathing air
- Major arrhythmias or significant poisoning with a drug known to have a high risk of causing arrhythmias (e.g. tricyclics)
- Recurrent seizures
- Hypotension not responsive to IV fluid

**2 Monitoring after severe poisoning:**
- Conscious level (initially hourly)
- Respiratory rate (initially every 15 min)
- Arterial oxygen saturation by pulse oximeter (continuous display)
- ECG monitor (continuous display)
- Blood pressure (initially every 15 min)
- Temperature (initially hourly)
- Urine output (put in a bladder catheter if the poison is potentially nephrotoxic or if the patient is unconscious)
- Arterial blood gases and pH (initially 2-hourly) if the poison can cause metabolic acidosis (Table 11.1) or there is suspected acute respiratory distress syndrome (Tables 29.1, 29.4) or after inhalation injury
- Blood glucose if the poison may cause hypo- or hyperglycemia (initially hourly) or in paracetamol poisoning presenting after 16 h (initially 4-hourly)

---

ITU, intensive therapy unit.
\* Unconscious patients not requiring endotracheal intubation or transfer to ITU should be nursed in the recovery position in a high-dependency area.

**TABLE 11.8** Management of problems commonly seen after poisoning

| Problem | Comment and management |
|---------|------------------------|
| **Coma** | If associated with focal neurological signs or evidence of head injury, CT must be done to exclude intracranial hematoma |
| **Cerebral edema** | May occur after cardiac arrest, in severe carbon monoxide poisoning, in fulminant hepatic failure from paracetamol (p. 402), and in MDMA poisoning, due to hyponatremia. Results in coma, hypertension and dilated pupils Secure the airway with an endotracheal tube and ventilate to maintain a normal arterial $PO_2$ and $PCO_2$. Consider mannitol to reduce intracranial pressure. See p. 362 |
| **Fits** | Due to toxin or metabolic complications Check blood glucose, arterial gases and pH, plasma sodium, potassium and calcium. Treat prolonged or recurrent major fits with diazepam IV up to 10 mg. |
| **Respiratory depression** | Half-life of most opioids is longer than that of naloxone and repeated doses or an infusion may be required. Elective ventilation may be preferable. |
| **Inhalation pneumonia** | See Table 42.2. Treatment includes tracheobronchial suction, consideration of bronchoscopy to remove particulate matter from the airways, physiotherapy and antibiotic therapy |

*Continued*

| Problem | Comment and management |
|---------|------------------------|
| **Hypotension** | Usually reflects vasodilatation, but always consider other causes (e.g. gastrointestinal bleeding). Record an ECG if the patient has taken a cardiotoxic poison, has known cardiac disease or is aged >60 years |
| **Arrhythmias** | Due to toxin or metabolic complications Check arterial gases and pH, and plasma potassium, calcium and magnesium. |
| **Renal failure** | May be due to prolonged hypotension, nephrotoxic poison, hemolysis or rhabdomyolysis. See p. 410 for management |
| **Gastric stasis** | Place a nasogastric tube in comatose patients to reduce the risk of regurgitation and inhalation |
| **Hypothermia** | Manage by passive rewarming (p. 567) |

MDMA, methylene dioxymethamfetamine ('ecstasy').

## Further reading

American Academy of Clinical Toxicology, European Association of Poisons Centres and Clinical Toxicologists. Position paper: gastric lavage. *Clin Toxicol* 2004; 42: 933–43.
American Academy of Clinical Toxicology, European Association of Poisons Centres and Clinical Toxicologists. Position paper: single-dose activated charcoal. *Clin Toxicol* 2005; 43: 61–87.

# 12 Poisoning with aspirin, paracetamol and carbon monoxide

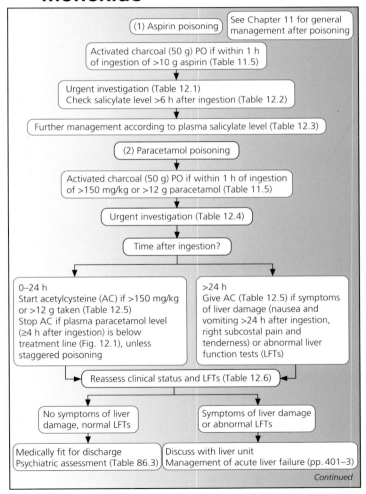

(1) Aspirin poisoning — See Chapter 11 for general management after poisoning

Activated charcoal (50 g) PO if within 1 h of ingestion of >10 g aspirin (Table 11.5)

Urgent investigation (Table 12.1)
Check salicylate level >6 h after ingestion (Table 12.2)

Further management according to plasma salicylate level (Table 12.3)

(2) Paracetamol poisoning

Activated charcoal (50 g) PO if within 1 h of ingestion of >150 mg/kg or >12 g paracetamol (Table 11.5)

Urgent investigation (Table 12.4)

Time after ingestion?

**0–24 h**
Start acetylcysteine (AC) if >150 mg/kg or >12 g taken (Table 12.5)
Stop AC if plasma paracetamol level (≥4 h after ingestion) is below treatment line (Fig. 12.1), unless staggered poisoning

**>24 h**
Give AC (Table 12.5) if symptoms of liver damage (nausea and vomiting >24 h after ingestion, right subcostal pain and tenderness) or abnormal liver function tests (LFTs)

Reassess clinical status and LFTs (Table 12.6)

No symptoms of liver damage, normal LFTs

Symptoms of liver damage or abnormal LFTs

Medically fit for discharge
Psychiatric assessment (Table 86.3)

Discuss with liver unit
Management of acute liver failure (pp. 401–3)

*Continued*

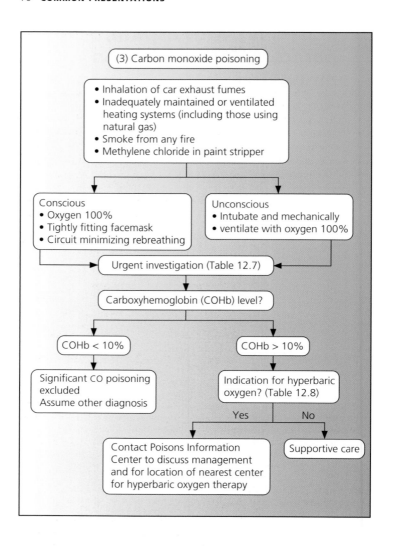

(3) Carbon monoxide poisoning

- Inhalation of car exhaust fumes
- Inadequately maintained or ventilated heating systems (including those using natural gas)
- Smoke from any fire
- Methylene chloride in paint stripper

Conscious
- Oxygen 100%
- Tightly fitting facemask
- Circuit minimizing rebreathing

Unconscious
- Intubate and mechanically
- ventilate with oxygen 100%

Urgent investigation (Table 12.7)

Carboxyhemoglobin (COHb) level?

COHb < 10%

COHb > 10%

Significant CO poisoning excluded
Assume other diagnosis

Indication for hyperbaric oxygen? (Table 12.8)

Yes          No

Contact Poisons Information Center to discuss management and for location of nearest center for hyperbaric oxygen therapy

Supportive care

---

**TABLE 12.1** Urgent investigations in aspirin poisoning

- Full blood count
- Prothrombin time (may be prolonged)
- Blood glucose (hypoglycemia may occur)
- Sodium, potassium and creatinine (hypokalemia is common)
- Arterial blood gases and pH (respiratory alkalosis in early stage, progressing to metabolic acidosis)
- Plasma salicylate level (sample taken >6h after ingestion) (Table 12.2)
- Chest X-ray (pulmonary edema may occur from increased capillary permeability)

---

**TABLE 12.2** Plasma salicylate level: interpretation and management

| Plasma level | | Interpretation | Action |
|---|---|---|---|
| **(mg/L)** | **(mmol/L)** | **Interpretation** | **Action** |
| **150–250** | **1.1–2.8** | Therapeutic level | None required |
| **250–350** | **1.8–3.6** | Mild poisoning | Fluid replacement |
| **500–750** | **3.6–5.4** | Moderate poisoning | Urinary alkalinization |
| **>750** | **>5.4** | Severe poisoning | Hemodialysis or peritoneal dialysis |

---

**TABLE 12.3** Management of aspirin poisoning

**Mild poisoning**
- Fluid replacement (oral or IV glucose 5% or normal saline)

**Moderate poisoning**
- Management is with urinary alkalinization (aim for urine pH over 7.0)
- Transfer the patient to HDU. Put in a bladder catheter to monitor urine output, arterial line to monitor pH, and, in patients over 60 or with cardiac disease, a central venous catheter so that CVP can be monitored to guide fluid replacement

*Continued*

- Give sodium bicarbonate 1.26% 500 ml + glucose 5% 500 ml initially over 1 h IV. Check the urinary and arterial pH and CVP and adjust the infusion rate accordingly. Stop the infusion of bicarbonate if arterial pH rises above 7.55
- Correct hypokalemia with IV potassium (p. 447)
- Give vitamin K 10 mg IV to reverse hypoprothrombinemia

**Severe poisoning**
- Defined as a plasma level >750 mg/L (>5.4 mmol/L), renal failure or pulmonary edema
- These patients should be referred for hemodialysis. Peritoneal dialysis can be used but is less effective
- Correct hypokalemia with IV potassium (p. 447)
- Give vitamin K 10 mg IV to reverse hypoprothrombinemia

CVP, central venous pressure; HDU, high-dependency unit.

---

**TABLE 12.4** Urgent investigations in paracetamol poisoning

- Full blood count
- Prothrombin time
- Blood glucose
- Sodium, potassium and creatinine (acute renal failure due to acute tubular necrosis may occur with severe poisoning, at 36–72 h after ingestion)
- Liver function tests
- Arterial blood gases and pH (respiratory alkalosis in early stage, progressing to metabolic acidosis)
- Plasma paracetamol level (sample taker >4 h after ingestion) (Fig. 12.1)

**TABLE 12.5** Acetylcysteine (AC) for paracetamol poisoning*

**Regimen**
- 150 mg/kg AC in 200 ml glucose 5% IV over 15 min, *then*
- 50 mg/kg AC in 500 ml glucose 5% IV over 4 h, *then*
- 100 mg/kg AC in 1 L glucose 5% IV over 16 h

**Problems**
- Minor reactions to AC (nausea, flushing, urticaria and pruritus) are relatively common, and usually settle when the peak rate of infusion is passed
- If there is a severe reaction (angioedema, wheezing, respiratory distress, hypotension or hypertension), stop the infusion and give an antihistamine (chlorphenamine 10 mg IV over 10 min)

* Acetylcysteine replenishes mitochondrial and cytosolic glutathione and is the preferred antidote for paracetamol poisoning. Oral methionine may be used if AC is not available, or if there is a risk that the patient will otherwise leave without any treatment.

**TABLE 12.6** Paracetamol poisoning: indications of severe hepatotoxicity

- Rapid development of grade 2 encephalopathy (confused but able to answer questions)
- Prothrombin time >20 s at 24 h, >45 s at 48 h or >50 s at 72 h
- Increasing plasma bilirubin
- Increasing plasma creatinine
- Falling plasma phosphate
- Arterial pH < 7.3 more than 24 h after ingestion

Poisoning with aspirin, paracetamol and carbon monoxide

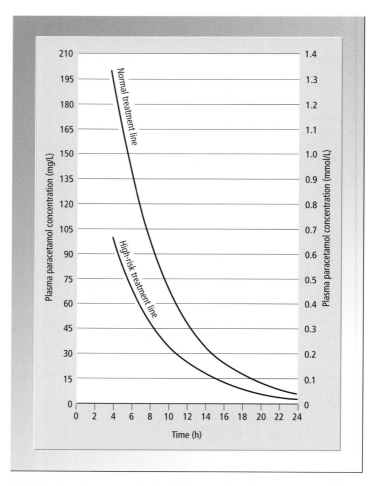

**FIGURE 12.1** Treatment thresholds in paracetamol poisoning. Use the high-risk (lower) treatment line in patients with: (i) chronic alcohol abuse; (ii) hepatic enzyme induction from therapy with carbamazepine, phenobarbitone, phenytoin or rifampicin; (iii) chronic malnutrition or recent starvation (within 24 h); or (iv) HIV/AIDS. (Reproduced with permission of the University of Wales College of Medicine Therapeutics and Toxicology Centre.)

**TABLE 12.7** Urgent investigation in carbon monoxide poisoning

- ECG (severe poisoning may result in myocardial ischemia, with anginal chest pain, ST segment depression and arrhythmias)
- Arterial blood gases and pH (metabolic acidosis is usually present)
- Chest X-ray
- Carboxyhemoglobin (COHb) level in venous blood (heparinized sample)

| Blood level of COHb (%) | Clinical features which may be seen |
|---|---|
| <10 | No symptoms. Acute poisoning excluded if exposure was within 4h |
| 10–50 | Headache, nausea, vomiting, tachycardia, tachypnea |
| >50 | Coma, fits, cardiorespiratory arrest |

**TABLE 12.8** Indications for hyperbaric oxygen therapy in carbon monoxide poisoning

- Carboxyhemoglobin level >40% at any time
- Coma
- Neurological symptoms or signs other than mild headache
- Evidence of myocardial ischemia or arrhythmias
- Pregnancy

## Further reading

Dargan Pl, et al. An evidence based flowchart to guide the management of acute salicylate (aspirin) overdose. *Emerg Med J* 2002; 19: 206–9.

Satran D, et al. Cardiovascular manifestations of moderate to severe carbon monoxide poisoning. *J Am Coll Cardiol* 2005; 45:1513–16.

Wallace CI, et al. Paracetamol overdose: an evidence based flowchart to guide management. *Emerg Med J* 2002; 19: 202–5.

Weaver L, et al. Hyperbaric oxygen for acute carbon monoxide poisoning. *N Engl J Med* 2002; 347: 1057–67.

# 13 Acute chest pain

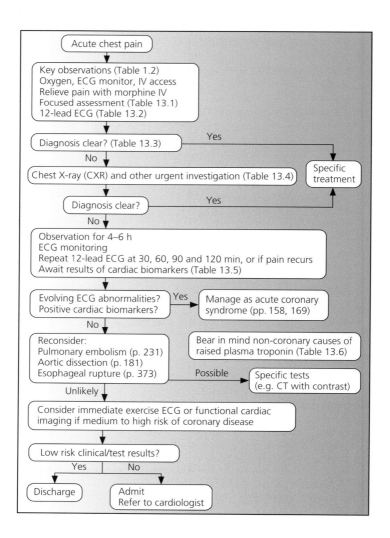

**TABLE 13.1** Focused assessment in acute chest pain

**History**

**1** *Onset and characteristics of the chest pain*
- Instantaneous onset suggests aortic dissection (p. 181)
- Onset following vomiting suggests esophageal rupture (p. 373)
- Radiation along the course of the aorta or its major branches (to neck, ear, back or abdomen) suggests aortic dissection. Radiation to the back alone is a non-specific feature which may occur in myocardial ischemia, and esophageal and musculoskeletal disorders
- Pleuritic pain is found in chest wall disorders, pleuropulmonary disorders (including pneumothorax, pneumonia and pulmonary infarction) and pericarditis

**2** *Background*
- Previous similar pain due to acute coronary syndrome?
- Known coronary disease or risk factors for coronary disease?
- Previous venous thromboembolism or risk factors for thromboembolism?
- Risk factors for aortic dissection (hypertension, Marfan syndrome, pregnancy)?

**Examination**

- Blood pressure in both arms (>15 mmHg difference in systolic pressure is abnormal), and the presence and symmetry of major pulses (if abnormal, consider aortic dissection)
- Jugular venous pressure (if raised, consider pulmonary embolism or pericardial effusion with tamponade)
- Murmur (if you hear the early diastolic murmur of aortic regurgitation, aortic dissection must be excluded)
- Pericardial or pleural rub?
- Signs of pneumothorax, pneumonia or pleural effusion?
- Localized chest wall or spinal tenderness (significant only if pressure exactly reproduces the spontaneous pain)?
- Subcutaneous emphysema around the neck (which may occur with esophageal rupture and pneumothorax)?

Acute chest pain

TABLE 13.2 ECG appearances in ST elevation myocardial infarction, benign early repolarization (normal variant) and acute pericarditis

| ECG feature | ST elevation myocardial infarction | Benign early repolarization (BER) (Fig. 13.1) | Acute pericarditis (Fig. 13.2) |
|---|---|---|---|
| ST segment morphology | Convex upwards | Concave upwards J point elevation Notching or irregular contour of J point | Concave upwards |
| Typical magnitude of ST elevation | 1–10 mm | 1–2 mm | 1–5 mm |
| Distribution of ST elevation | Inferior, anterior and lateral patterns seen depending on the involved coronary artery | More marked in chest leads than in limb leads | Seen in both limb and chest leads |
| ST depression in V1 | In posterior infarction | Rare | Common |
| ST elevation in V6 | In anterolateral infarction | May be seen | Common |

*Continued*

| ECG feature | ST elevation myocardial infarction | Benign early repolarization (BER) (Fig. 13.1) | Acute pericarditis (Fig. 13.2) |
|---|---|---|---|
| **T wave morphology** | Peaking of T waves in hyperacute phase, with subsequent inversion | Large amplitude concordant T waves | T wave inversion may develop, typically after ST segments have become isoelectric |
| **ST/T wave evolution** | Uniform in all involved leads | Does not occur | Various stages occur concurrently |
| **Depression of PR segment** | Does not occur | Does not occur | May be seen |
| **Pathological Q waves** | Commonly develop | Never develop | Never develop |
| **Rhythm disturbances** | May occur | Do not occur | Supraventricular tachyarrhythmias may occur |
| **Echocardiographic findings** | Left ventricular regional wall motion abnormality (hypokinesis/akinesis) | Normal appearances of left ventricle No pericardial effusion | Normal appearances of left ventricle (unless associated myocarditis) Pericardial effusion may be present |

**Acute chest pain**

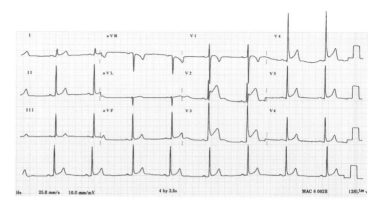

**FIGURE 13.1** ECG showing marked benign early repolarization (normal variant).

**ALERT**

Benign early repolarization, a normal variant, is found in ~1% of the population, and is most common in African or Afro-Caribbean men between the ages of 20 and 40.

**ALERT**

Esophageal rupture is rare and easily missed. Typically the pain follows vomiting (while in acute myocardial infarction, vomiting follows pain). A small pleural effusion is an important clue.

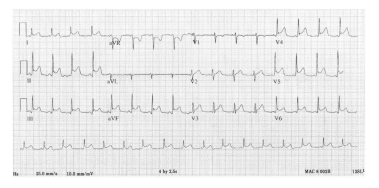

**FIGURE 13.2** ECG of acute pericarditis. There is ST elevation in all arterial territories.

> **ALERT**
> Consider aortic dissection in any patient with chest or upper abdominal pain of abrupt onset.

**TABLE 13.3** Causes of acute chest pain

| Cause | Common | Less common or rare |
|---|---|---|
| **Coronary disease** | Acute coronary syndrome (pp. 158, 169) | Angina due to tachyarrhythmia |
| **Other cardiovascular disorders** | Pulmonary embolism (p. 231) | Aortic dissection (p. 181) Aortic intramural hematoma (p. 184) Pericarditis (p. 212) |
| **Esophageal disorders** | Gastroesophageal reflux Esophageal motility disorder | Infective esophagitis Esophageal rupture (p. 373) |

*Continued*

| Cause | Common | Less common or rare |
|---|---|---|
|  |  | Esophageal hematoma (spontaneous (risk increased by anticoagulation) or due to food bolus or foreign body) |
| **Pulmonary and pleural disorders** | Pneumonia (p. 268)<br>Pleurisy | Pneumothorax (p. 280)<br>Pneumomediastinum |
| **Musculoskeletal disorders** | Pain arising from costochondral or chondrosternal joints<br>Rib fractures<br>Pain arising in intercostal or shoulder girdle muscles | Crush fracture of thoracic vertebra |
| **Others** | Panic attack | Biliary tract disease (p. 406)<br>Acute pancreatitis (p. 408)<br>Perforated peptic ulcer<br>Herpes zoster<br>Vaso-occlusive crisis (p. 514) of sickle cell disease |

**TABLE 13.4** Urgent investigation in acute chest pain

- ECG on admission, repeated at 30, 60, 90 and 120min, and if pain recurs
- Chest X-ray (consider pulmonary embolism, aortic dissection and esophageal rupture if there is a small pleural effusion)
- Arterial blood gases and pH
- Cardiac biomarkers (Table 13.5)
- Full blood count
- Blood glucose
- Sodium, potassium and creatinine

**TABLE 13.5** Cardiac biomarkers

| Marker | Rises after: | Peaks at: | Returns to normal: |
|---|---|---|---|
| **Myoglobin** | 1–4 h | 6–7 h | 24 h |
| **Troponin I** | 3–12 h | 24 h | 5–10 days |
| **Troponin T** | 3–12 h | 12–48 h | 5–14 days |
| **Creatine kinase** | 4–8 h | 12–24 h | 3–4 days |
| **CK-MB** | 4–8 h | 12–20 h | 2–3 days |

CK-MB, creatine kinase–MB fraction.

**TABLE 13.6** Non-coronary causes of raised plasma troponins

**Cardiac disorders**
- Supraventricular tachycardia/atrial fibrillation
- Left ventricular hypertrophy
- Intracranial hemorrhage or stroke
- Ingestion of sympathomimetic agents
- Cardiac contusion
- DC cardioversion
- Cardiac infiltrative disorders
- Chemotherapy
- Myocarditis
- Pericarditis
- Cardiac transplantation
- Congestive heart failure

**Non-cardiac disorders**
- Sepsis
- Hypotension
- Hypovolemia
- Pulmonary embolism
- Pulmonary hypertension
- Emphysema
- Strenuous exercise
- Chronic renal failure

Acute chest pain

**ALERT**

If you cannot make a confident diagnosis of a minor and self-limiting disorder, admit the patient with acute chest pain for observation (>6 h) and further investigation.

**ALERT**

The first sign of acute myocardial infarction may be hyperacute peaking of the T wave, which is often overlooked.

## Further reading

European Society of Cardiology Task Force on the Management of Chest Pain (2002). European Society of Cardiology website (http://www.escardio.org/knowledge/guidelines/Guidelines_list.htm?hit=quick).

Goldman L, Kirtane AJ. Triage of patients with acute chest pain and possible cardiac ischemia: the elusive search for diagnostic perfection. *Ann Intern Med* 2003; 139: 987–95.

Jeremias A, Gibson CM. Narrative review: alternative causes for elevated cardiac troponin levels when acute coronary syndromes are excluded. *Ann Intern Med* 2005; 142: 786–91.

Korff S, et al. Differential diagnosis of elevated troponins. *Heart* 2006; 92: 987–93.

Lange RA, Hillis LD. Cardiovascular complications of cocaine use. *N Engl J Med* 2001; 345: 351–8.

Sanchis J, et al. New risk score for patients with acute chest pain, non-ST-segment deviation, and normal troponin concentrations: a comparison with the TIMI risk score. *J Am Coll Cardiol* 2005; 46: 4443–9.

Swap CJ, Nagurney JT. Value and limitations of chest pain history in the evaluation of patients with suspected acute coronary syndromes. *JAMA* 2005; 294: 2623–9.

Turnipseed SD, et al. Electrocardiogram differentiation of benign early repolarization versus acute myocardial infarction by emergency physicians and cardiologists. *Acad Emerg Med* 2006; 13: 961–7.

# 14 Acute breathlessness

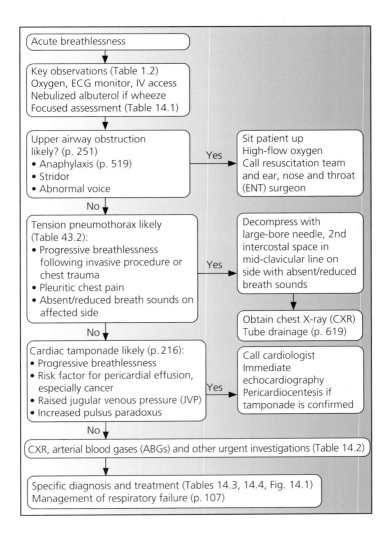

Acute breathlessness

↓

Key observations (Table 1.2)
Oxygen, ECG monitor, IV access
Nebulized albuterol if wheeze
Focused assessment (Table 14.1)

↓

Upper airway obstruction likely? (p. 251)
• Anaphylaxis (p. 519)
• Stridor
• Abnormal voice

—Yes→ Sit patient up
High-flow oxygen
Call resuscitation team and ear, nose and throat (ENT) surgeon

No ↓

Tension pneumothorax likely (Table 43.2):
• Progressive breathlessness following invasive procedure or chest trauma
• Pleuritic chest pain
• Absent/reduced breath sounds on affected side

—Yes→ Decompress with large-bore needle, 2nd intercostal space in mid-clavicular line on side with absent/reduced breath sounds

↓

Obtain chest X-ray (CXR)
Tube drainage (p. 619)

No ↓

Cardiac tamponade likely (p. 216):
• Progressive breathlessness
• Risk factor for pericardial effusion, especially cancer
• Raised jugular venous pressure (JVP)
• Increased pulsus paradoxus

—Yes→ Call cardiologist
Immediate echocardiography
Pericardiocentesis if tamponade is confirmed

No ↓

CXR, arterial blood gases (ABGs) and other urgent investigations (Table 14.2)

↓

Specific diagnosis and treatment (Tables 14.3, 14.4, Fig. 14.1)
Management of respiratory failure (p. 107)

**TABLE 14.1** Focused assessment in acute breathlessness

**History**
- Breathlessness: usual and recent change
- Wheeze: usual and recent change
- Sputum: usual volume/purulence and recent change
- Chest pain: pleuritic/non-pleuritic
- Effort tolerance: usual (e.g. distance walked on the flat; number of stairs climbed without stopping; ability to manage activities of daily living unaided) and recent change
- Known respiratory disease?
  - Previous acute exacerbations of chronic obstructive pulmonary disease (COPD) requiring hospital admission/ventilation?
  - Previous lung function tests and arterial blood gases (check notes): an $FEV_1$ 60–80% of predicted signifies mild COPD; 40–60%, moderate COPD; less than 40%, severe COPD
  - Requirement for home nebulized bronchodilator and/or oxygen therapy?
- Known cardiac disease?
- Coronary disease (check notes for angiography report)?
- Myocardial or valve disease (check notes for echo report)?
- Risk factors for venous thromboembolism (see Table 35.2)?

**Examination**
- See assessment of airway (Table 1.3), breathing (Table 1.4) and circulation (Table 1.6)

---

**TABLE 14.2** Urgent investigation in acute breathlessness

- Chest X-ray
- Arterial blood gases and pH
- ECG (except in patients under 40 with pneumothorax or acute asthma)
- Full blood count
- Blood glucose
- Sodium, potassium and creatinine
- Biomarkers:
    - D-dimer if pulmonary embolism is suspected
    - Troponin if acute coronary syndrome is suspected
    - Brain natriuretic peptide (BNP) if heart failure is suspected (send in EDTA tube)

EDTA, ethylene diaminetetra-acetic acid.

---

**TABLE 14.3** Causes of acute breathlessness

| Diagnosis | Features |
| --- | --- |
| **Acute asthma (p. 253)** | Wheeze with reduced peak flow rate<br>Previous similar episodes responding to bronchodilator therapy<br>Diurnal and seasonal variation in symptoms<br>Symptoms provoked by allergen exposure or exercise<br>Sleep disturbance by breathlessness and wheeze |
| **Cardiogenic pulmonary edema (p. 185)** | Cardiac disease<br>Abnormal ECG<br>Bilateral interstitial or alveolar shadowing on chest X-ray |

*Continued*

| Diagnosis | Features |
|---|---|
| **Acute respiratory distress syndrome (p. 192)** | Antecedent history of precipitating condition<br>Refractory hypoxemia ($PaO_2$ <8 kPa despite $FiO_2$ >40%)<br>Bilateral pulmonary infiltrates on chest X-ray<br>No evidence of cardiac cause for pulmonary edema on echocardiography |
| **Pneumonia (p. 268)** | Fever<br>Productive cough<br>Pleuritic chest pain<br>Focal shadowing on chest X-ray |
| **Exacerbation of chronic obstructive pulmonary disease (p. 261)** | Increase in sputum volume, tenacity or purulence<br>Previous chronic bronchitis: sputum production daily for 3 months of the year, for two or more consecutive years<br>Wheeze with reduced peak flow rate |
| **Pulmonary embolism (p. 231)** | Pleuritic or non-pleuritic chest pain<br>Risk factors for venous thromboembolism present (signs of DVT commonly absent) |
| **Pneumothorax (p. 280)** | Sudden breathlessness in young, otherwise fit adult<br>Breathlessness following invasive procedure, e.g. subclavian vein puncture<br>Pleuritic chest pain<br>Visceral pleural line on chest X-ray, with absent lung markings between this line and the chest wall |

*Continued*

| Diagnosis | Features |
|---|---|
| **Tension pneumothorax (p. 282)** | Respiratory distress<br>Ipsilateral hyperexpansion, hypomobility, and hyperresonance with decreased breath sounds<br>Tracheal deviation (inconsistent finding)<br>Elevated jugular venous pressure (inconsistent finding) |
| **Cardiac tamponade (p. 216)** | Raised jugular venous pressure<br>Pulsus paradoxus >10 mmHg<br>Enlarged cardiac silhouette on chest X-ray<br>Known carcinoma of bronchus or breast |
| **Laryngeal obstruction (p. 245)** | History of smoke inhalation or the ingestion of corrosives<br>Palatal or tongue edema<br>Anaphylaxis |
| **Tracheobronchial obstruction (p. 245)** | Stridor (inspiratory noise) or monophonic wheeze (expiratory 'squeak')<br>Known carcinoma of the bronchus<br>History of inhaled foreign body<br>$PaCO_2$ >6 kPa in the absence of chronic obstructive pulmonary disease<br>Wheeze unresponsive to bronchodilators |
| **Large pleural effusion (p. 283)** | Distinguished from pulmonary consolidation on chest X-ray by: shadowing higher laterally than medially; shadowing does not conform to that of a lobe or segment; no air bronchogram; trachea and mediastinum pushed to opposite side<br>If in doubt, use ultrasound to confirm effusion and establish if loculated |

DVT, deep vein thrombosis.

**TABLE 14.4** Arterial blood gases and pH in the breathless patient with clear lungs on chest X-ray

| Disorder | $PaO_2$ | $PaCO_2$ | pHa* |
|---|---|---|---|
| **Acute asthma** | Normal/low | Low | High |
| **Acute exacerbation of chronic obstructive pulmonary disease** | Usually low | May be high | Normal or low |
| **Pulmonary embolism (without pre-existing cardiopulmonary disease)** | Normal/low | Low | High |
| **Preradiological pneumonia[†]** | Low | Low | High |
| **Sepsis** | Normal/low | Low | Low |
| **Metabolic acidosis** | Normal | Low | Low |
| **Hyperventilation without organic disease[‡]** | High/normal | Low | High |

* Respiratory alkalosis may be offset by a metabolic acidosis. Figure 17.1, p. 113 allows identification of mixed acid–base disturbances.
† Most commonly due to viruses or *Pneumocystis carinii* (p. 539).
‡ Before diagnosing primary hyperventilation, exclude an underlying organic cause of tachypnea including diabetic ketoacidosis and acute asthma. Arterial blood gases and pH should be checked, and the patient admitted for further investigation if these are abnormal.

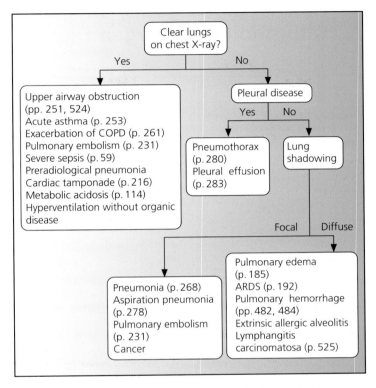

**Acute breathlessness**

**FIGURE 14.1** Causes of acute breathlessness according to chest X-ray appearances. ARDS, acute respiratory distress syndrome; COPD, chronic obstructive pulmonary disease.

## Further reading

Gehlbach BK, Geppert E. The pulmonary manifestations of left heart failure. *Chest* 2004; 125: 669–82.

Mueller C, et al. Cost-effectiveness of B-type natriuretic peptide testing in patients with acute dyspnea. *Arch Intern Med* 2006; 166: 1081–87.

# 15 Arterial blood gases, oxygen saturation and oxygen therapy

**TABLE 15.1** Overview

| Feature | Comment |
|---|---|
| **Normal values** | In a person breathing air ($FiO_2$ 21%), normal arterial oxygen tension ($PaO_2$) is >10.7 kPa and normal arterial oxygen saturation ($SaO_2$) is >93%<br><br>Arterial oxygen tension and oxygen saturation are related by the oxyhemoglobin dissocation curve<br><br>Normal arterial carbon dioxide tension ($PaO_2$) is 4.7–6.0 kPa |
| **Determinants of arterial oxygen tension** | • Inspired oxygen concentration ($FiO_2$)<br>• Alveolar ventilation (determined by tidal volume, dead space and respiratory rate)<br>• Diffusion of oxygen from alveoli to pulmonary capillaries<br>• Distribution and matching of lung ventilation and pulmonary blood flow ($V/Q$ matching). (see Table 15.2) |
| **Pulse oximetry** | • Arterial oxygen saturation can be measured non-invasively by pulse oximetry, although this method does not always give accurate readings (Table 15.3)<br>• Remember that pulse oximetry does not give information about arterial $PCO_2$ or pH<br>• Arterial blood gases and pH should be checked if arterial oxygen saturation by oximetry is <92%, or if there are clinical features of respiratory failure (Table 16.1) |

*Continued*

| Feature | Comment |
|---|---|
| **Respiratory failure** | Arterial hypoxemia is defined as an arterial $PO_2$ <10.7 kPa, and respiratory failure as an arterial $PO_2$ <8 kPa, breathing air<br>Respiratory failure is subdivided according to the arterial carbon dioxide tension ($PaCO_2$). Type 1 respiratory failure is when arterial $PCO_2$ is normal or low (<6 kPa), and type 2 respiratory failure is when arterial $PCO_2$ is high (>6 kPa)<br>See Chapter 16 |
| **Oxygen therapy and delivery devices** | Oxygen should be given to patients with hypoxemia (oxygen saturation by oximetry <92%), hypotension, low cardiac output, respiratory distress or cardiorespiratory arrest<br>Where possible, arterial blood gases should be measured before oxygen is started<br>Oxygen should be prescribed as carefully as any other drug, specifying the delivery device to be used and the oxygen flow rate<br>Commonly used oxygen delivery devices are described in Table 15.4<br>Initial $FiO_2$ should be 40–60%, except for patients with type 2 respiratory failure ($PaCO_2$ >6 kPa) who should start with 24% oxygen, and patients with cardiorespiratory arrest who should receive ~100% oxygen<br>Arterial blood gases should be checked within 2 h of starting oxygen, and $FiO_2$ adjusted accordingly. The target is a $PaO_2$ of >8 kPa or $SaO_2$ >92% |
| **Ventilatory support** | See Table 16.5 |

Arterial blood gases, oxygen saturation and oxygen therapy

## Further reading

Lee WW, et al. The accuracy of pulse oximetry in the emergency department. *Am J Emerg Med* 2000; 18: 427–31.

Soubani S. Noninvasive monitoring of oxygen and carbon dioxide. *Am J Emerg Med* 2001; 19: 141–6.

**TABLE 15.2** Estimation of the alveolar–arterial oxygen difference

**1** Establish $FiO_2$, the fractional concentration of oxygen in inspired gas (0.21 in air)

**2** Measure $PaO_2$ and $PaCO_2$, the partial pressures of oxygen and carbon dioxide (in kPa) in arterial blood

**3** Estimate the partial pressure of oxygen in alveolar gas ($PAO_2$) from the simplified form of the alveolar gas equation:

$PAO_2 = [PiO_2 - (PaCO_2/R)] = [(94.8 \times FiO_2) - (PaCO_2/R)]$

where $PiO_2$ is the partial pressure of inspired oxygen and $R$ is the respiratory quotient (can be taken to be 1). The table below shows the $PiO_2$ for a given $FiO_2$:

| $FiO_2$ | 0.21 | 0.24 | 0.28 | 0.31 | 0.35 | 0.40 | 0.60 | 1.0 |
|---------|------|------|------|------|------|------|------|-----|
| $PiO_2$ | 19.9 | 22.8 | 26.5 | 29.4 | 33.2 | 37.9 | 56.9 | 94.8 |

**4** Subtract $PaO_2$ from $PAO_2$ to give the alveolar–arterial oxygen difference (A–a gradient). Normal values are given below:

| Age (years) | Normal $PaO_2$ (kPa) | Normal A–a gradient (kPa) |
|-------------|----------------------|---------------------------|
| 20 | 13.2 | 1.8 |
| 40 | 12.5 | 2.5 |
| 60 | 11.9 | 3.1 |
| 80 | 11.3 | 3.7 |

**5** An increased alveolar–arterial oxygen difference indicates $V/Q$ mismatching: this may reflect a range of pulmonary and pulmonary vascular disorders, e.g. acute asthma, pneumonia, pulmonary edema and pulmonary embolism

---

**TABLE 15.3** Pulse oximetry: causes of inaccurate reading

- Probe not properly on finger
- Motion artifact
- Poor perfusion of finger
- Venous congestion
- Hypothermia
- Intense ambient light
- Abnormal hemoglobin (carboxyhemoglobin, methemoglobin, sickle hemoglobin)
- Severe anemia (Hb <5 g/dl)

**TABLE 15.4** Oxygen delivery devices

| Device | Indication | Concentration of $O_2$ delivered | Advantages | Disadvantages |
| --- | --- | --- | --- | --- |
| **Facemask with reservoir bag ($O_2$ flow rate 10–15 L/min)** | Cardiorespiratory arrest or peri-arrest, when high concentration of $O_2$ essential | >80% | Highest $O_2$ concentration delivered | Some rebreathing of $CO_2$, with risk of $CO_2$ retention in type 2 respiratory failure |
| **Low-flow mask (e.g. Hudson)** | Type 1 respiratory failure | 28–60%, depending on the $O_2$ flow rate, degree of leakage between the mask and face, and ventilatory minute volume | Simple and cheap No need to change mask if $FIO_2$ has to be changed | $FIO_2$ provided by a given $O_2$ flow rate is variable At flow rates <5 L/min, significant rebreathing may occur, with risk of $CO_2$ retention in type 2 respiratory failure |

*Continued*

**Arterial blood gases, oxygen saturation and oxygen therapy**

| Device | Indication | Concentration of $O_2$ delivered | Advantages | Disadvantages |
|---|---|---|---|---|
| **High-flow mask (Venturi principle)** | Type 2 respiratory failure, and when accurate $FiO_2$ is needed | 24%, 28%, 35%, 40% and 60%, determined by the Venturi valve (color coded) used and the $O_2$ flow rate | Delivers an accurate $FiO_2$. Reduces the risk of $CO_2$ retention in type 2 respiratory failure. 60% mask is useful in type 1 respiratory failure when hypoxemia persists despite 10 L/min $O_2$ flow rate via low-flow mask | Uncomfortable to wear for long periods New valve needed if $FiO_2$ has to be changed |

*Continued*

Arterial blood gases, oxygen saturation and oxygen therapy

| Device | Indication | Concentration of $O_2$ delivered | Advantages | Disadvantages |
|---|---|---|---|---|
| **Nasal cannulae** | Patients with COPD or recovering from other causes of respiratory failure | Depends on the $O_2$ flow rate and ventilatory minute volume; 2 L/min gives an $FiO_2$ of roughly 25–30% | Prevents rebreathing and so reduces the risk of $CO_2$ retention in type 2 respiratory failure. Comfortable to wear for long periods | Nasal irritation with flow rates >3 L/min |

COPD, chronic obstructive pulmonary disease.

# 16 Respiratory failure

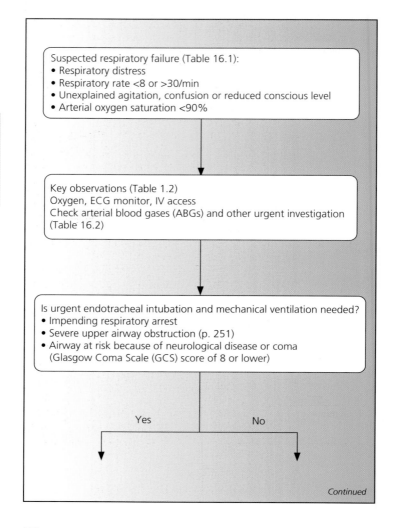

Suspected respiratory failure (Table 16.1):
- Respiratory distress
- Respiratory rate <8 or >30/min
- Unexplained agitation, confusion or reduced conscious level
- Arterial oxygen saturation <90%

Key observations (Table 1.2)
Oxygen, ECG monitor, IV access
Check arterial blood gases (ABGs) and other urgent investigation
(Table 16.2)

Is urgent endotracheal intubation and mechanical ventilation needed?
- Impending respiratory arrest
- Severe upper airway obstruction (p. 251)
- Airway at risk because of neurological disease or coma
  (Glasgow Coma Scale (GCS) score of 8 or lower)

Yes                No

*Continued*

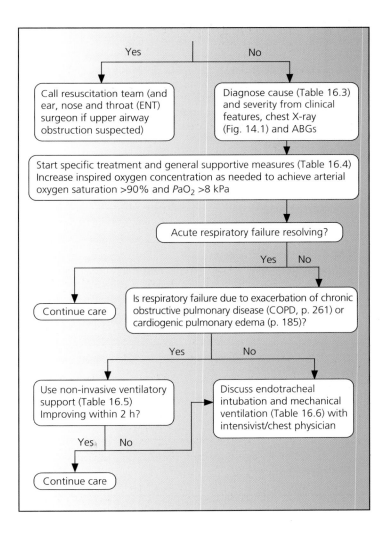

---

**TABLE 16.1** Clinical features of acute respiratory failure

- Respiratory distress (dyspnea, tachypnea, ability to speak only in short sentences or single words, agitation, sweating)
- Respiratory rate <8 or >30/min
- Accessory muscles of breathing active
- Feeble respiratory efforts, silent chest
- Tremor, asterixis
- Cyanosis
- Agitation, confusion
- Reduced conscious level, coma
- Bradycardia or hypotension

---

**ALERT**
Acute respiratory failure developing in hospital is usually due to pneumonia, aspiration of secretions or gastric contents, pulmonary edema or sedative drugs.

---

**TABLE 16.2** Urgent investigation in acute respiratory failure

- Chest X-ray
- Arterial blood gases and pH
- ECG
- Full blood count
- Blood glucose
- Sodium, potassium and creatinine
- Blood culture
- Sputum culture

---

## Further reading

British Thoracic Society Standards of Care Committee. Non-invasive ventilation in acute respiratory failure. *Thorax* 2002; 57: 192–211.

---

**TABLE 16.3** Common causes of acute respiratory failure

**Primary cause**
- Airway obstruction in the unconscious patient (p. 7)
- Acute severe asthma (p. 253)
- Acute exacerbation of chronic obstructive pulmonary disease (p. 261)
- Pneumonia (p. 268)
- Pulmonary embolism (p. 231)
- Cardiogenic pulmonary edema (p. 185)
- Acute respiratory distress syndrome (p. 192)
- Poisoning with psychotropic drugs or alcohol (p. 112)

**Contributory factors**
- Aspiration of secretions or gastric contents (p. 278)
- Respiratory muscle fatigue (p. 347)
- Severe obesity
- Chest wall abnormality, e.g. kyphoscoliosis
- Large pleural effusion (p. 283)
- Pneumothorax (p. 280)
- Sedative drugs: benzodiazepines, opioids

---

**TABLE 16.4** Management of respiratory failure: general principles

- Maintain patent airway (pp. 245–9)
- Increase inspired oxygen concentration if needed to achieve target arterial oxygen saturation >90% (>88% in acute exacerbation of COPD)
- Treat underlying cause and contributory factors (Table 16.3)
- If feasible, sit the patient up to improve diaphragmatic descent and increase tidal volume
- Clear secretions: encourage cough, physiotherapy, aspiration
- Drain large pleural effusion if present
- Drain pneumothorax if present (Table 43.3; p. 619)
- Optimize cardiac output: treat hypotension and heart failure
- Consider ventilatory support (Table 16.5)

Respiratory failure

Respiratory failure

**TABLE 16.5** Management of respiratory failure: non-invasive ventilatory support

| Mode of ventilation | Indications | Contraindications | Disadvantages and complications |
|---|---|---|---|
| **Continuous positive airways pressure (CPAP)** | Cardiogenic pulmonary edema | Recent facial, upper airway, or upper gastrointestinal tract surgery | Discomfort from tightly fitting facemask |
| **Bilevel positive airways pressure (BiPAP)** | Acute exacerbation of COPD with $PaO_2$ <7.5–8 kPa despite supplemental oxygen, and arterial pH 7.25–7.35 | Vomiting or bowel obstruction | Discourages coughing and clearing of secretions |
| | | Copious secretions* | |
| | | Hemodynamic instability | |
| | Pneumonia | Impaired consciousness, confusion or agitation* | |

COPD, chronic obstructive pulmonary disease; * relative contraindication.

**TABLE 16.6** Management of respiratory failure: invasive ventilatory support

| Mode of ventilation | Indications | Contraindications | Disadvantages and complications |
|---|---|---|---|
| **Endotracheal intubation and mechanical ventilation** | Upper airway obstruction<br><br>Impending respiratory arrest<br><br>Airway at risk because of neurological disease or coma (GCS of 8 or lower)<br><br>Oxygenation failure: $PaO_2$ <7.5–8 kPa despite supplemental oxygen/NIV<br><br>Ventilatory failure: respiratory acidosis with arterial pH <7.25 | Known severe COPD with severely impaired functional capacity and/or severe comorbidity<br><br>Patient has expressed wish not to be ventilated | Adverse hemodynamic effects<br><br>Pharyngeal, laryngeal and tracheal injury<br><br>Pneumonia<br><br>Ventilator-induced lung injury (e.g. pneumothorax)<br><br>Complications of sedation and neuromuscular blockade |

COPD, chronic obstructive pulmonary disease; GCS, Glasgow Coma Scale (see p. 297); NIV, non-invasive ventilation.

Respiratory failure

# 17 Acid–base disorders

**TABLE 17.1** Grading of severity of acid–base disorders

| Arterial pH | Acid–base status | Arterial hydrogen ion concentration (nmol/L) |
|---|---|---|
| <7.2 | Severe acidosis | >60 |
| 7.2–7.3 | Moderate acidosis | 50–60 |
| 7.3–7.35 | Mild acidosis | 45–50 |
| 7.35–7.45 | Normal range | 35–45 |
| 7.45–7.5 | Mild alkalosis | 30–35 |
| 7.5–7.6 | Moderate alkalosis | 20–30 |
| >7.6 | Severe alkalosis | <20 |

**TABLE 17.2** Acidity of arterial blood: conversion of pH units to hydrogen ion concentration (nmol/L)

| | 0 | 1 | 2 | 3 | 4 | 5 | 6 | 7 | 8 | 9 |
|---|---|---|---|---|---|---|---|---|---|---|
| **7.0** | 99 | 97 | 95 | 93 | 91 | 89 | 87 | 85 | 83 | 81 |
| **7.1** | 79 | 78 | 76 | 74 | 72 | 71 | 69 | 68 | 66 | 65 |
| **7.2** | 63 | 62 | 60 | 59 | 58 | 56 | 55 | 54 | 53 | 51 |
| **7.3** | 50 | 49 | 48 | 47 | 46 | 45 | 44 | 43 | 42 | 41 |
| **7.4** | 40 | 39 | 38 | 37 | 36 | 35 | 35 | 34 | 33 | 32 |
| **7.5** | 31 | 30 | 30 | 30 | 29 | 28 | 28 | 27 | 26 | 26 |
| **7.6** | 25 | 25 | 24 | 23 | 23 | 22 | 22 | 21 | 21 | 20 |

TABLE 17.3 Classification of acid–base disorders according to arterial hydrogen ion concentration/pH and $PCO_2$ (Fig. 17.1)

| Arterial $PCO_2$ (kPa) | Arterial hydrogen ion concentration (nmol/L) or pH | | |
|---|---|---|---|
| | [H+] >45<br>pH < 7.35 | 35–45<br>7.35–7.45 | <35<br>>7.45 |
| <4.7 | Metabolic acidosis with respiratory compensation<br>*or*<br>Metabolic acidosis + respiratory alkalosis, e.g.:<br>• Pulmonary edema<br>• Salicylate poisoning<br>• Hepatorenal syndrome | Respiratory alkalosis with metabolic compensation | Respiratory alkalosis *or* Respiratory alkalosis + metabolic alkalosis, e.g.:<br>• Acute liver failure with vomiting, nasogastric drainage or severe hypokalemia<br>• Peritoneal dialysis for chronic renal failure<br>*Continued* |

Acid–base disorders

**Acid–base disorders**

| Arterial $PCO_2$ (kPa) | Arterial hydrogen ion concentration (nmol/L) or pH | | |
|---|---|---|---|
| | [H+] >45<br>pH < 7.35 | 35–45<br>7.35–7.45 | <35<br>>7.45 |
| 4.7–6.0 | Metabolic acidosis | Normal acid–base status | Metabolic alkalosis |
| >6.0 | Respiratory acidosis with partial metabolic compensation or<br>Respiratory acidosis + metabolic acidosis, e.g.:<br>• Cardiopulmonary arrest<br>• COPD complicated by circulatory failure or sepsis<br>• Severe pulmonary edema<br>• Combined respiratory and renal failure<br>• Severe tricyclic poisoning | Respiratory acidosis with metabolic compensation, e.g.:<br>• COPD with chronic $CO_2$ retention | Metabolic alkalosis +<br>respiratory acidosis, e.g.:<br>• Diuretic therapy + COPD with chronic $CO_2$ retention |

COPD, chronic obstructive pulmonary disease.

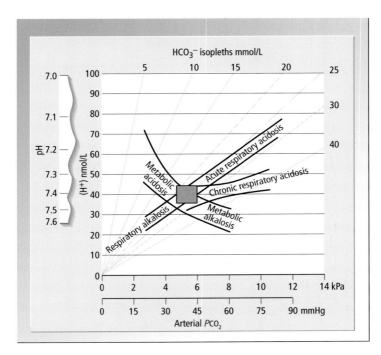

**FIGURE 17.1** Acid–base diagram relating arterial hydrogen ion concentration (nmol/L) or pH to $PaCO_2$. The shaded rectangle is the normal range. The 95% confidence limits of hydrogen ion concentration/$PaCO_2$ relationships in single disturbances of acid–base balance are shown. (From Flenley, D.C. *Lancet* 1971; **1**: 961.)

**TABLE 17.4**  Causes of metabolic acidosis

- Lactic acidosis
  - Inadequate tissue perfusion due to hypotension, low cardiac output or sepsis
  - Prolonged hypoxemia
  - Muscle contraction: status epilepticus
  - Metformin
- Diabetic, alcoholic* and starvation ketoacidosis
- Poisoning
  - Carbon monoxide (p. 76)
  - Ethanol
  - Ethylene glycol
  - Methanol
  - Paracetamol (p. 75)
  - Salicylates (p. 75)
  - Tricyclics (p. 112)
  - Toluene (glue sniffing)
- Renal failure (p. 410)
- Renal tubular acidosis
- Loss of bicarbonate from the gut
  - Severe diarrhea (p. 376)
  - Tube drainage

* Alcoholic ketoacidosis is due to alcohol binge plus starvation, and often associated with pancreatitis; hyperglyaemia may occur but is mild (<15 mmol/L); treat with IV glucose infusion; for other supportive therapy see p. 434.

**TABLE 17.5** Causes of respiratory acidosis (inadequate alveolar ventilation resulting in a raised arterial $PCO_2$)

| Site of lesion | Causes |
| --- | --- |
| **Brain** | Stroke (p. 303)<br>Mass lesion with brainstem compression<br>Encephalitis (p. 334)<br>Sedative drugs<br>Status epilepticus |
| **Spinal cord** | Cord compression (p. 339)<br>Transverse myelitis<br>Poliomyelitis, rabies |
| **Peripheral nerve** | Guillain–Barré syndrome (p. 342)<br>Critical illness polyneuropathy<br>Toxins<br>Acute intermittent porphyria<br>Vasculitis, e.g. systemic lupus erythematosus<br>Diphtheria |
| **Neuromuscular junction** | Myasthenia gravis<br>Eaton–Lambert syndrome<br>Botulism<br>Toxins |
| **Muscle** | Hypokalamia<br>Hypophosphatemia<br>Rhabdomyolysis (see Table 65.4) |
| **Thoracic cage and pleura** | Crushed chest<br>Morbid obesity<br>Kyphoscoliosis<br>Ankylosing spondylitis<br>Large pleural effusion (p. 283) |
| **Lungs and airways** | Upper airway obstruction (p. 251)<br>Severe acute asthma (p. 253)<br>Chronic obstructive pulmonary disease (p. 261)<br>Severe pneumonia (p. 268)<br>Severe pulmonary edema (p. 185) |

Acid-base disorders

---

**TABLE 17.6** Causes of respiratory alkalosis

- Pulmonary disorders with hyperventilation
  - Acute asthma (p. 253)
  - Pneumonia (p. 268)
  - Pulmonary embolism (p. 231)
  - Pulmonary edema (p. 185)
- Primary hyperventilation
  - Anxiety and pain
  - Central nervous system disorders, e.g. stroke (p. 303), bacterial meningitis (p. 327)
- Liver failure (p. 394)
- Sepsis (p. 59)
- Salicylate poisoning (p. 75)

---

**TABLE 17.7** Causes of metabolic alkalosis

- Loss of gastric acid
  - Prolonged vomiting
  - Gastric aspiration
- Diuretic therapy
- Severe and prolonged potassium deficiency (p. 447)
- Mineralocorticoid and glucocorticoid excess

---

## Further reading

Maccari C, et al. The patient with a severe degree of metabolic acidosis: a deductive analysis. *Q J Med* 2006; 99: 475–85.

# 18 The unconscious patient

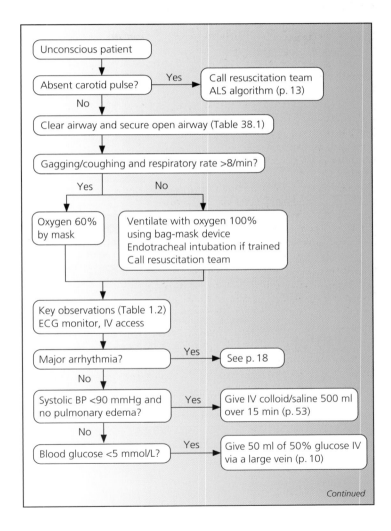

Unconscious patient

Absent carotid pulse? → **Yes** → Call resuscitation team ALS algorithm (p. 13)

**No**

Clear airway and secure open airway (Table 38.1)

Gagging/coughing and respiratory rate >8/min?

**Yes** — Oxygen 60% by mask

**No** — Ventilate with oxygen 100% using bag-mask device
Endotracheal intubation if trained
Call resuscitation team

Key observations (Table 1.2)
ECG monitor, IV access

Major arrhythmia? → **Yes** → See p. 18

**No**

Systolic BP <90 mmHg and no pulmonary edema? → **Yes** → Give IV colloid/saline 500 ml over 15 min (p. 53)

**No**

Blood glucose <5 mmol/L? → **Yes** → Give 50 ml of 50% glucose IV via a large vein (p. 10)

*Continued*

The unconscious patient

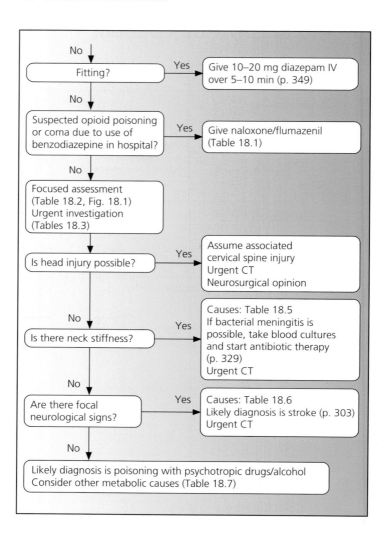

No ↓

Fitting? — Yes → Give 10–20 mg diazepam IV over 5–10 min (p. 349)

No ↓

Suspected opioid poisoning or coma due to use of benzodiazepine in hospital? — Yes → Give naloxone/flumazenil (Table 18.1)

No ↓

Focused assessment (Table 18.2, Fig. 18.1) Urgent investigation (Tables 18.3)

↓

Is head injury possible? — Yes → Assume associated cervical spine injury Urgent CT Neurosurgical opinion

No ↓

Is there neck stiffness? — Yes → Causes: Table 18.5 If bacterial meningitis is possible, take blood cultures and start antibiotic therapy (p. 329) Urgent CT

No ↓

Are there focal neurological signs? — Yes → Causes: Table 18.6 Likely diagnosis is stroke (p. 303) Urgent CT

No ↓

Likely diagnosis is poisoning with psychotropic drugs/alcohol Consider other metabolic causes (Table 18.7)

---

**TABLE 18.1** Naloxone and flumazenil

**Naloxone**
- If the respiratory rate is <12/min, or the pupils are pinpoint, or there is another reason to suspect opioid poisoning, give naloxone
- Give 0.4–2 mg IV every 2–3 min, to a maximum of 10 mg, until the respiratory rate is around 15/min.
- If there is a response, start an IV infusion: add 4 mg to 500 ml glucose 5% or saline (8 μg/ml) and titrate against the respiratory rate and conscious level. The plasma half-life of naloxone is 1 h, shorter than that of most opioids
- If there is no response to naloxone, opioid poisoning is excluded

**Flumazenil**
- If coma is a complication of the therapeutic use of benzodiazepine in hospital, give flumazenil 200 μg IV over 15 s; if needed, further doses of 100 μg can be given at 1 min intervals up to a total dose of 2 mg
- Flumazenil should not be given to other patients because of the risk of precipitating fits if there is mixed poisoning with benzodiazepines and tricyclics

---

**TABLE 18.2** Focused assessment of the unconscious patient

**Priorities**
- Stabilize the airway, breathing and circulation
- Exclude/treat hypoglycemia
- Consider naloxone (and flumazenil if the patient has received benzodiazepine in hospital) (Table 18.1)

**History**
Obtain the history from all available sources: ambulance personnel, friends and family, general practitioner and hospital records, patient's belongings. Establish:
- Time course of loss of consciousness? Abrupt (e.g. subarachnoid hemorrhage, seizure), gradual (e.g. poisoning, bacterial meningitis) or fluctuating (e.g. recurring seizures, subdural hematoma, metabolic encephalopathy)?

*Continued*

The unconscious patient

- Focal neurological features before loss of consciousness?
- Known neurological disorder?
- Recent systemic symptoms?
- Recent foreign travel?
- Known physical or psychiatric illness?
- Alcohol or substance abuse?
- Current medications

**Examination**
- Document the level of consciousness in objective terms, e.g. using the Glasgow Coma Scale (see Table 46.2)
- Assess carefully the respiratory rate and pattern. Causes of coma with hyperventilation are given in Table 18.4
- Examine for signs of head injury (e.g. scalp laceration, bruising, bleeding from an external auditory meatus or from the nose). If there are signs of head injury, assume additional cervical spine injury until proven otherwise: the neck must be immobilized in a collar and X-rayed before you check for neck stiffness and the oculocephalic response
- Check for neck stiffness
- Check the position of the eyes, the size and symmetry of the pupils and their response to bright light (Fig. 18.1)
- Check the oculocephalic response. This is a simple but important test of an intact brainstem. Rotate the head to left and right. In an unconscious patient with an intact brainstem, both eyes rotate counter to movement of the head
- Examine the limbs: tone, response to a painful stimulus (nailbed pressure), tendon reflexes and plantar responses
- Examine the fundi
- Complete a systematic examination of the patient (see Table 1.9). Check for possible complications of coma (hypothermia, pressure necrosis of skin or muscle, corneal abrasions, inhalation pneumonia)
- In patients with suspected poisoning, the clinical features may give clues to the poison (see Table 11.1)

## Further reading

Bateman DE. Neurological assessment of coma. *J Neurol Neurosurg Psychiatry* 2001; 71 (suppl I): i13–i17.

Wijdicks EFM, et al. Validation of a new coma scale: the FOUR score. *Ann Neurol* 2005; 58: 585–93.

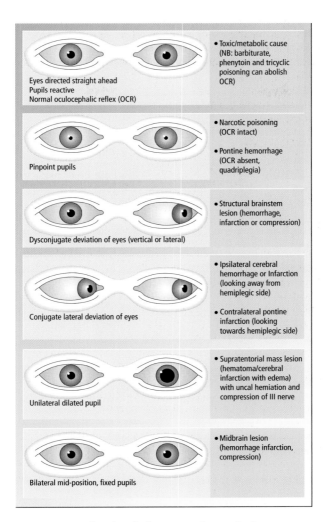

The unconscious patient

**FIGURE 18.1** Eye signs in the unconscious patient.

---

**TABLE 18.3** Urgent investigation of the unconscious patient

- Blood glucose
- Sodium, potassium and creatinine
- Liver function tests, albumin and calcium
- Plasma osmolality (see Table 11.3) if poisoning suspected[†] or coma remains unexplained
- Full blood count
- Prothrombin time if liver failure suspected or coma remains unexplained
- Blood culture if temperature <36 or >38°C
- Arterial blood gases and pH (Table 17.5)
- Chest X-ray
- ECG if there is hypotension, coexistent heart disease or suspected ingestion of cardiotoxic drugs (antiarrhythmics, tricyclics)
- Cranial CT if metabolic cause of coma is not evident

[†] If poisoning is suspected: save serum (10 ml), urine (50 ml) and vomit or gastric aspirate (50 ml) at 4°C for subsequent analysis.

---

**TABLE 18.4** Causes of coma with hyperventilation (low $PaCO_2$)

- Ketoacidosis: diabetic or alcoholic
- Liver failure
- Renal failure
- Bacterial meningitis
- Poisoning with aspirin, carbon monoxide, ethanol, ethylene glycol, methanol, paracetamol or tricyclics
- Stroke complicated by pneumonia or pulmonary edema
- Brainstem stroke

---

**TABLE 18.5** Causes of coma with neck stiffness*

- Bacterial meningitis (p. 327)
- Encephalitis (p. 334)
- Subarachnoid hemorrhage (p. 321)
- Cerebral or cerebellar hemorrhage with extension into the subarachnoid space
- Cerebral malaria (p. 546)

* In any of these conditions, neck stiffness may be lost with increasing coma

---

**TABLE 18.6** Causes of coma with focal neurological signs

**With brainstem signs** (deviation of the eyes/abnormal pupils)
- Brainstem compression due to large intracerebral hemorrhage or infarction with edema
- Brainstem stroke
- Cerebellar stroke
- Head injury
- Cerebral malaria (p. 546)

**Without brainstem signs**
- Hypoglycemia (in some cases) (p. 423)
- Liver failure (in some cases) (p. 394)
- Head injury
- Cerebral malaria (p. 546)

---

**TABLE 18.7** Metabolic causes of coma

- Poisoning with psychotropic drugs or alcohol (p. 112)
- Hypoglycemia (p. 423)
- Hypoxic ischemic brain injury
- Septic encephalopathy
- Liver failure (p. 394)
- Respiratory failure (p. 104)
- Renal failure (p. 410)
- Diabetic ketoacidosis (p. 429)
- Hyperosmolar non-ketotic hyperglycemia (p. 436)
- Myxedema coma (p. 464)
- Acute adrenal insufficiency (p. 457)
- Severe hyponatremia (p. 440)
- Central pontine myelinolysis
- Severe hypercalcemia (p. 451)
- After major tonic-clonic seizure (p. 355)

**The unconscious patient**

# 19 Transient loss of consciousness

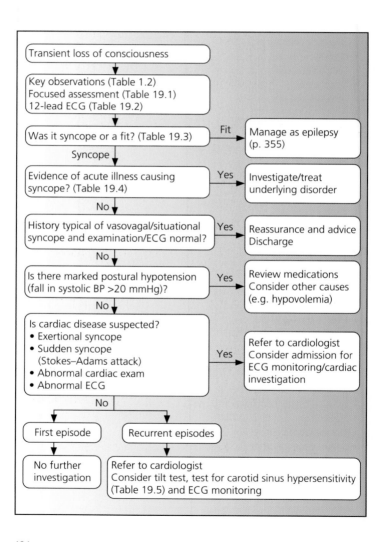

**TABLE 19.1** Focused assessment after transient loss of consciousness

**History**

**1** *Background*
- Any previous similar attacks
- Previous significant head injury (i.e. with skull fracture or loss of consciousness)
- Birth injury, febrile convulsions in childhood, meningitis or encephalitis
- Family history of epilepsy
- Cardiac disease associated with ventricular arrhythmia (previous myocardial infarction, hypertrophic or dilated cardiomyopathy, heart failure)
- Medications
- Alcohol or substance abuse
- Sleep deprivation

**2** *Before the attack*
- Prodromal symptoms: were these cardiovascular (e.g. dizziness, palpitation, chest pain) or focal neurological symptoms (aura)?
- Circumstances, e.g. exercising, standing, sitting or lying, asleep
- Precipitants, e.g. coughing, micturition, head-turning

**3** *The attack*
- Were there any focal neurological features at the onset: sustained deviation of the head or eyes or unilateral jerking of the limbs?
- Was there a cry (may occur in tonic phase of fit)?
- Duration of loss of consciousness
- Associated tongue biting, urinary incontinence or injury
- Facial color changes (pallor common in syncope, uncommon with a fit)
- Abnormal pulse (must be assessed in relation to the reliability of the witness)

**4** *After the attack*
- Immediately well or delayed recovery with confusion or headache?

*Continued*

Transient loss of consciousness

**Examination**

- Conscious level and mental state (confirm the patient is fully oriented)
- Pulse, blood pressure, respiratory rate, arterial oxygen saturation, temperature
- Systolic BP sitting or lying and after 2 min standing (a fall of >20 mmHg is abnormal; note if symptomatic or not)
- Arterial pulses (check major pulses for asymmetry or bruits)
- Jugular venous pressure (if raised, consider pulmonary embolism, pulmonary hypertension or cardiac tamponade)
- Heart murmurs (aortic stenosis and hypertrophic cardiomyopathy may cause exertional syncope; atrial myxoma may simulate mitral stenosis)
- Neck mobility (does neck movement induce presyncope? Is there neck stiffness?)
- Presence of focal neurological signs: as a minimum, check visual fields, limb power, tendon reflexes and plantar responses
- Fundi (for hemorrhages or papilledema)

**TABLE 19.2** The ECG after syncope

| ECG feature | Possible significance |
|---|---|
| **Sinus bradycardia (rate <50/min) or sinus pauses** | May reflect sinoatrial disorder. Accept as the cause of syncope if definitely related to symptoms |
| **First degree AV block** | Raises the possibility of intermittent second or third degree AV block, but as an isolated abnormality is usually of no significance |
| **Second degree AV block** | Likely to be the cause of syncope: indication for pacing |
| **Third degree (complete) AV block** | Likely to be the cause of syncope: indication for pacing |
| **Atrial fibrillation** | May reflect sinoatrial disorder or underlying structural heart disease |

*Continued*

| ECG feature | Possible significance |
|---|---|
| **Paced rhythm** | Pacemaker failure is rare but should be excluded (p. 236) |
| **Short PR interval (<120 ms)** | Look for other features of WPW syndrome (delta wave, widened QRS complex): if WPW present, discuss management with a cardiologist |
| **Right axis deviation (QRS predominantly negative in lead I and positive in lead II)** | Consider pulmonary hypertension or pulmonary embolism |
| **Left axis deviation (QRS predominantly positive in lead I and negative in lead II)** | As an isolated abnormality, usually of no significance |
| **Right bundle branch block (RBBB)** | Consider pulmonary embolism |
| **Left bundle branch block (LBBB)** | May reflect structural heart disease or conducting system disease |
| **Bifascicular block (RBBB– left axis deviation) with or without first degree AV block** | Significantly increases the likelihood that syncope was due to intermittent AV block |

*Continued*

| ECG feature | Possible significance |
| --- | --- |
| **Pathological Q waves** | Usually reflect previous myocardial infarction<br>May also be seen in hypertrophic cardiomyopathy or WPW syndrome (pseudoinfarct pattern) |
| **Left ventricular hypertrophy** | Consider aortic stenosis, hypertrophic cardiomyopathy or hypertension |
| **Dominant R wave in V1** | May be due to:<br>• Right ventricular hypertrophy<br>• RBBB<br>• WPW syndrome<br>• Posterior myocardial infarction<br>• Normal variant |
| **Right ventricular hypertrophy** | Consider pulmonary hypertension |
| **Long QT interval** | QT inverval >500 ms is associated with high risk of polymorphic ventricular tachycardia (torsade de pointes)<br>Usually due to drugs, may be exacerbated by bradycardia and hypokalemia |

AV, atrioventricular; WPW, Wolff–Parkinson–White.

TABLE 19.3 Features differentiating a generalized fit from vasovagal and cardiac syncope (Stokes–Adams attack)

| | Generalized fit | Vasovagal syncope | Cardiac syncope (Stokes–Adams attack) |
|---|---|---|---|
| **Occurrence when sitting or lying** | Common | Rare | May occur |
| **Occurrence during sleep** | Common | Does not occur | May occur |
| **Prodromal symptoms** | May occur, with focal neurological symptoms, head turning, automatisms | Typical, with dizziness, sweating, nausea, blurring of vision, disturbance of hearing, yawning | Often none. Palpitation may precede syncope in tachyarrhythmias |
| **Focal neurological features at onset** | May occur (and signify focal cerebral lesion) | Never occur | Never occur |
| **Tonic-clonic movments** | Characteristic, occur within 30s of onset | May occur after 30s of syncope (secondary anoxic seizure) | May occur after 30s of syncope (secondary anoxic seizure) |

*Continued*

**Transient loss of consciousness**

**Transient loss of consciousness**

|  | Generalized fit | Vasovagal syncope | Cardiac syncope (Stokes–Adams attack) |
|---|---|---|---|
| **Facial color** | Flush or cyanosis at onset | Pallor at onset and after syncope | Pallor at onset, flush on recovery |
| **Tongue biting** | Common | Rare | Rare |
| **Urinary incontinence** | Common | May occur | May occur |
| **Injury** | May occur | Uncommon | May occur |
| **Postictal confusion** | Common (wakes in ambulance) | Uncommon (wakes on floor) | Uncommon (wakes on floor) |

**TABLE 19.4** Causes of syncope

| Common | Less common or rare |
|---|---|
| **Cardiovascular** | |
| Vasovagal syncope | Aortic stenosis |
| Situational syncope* | Pulmonary embolism (p. 231) |
| Postural hypotension due to drugs | Carotid sinus hypersensitivity (Table 19.5) |
| Arrhythmias | Pulmonary hypertension |
| | Aortic dissection (p. 181) |
| | Acute myocardial infarction (p. 158) |
| | Hypertrophic cardiomyopathy |
| | Atrial myxoma |
| | Postural hypotension due to other causes |
| | Cardiac tamponade (p. 216) |
| **Neurological** | |
| Epilepsy (p. 349) | Subarachnoid hemorrhage (p. 321) |
| | Subclavian steal syndrome |
| | Vertebrobasilar TIA |
| | Migraine |
| **Others** | |
| | Rapid hemorrhage (e.g. variceal bleeding) |
| | Hypoglycemia (p. 423) |
| | Hyperventilation |

TIA, transient ischemic attack.
* Situational syncope: syncope occurring in relation to coughing, micturition, defecation or swallowing, without another cause apparent on examination or ECG.

Transient loss of consciousness

---

**TABLE 19.5** Testing for carotid sinus hypersensitivity

- Indicated in patients aged 60 and over with unexplained syncope
- Contraindications include the presence of a carotid bruit, recent myocardial infarction, recent stroke or a history of ventricular tachycardia
- Begin with the patient lying
- Attach an ECG monitor with a printer and check the blood pressure
- The carotid sinus lies at the level of the upper border of the thyroid cartilage just below the angle of the jaw
- Perform carotid sinus massage for up to 15s whilst recording a rhythm strip. Press posteriorly and medially over the artery (first on the right, and if this is negative on the left) with your thumb or index and middle fingers
- If the test is negative, repeat with the patient sitting
- An abnormal response is defined by a sinus pause >3s or a drop in systolic blood pressure >50 mmHg. If these occur, discuss with a cardiologist whether pacemaker implantation is indicated

---

## Further reading

American Heart Association and American College of Cardiology. Foundation scientific statement on the evaluation of syncope. *Circulation* 2006; 113: 316–27.

Bergfeldt L. Differential diagnosis of cardiogenic syncope and seizure disorders. *Heart* 2003; 89: 353–58.

Brignole M. Diagnosis and treatment of syncope. *Heart* 2007; 93: 130–6.

Goldschlager N, et al. Etiologic considerations in the patients with syncope and an apparently normal heart. *Arch Intern Med* 2003; 163: 151–62.

Grubb BP. Neurocardiogenic syncope. *N Engl J Med* 2005; 352: 1004–10.

Harbison J, et al. Stokes Adams attacks and cardiovascular syncope. *Lancet* 2002; 359: 158–60.

**Transient loss of consciousness**

# 20 Acute confusional state

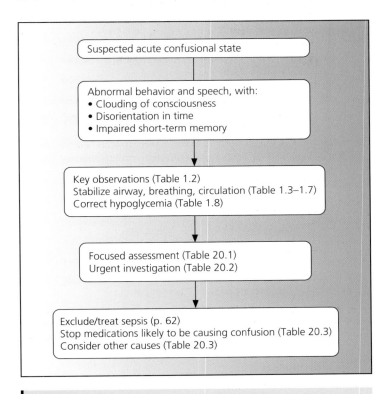

Suspected acute confusional state

Abnormal behavior and speech, with:
- Clouding of consciousness
- Disorientation in time
- Impaired short-term memory

Key observations (Table 1.2)
Stabilize airway, breathing, circulation (Table 1.3–1.7)
Correct hypoglycemia (Table 1.8)

Focused assessment (Table 20.1)
Urgent investigation (Table 20.2)

Exclude/treat sepsis (p. 62)
Stop medications likely to be causing confusion (Table 20.3)
Consider other causes (Table 20.3)

**ALERT**
Vivid visual or auditory hallucinations suggest alcohol withdrawal as the cause of an acute confusional state.

**ALERT**
Consider non-convulsive status epilepticus as the cause of an acute confusional state if there are mild clonic movements of the eyelids, face or hands, or simple automatisms. Diazepam (10 mg IV) may terminate the status with improvement in conscious level.

---

**TABLE 20.1** Focused assessment in acute confusional state

**1 Assess the mental state** (see Tables 46.3, 46.4)
- Does the patient really have an acute confusional state (and not dementia, a functional psychosis or severe depression)? Acute confusional state is characterized by:
  - Clouding of consciousness (reduced alertness, impaired attention and concentration)
  - Disorientation in time (and often also for place and person)
  - Impaired short-term memory
- The duration of the patient's abnormal mental state, as assessed by a reliable witness, often helps distinguish acute confusional state from dementia (which may of course coexist). Other features which differentiate between these diagnoses are given in Table 86.1

**2 Check the drug chart**
- Many drugs may cause an acute confusional state in the elderly, notably benzodiazepines, tricyclics, analgesics (including NSAIDs, particularly indomethacin), lithium, corticosteroids, and drugs for parkinsonism
- If the patient was admitted with an acute confusional state, find out exactly what medications were being taken prior to admission (if necessary, contact the patient's general practioner to check which drugs were prescribed, and ask relatives to collect all medications in the home)

**3 Are there signs of sepsis or other illness which may cause acute confusion?**
- Key observations (see Table 1.2) and systematic examination (see Table 1.9)

---

NSAIDs, non-steroidal anti-inflammatory drugs.

## Further reading

British Geriatrics Society. Guidelines for the prevention, diagnosis and management of delirium in older people in hospital (2005). British Geriatrics Society website (http://www.bgs.org.uk).

Johnson MH. Assessing confused patients. *J Neurol Neurosurg Psychiatry* 2001; 71 (suppl I): i7–i12.

---

**TABLE 20.2** Urgent investigation in acute confusional state

- Blood glucose
- Sodium, potassium and creatinine
- Liver function tests, albumin and calcium
- Full blood count
- Prothrombin time if suspected liver disease
- C-reactive protein
- Blood culture if temperature <36 or >38°C
- Urine stick test, microscopy and culture
- ECG
- Chest X-ray
- Arterial blood gases if arterial oxygen saturation <92% or new chest signs
- Cranial CT if:
  - Confusional state followed a fall or head injury
  - There are new focal neurological signs
  - There is papilledema or other evidence of raised intracranial pressure

---

**ALERT**

Consider acute confusional state in any patient labeled difficult, uncooperative or a 'poor historian'.

---

**TABLE 20.3** Causes of acute confusional state

**Infection**
- Urinary or respiratory tract infections are the commonest causes
- Bacterial meningitis (p. 327), infective endocarditis (p. 203) and intra-abdominal sepsis (e.g. cholangitis (p. 407)) should be considered in the febrile patient without localizing signs
- Exclude malaria if there has been recent travel to an endemic region (p. 546).

**Drug-related**
- Many drugs may cause an acute confusional state in the elderly, notably benzodiazepines, tricyclics, analgesics (including NSAIDs, particularly indomethacin), lithium, steroids, and drugs for parkinsonism

*Continued*

- Consider poisoning with amphetamine, cocaine and other psychotropic drugs in younger patients with acute confusional state (see Table 11.1)
- Benzodiazepine withdrawal may also cause a confusional state
- Consider neuroleptic malignant syndrome if the patient is taking neuroleptics (see Table 51.5)

**Alcohol-related**
- Intoxication or withdrawal (see p. 563)
- Wernicke encephalopathy: confusional state, nystagmus, sixth nerve palsy (unable to abduct the eye) and ataxia (wide-based gait; may be unable to stand or walk)

**Primary neurological disorders**
- Head injury
- Postictal state
- Non-dominant parietal lobe stroke
- Subdural hematoma (p. 303)
- Subarachnoid hemorrhage (p. 321)
- Non-convulsive status epilepticus
- Meningitis (p. 327)
- Encephalitis (p. 334)
- Raised intracranial pressure (p. 360)

**Other systemic disorders**
- Hypoglycemia (p. 423)
- Hyperglycemic states: ketoacidosis (p. 429) and non-ketotic hyperglycemia (p. 436)
- Respiratory failure (p. 104)
- Heart failure
- Acute liver failure (p. 394)
- Advanced renal failure (p. 410)
- Hypertensive encephalopathy (p. 221)
- Acute adrenal insufficiency (p. 457)
- Severe hypothyroidism (p. 464) or thyrotoxicosis (p. 462)
- Porphyria
- Hypernatremia or hyponatremia (p. 439)
- Hypercalcemia (p. 451)
- Hypothermia (p. 566)

NSAIDs, non-steroidal anti-inflammatory drugs.

# 21 Falls and 'off legs'

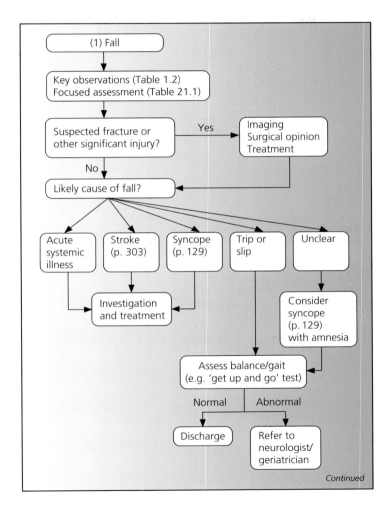

(1) Fall

→

Key observations (Table 1.2)
Focused assessment (Table 21.1)

↓

Suspected fracture or
other significant injury? —Yes→ Imaging
Surgical opinion
Treatment

↓ No

Likely cause of fall? ←

- Acute systemic illness
- Stroke (p. 303)
- Syncope (p. 129)
- Trip or slip
- Unclear

Investigation and treatment

Consider syncope (p. 129) with amnesia

Assess balance/gait
(e.g. 'get up and go' test)

Normal → Discharge

Abnormal → Refer to neurologist/geriatrician

*Continued*

137

Falls and 'off legs'

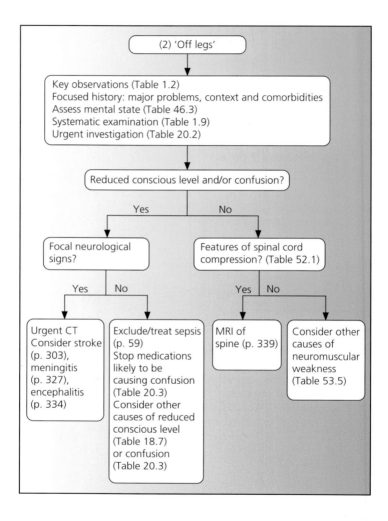

(2) 'Off legs'

Key observations (Table 1.2)
Focused history: major problems, context and comorbidities
Assess mental state (Table 46.3)
Systematic examination (Table 1.9)
Urgent investigation (Table 20.2)

Reduced conscious level and/or confusion?

Yes — No

Focal neurological signs?

Features of spinal cord compression? (Table 52.1)

Yes — No    Yes — No

Urgent CT
Consider stroke
(p. 303),
meningitis
(p. 327),
encephalitis
(p. 334)

Exclude/treat sepsis
(p. 59)
Stop medications
likely to be
causing confusion
(Table 20.3)
Consider other
causes of reduced
conscious level
(Table 18.7)
or confusion
(Table 20.3)

MRI of
spine (p. 339)

Consider other
causes of
neuromuscular
weakness
(Table 53.5)

**TABLE 21.1** Focused assessment after a fall

**History**
- Circumstances of fall (e.g. place, time of day, witnessed)
- Symptoms before fall (e.g. presyncope/syncope, palpitations)
- Injuries sustained
- Contributory factors (e.g. dementia, previous stroke, parkinsonism, lower limb joint disorders, foot disorders)
- Previous falls (how many in past year?)
- Previous syncope
- Usual effort tolerance (e.g. able to climb stairs; able to walk on flat; able to manage activities of daily living)
- Walking aids used
- If fall at home, are there environmental hazards (ask family/carer), e.g. loose rugs, poor lighting?
- Current medications (e.g. sedatives, hypnotics, antidepressants, antihypertensives, multiple drugs)
- Alcohol history
- Social history: living at home or residential/nursing home resident?

**Examination**
- Key observations (see Table 1.2) and systematic examination (see Table 1.9)
- Injuries sustained (check for head injury, fracture, joint dislocation, soft tissue bruising and laceration)
- Assess mental state (e.g. abbreviated mental status examination of the elderly, see Table 46.3)
- If the patient does not have evidence of acute illness or injury, screen for neurological and musculoskeletal disorders with the 'get up and go' test: ask the patient to stand up from a chair without using the arms, walk several paces and return: can this be done without difficulty or unsteadiness?

## Further reading

American Geriatrics Society, British Geriatrics Society and American Academy of Orthopaedic Surgeons Panel on Falls Prevention. Guideline for the prevention of falls in older persons. *J Am Geriatrics Soc* 2001; 49: 664–72.

Kannus P. Prevention of falls and consequent injuries in elderly people. *Lancet* 2005; 366: 1885–93.

Parker M, Johansen A. Hip fracture. *BMJ* 2006; 333: 27–30.

# 22 Acute headache

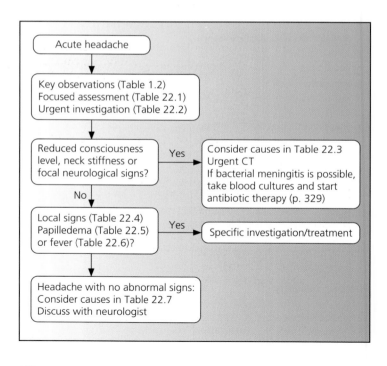

**TABLE 22.1** Focused assessment in acute headache

**History**
- How did the headache start? Instantaneous onset?
- Still present? How long has it lasted?
- Syncope at onset?
- How severe? Worst headache ever?
- Distribution (unilateral, diffuse, localized)
- Associated systemic, neurological or visual symptoms (e.g. syncope/presyncope, limb weakness, speech disturbance, blurring of vision, transient blindness, diplopia, scotomata, fortification spectra). Did these precede or follow the headache?

**Background**
- Medication history and possible exposure to toxins
- Recent travel abroad?
- Immunocompromised or known malignancy?
- Disorders associated with increased risk of aneurysmal subarachnoid hemorrhage: polycystic kidney disease, Ehlers–Danlos syndrome type IV, pseudoxanthoma elasticum, fibromuscular dysplasia, sickle cell disease, alfa-1 antitrypsin deficiency
- Family history of migraine or subarachnoid hemorrhage?

**Examination**
- Key observations: airway, respiratory rate, arterial oxygen saturation, heart rate, blood pressure, perfusion, consciousness level, temperature, blood glucose
- Neck stiffness (in both flexion and extension)?
- Focal neurological signs?
- Horner syndrome (partial ptosis and constricted pupil: if present, consider carotid artery dissection (p. 306))?
- Visual acuity and fields
- Fundi (papilledema or retinal hemorrhage?)
- Signs of dental, ENT or ophthalmic disease?
- Temporal artery tenderness or loss of pulsation?

ENT, ears, nose and throat.

> **ALERT**
>
> Most patients with acute headache have tension-type headache or migraine. A minority have life-threatening disorders such as subarachnoid hemorrhage or bacterial meningitis.

---

**TABLE 22.2** Urgent investigation in acute headache

- Full blood count
- Coagulation screen if suspected intracranial hemorrhage
- ESR and C-reactive protein
- Blood glucose
- Sodium, potassium and creatinine
- Skull X-ray if suspected sinus infection
- Blood culture if suspected bacterial meningitis
- CT scan if suspected intracranial hemorrhage (see p. 305) or meningitis/encephalitis with contraindication to LP (p. 328)
- LP if suspected subarachnoid hemorrhage (p. 321) or meningitis/encephalitis (pp. 327, 334), if there are no contraindications (p. 328)

ESR, erythrocyte sedimentation rate; LP, lumbar puncture.

---

**TABLE 22.3** Causes of acute headache with reduced conscious level, neck stiffness or focal neurological signs

- Stroke (p. 303)
- Subarachnoid hemorrhage (p. 321)
- Chronic subdural hematoma (p. 303)
- Raised intracranial pressure (p. 360)
- Meningitis (p. 327)
- Encephalitis (p. 334)
- Cerebral malaria (p. 546)
- Hypertensive encephalopathy (p. 221)

**TABLE 22.4** Causes of acute headache with local signs

- Acute sinusitis
- Acute angle closure glaucoma (usually unilateral; eye red and injected, visual acuity reduced, pupil dilated and unresponsive to light)
- Giant cell arteritis (Table 22.7)
- Temperomandibular joint dysfunction
- Cervicogenic headache (headache referred from disorder of the cervical spine)
- Mucormycosis (diabetes, orbital and facial pain, periorbital and orbital cellulitis, proptosis, purulent nasal discharge, mucosal necrosis)

**TABLE 22.5** Causes of acute headache with papilledema

- Accelerated-phase hypertension (p. 219)
- Hypertensive encephalopathy (p. 221)
- Cerebral venous sinus thrombosis (p. 145)
- Idiopathic intracranial hypertension (p. 360)
- Other causes of raised intracranial pressure (p. 360)

**TABLE 22.6** Causes of acute headache with fever but no focal neurological signs

- Meningitis (p. 327) (neck stiffness is not an invariable feature especially in cryptococcal meningitis (p. 332))
- Encephalitis (p. 334)
- Subarachnoid hemorrhage (p. 321)
- Systemic infectious disease (including malaria and typhoid in patients who have returned from abroad (p. 542))
- Local infection (e.g. sinusitis)

**TABLE 22.7** Acute headache with no abnormal signs

| Cause | Comment |
|---|---|
| **Tension-type headache** | Usually described as pressure or tightness around the head<br>Does not have the associated symptoms or aura of migraine (although some patients may have both types of headache) |
| **Medication-misuse headache** | Suspect in patients who have frequent or daily headaches despite (or because of) the regular use of medications for headache |
| **Migraine** | Headache lasting 4–72 h, which may be preceded or accompanied by transient focal neurological symptoms (aura), with at least two of the following characteristics: unilateral; pulsating; moderate to severe; aggravated by movement, and at least one associated symptom – nausea or vomiting, photophobia, phonophobia |
| **Drug-related** | E.g. nitrates, nicorandil, dihydropyridine calcium antagonists |
| **Toxin exposure** | E.g. carbon monoxide poisoning (p. 76) |
| **Giant cell arteritis** | Age >50 years, headache usually of days or a few weeks in duration<br>Associated symptoms include malaise, weight loss, jaw claudication, scalp tenderness and visual changes (amaurosis fugax, diplopia and partial or complete loss of vision)<br>If ESR is >50 mm/h and/or temporal artery is thickened or tender, start prednisolone. For patients without visual symptoms, give 40 mg daily; with visual symptoms, give 60–80 mg daily<br>Arrange for a temporal artery biopsy to be done within 48 h of starting prednisolone |

*Continued*

| Cause | Comment |
|---|---|
| **Subarachnoid hemorrhage** | Around 20% of patients with subarachnoid hemorrhage have acute headache with no other signs (p. 321) |
| **Cerebral venous sinus thrombosis** | Headache frequently precedes other symptoms, and rarely may be only symptom<br>Onset may be 'thunderclap', acute or progressive |
| **Pituitary apoplexy** | Usually associated with ophthalmoplegia and reduced visual acuity |
| **Carotid or vertebral arterial dissection** | Unilateral headache, which may be accompanied by neck pain. May follow neck manipulation or minor trauma<br>Usually accompanied by other signs (ischemic stroke, Horner syndrome or pusatile tinnitus) |
| **Spontaneous intracranial hypotension** | Due to leak of CSF from spinal meningeal defects or dural tears<br>Headache worse on standing and relieved by lying down (like post-LP headache)<br>May be accompanied by nausea and vomiting, dizziness, auditory changes, diplopia, visual blurring, interscapular pain and/or radicular pain in the arm |
| **Benign (idiopathic) 'thunderclap' headache** | Assumes subarachnoid hemorrhage and cerebral venous sinus thrombosis have been excluded |

CSF, cerebrospinal fluid; ESR, erythrocyte sedimentation rate; LP, lumbar puncture.

**ALERT**
Headache in the HIV-positive patient: See Table 83.5, p. 540.

Acute headache

> **ALERT**
> A first episode of severe headache cannot reliably be diagnosed
> as migraine or tension-type headache: diagnostic criteria require
> more than nine episodes for tension-type headache and more
> than four episodes for migraine without aura.

## Further reading

Dodick DW. Thunderclap headache. *J Neurol Neurosurg Psychiatry* 2002: 72: 6–11.
Edlow JA, Caplan LR. Avoiding pitfalls in the diagnosis of subarachnoid hemorrhage.
    *N Engl J Med* 2000; 342: 29–36.
Piccirillo JF. Acute bacterial sinusitis. *N Engl J Med* 2004; 351: 902–10.
Silberstein SD. Migraine. *Lancet* 2004; 363: 381–91.
Steiner TJ, Fontebasso M. Headache. *BMJ* 2002; 325: 81–6.

# 23 Acute vomiting

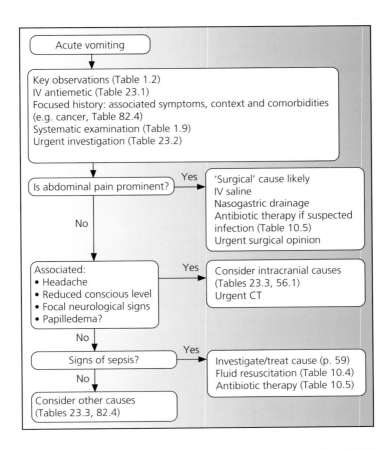

**ALERT**
Vomiting beginning in hospital is usually due to ileus or drugs.

**TABLE 23.1** Treatment of nausea and vomiting

| Drug | Comment | Dose |
|---|---|---|
| Cyclizine | Antihistamine<br>Can be coadministered with opioid to prevent vomiting | 50 mg 8-hourly IV/IM/PO |
| Prochlorperazine | Phenothiazine<br>Can be coadministered with opioid to prevent vomiting | 12.5 mg IM followed if needed after 6h by oral dose of 10 mg |
| Domperidone | Dopamine antagonist<br>Less likely to cause sedation and dystonic reaction than prochlorperazine and metoclopramide<br>Can be used to treat vomiting associated with chemotherapy | 12.5 mg IM |
| Metoclopramide | Has prokinetic as well as antiemetic effect and so may be more effective than phenothiazines for vomiting due to intra-abdominal disease<br>May cause acute dystonic reaction (treat with procyclidine 5 mg IV) | 5–10 mg 8-hourly IV/IM/PO |
| Ondansetron | $5HT_3$ antagonist<br>Used to treat vomiting associated with chemotherapy/radiotherapy and postoperative vomiting | 4 mg IV |

---

**TABLE 23.2** Investigation in acute severe vomiting

**All patients**
- Blood glucose
- Sodium, potassium and creatinine
- Liver function tests, albumin and calcium
- Full blood count

**Depending on clinical setting**
- ECG
- Arterial blood gases and pH
- Chest X-ray
- Abdominal X-ray if suspected intestinal obstruction/ileus (supine and erect or lateral decubitus)
- Cranial CT
- Blood culture

---

**TABLE 23.3** Causes of acute vomiting*

**Intracranial**
- Raised intracranial pressure (Table 56.1)
- Intracranial hemorrhage (subarachnoid hemorrhage or intracerebral hemorrhage)
- Cerebellar hemorrhage or infarction
- Acute labyrinthitis
- Acute migraine

**Intrathoracic**
- Inferior myocardial infarction

**Intra-abdominal**
- Acute gastroenteritis
- Gastroparesis
- Intestinal obstruction
- Ileus
- Biliary tract and pancreatic disorders (p. 406)
- After abdominal and pelvic surgery

*Continued*

**Systemic**
- Sepsis
- Drugs and toxins (including anesthetic agents and chemotherapy)
- Diabetic ketoacidosis (p. 429)
- Adrenal insufficiency (p. 457)
- Uremia (p. 410)
- Hypercalcemia (p. 453)
- Acute intermittent porphyria
- Pregnancy

\* See Table 82.4 for causes of vomiting in patients with cancer.

## Further reading

Baloh RW. Vestibular neuritis. *N Engl J Med* 2003; 348: 1027–32.

# 24 Acute abdominal pain

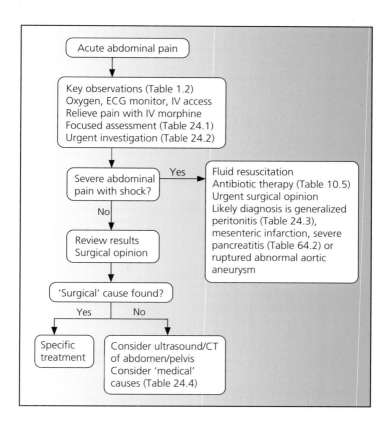

---

**TABLE 24.1** Focused assessment in acute abdominal pain

**History**
- When did the pain start and how did it start – gradually or abruptly?
- Where is the pain, and has it moved since its onset? Visceral pain arising from the gut, biliary tract or pancreas is poorly localized. Peritoneal pain (due to inflammation or infection) is well localized (unless there is generalized peritonitis), constant, and associated with abdominal tenderness.
- How severe is the pain?
- Has there been vomiting, and when did vomiting begin in relation to the onset of the pain?
- Previous abdominal surgery, and if so what for?
- Other medical problems?

**Examination**
- Key observations (Table 1.2)
- Abdominal distension?
- Presence of abdominal scars? If present, check what operations have been done; adhesions from previous surgery may cause obstruction
- Tenderness: localized or generalized?
- Palpable organs or masses?
- Hernial orifices (inguinal, femoral and umbilical) clear?
- Femoral pulses present and symmetrical?
- Bowel sounds
- Rectal examination
- Lungs: basal pneumonia?

---

**TABLE 24.2** Urgent investigation in acute abdominal pain

- Full blood count
- Clotting screen if there is purpura or jaundice, prolonged oozing from puncture sites, or a low platelet count
- C-reactive protein
- Group and save
- Blood glucose
- Sodium, potassium and creatinine

*Continued*

- Liver function tests
- Serum amylase (raised in pancreatitis, perforated ulcer, mesenteric ischemia and severe sepsis)
- Other tests to confirm or exclude pancreatitis if indicated (serum lipase; urine dipstick test for trypsinogen-2 (which has a high negative predictive value))
- Arterial gases and pH if hypotensive or oxygen saturation <90% (metabolic acidosis seen in generalized peritonitis, mesenteric infarction and severe pancreatitis)
- Blood culture if febrile or suspected peritonitis
- Urine stick test, microscopy and culture
- ECG if age >60 or known cardiac disease or unexplained upper abdominal pain
- Chest X-ray – looking for free gas under the diaphragm, indicating perforation, and evidence of basal pneumonia
- Abdominal X-ray (supine and erect or lateral decubitus) – looking for evidence of obstruction of large and/or small bowel; ischemic bowel (dilated and thickened loops of small bowel); cholangitis (gas in biliary tree); radiodense gall stones; radiodense urinary tract stones

**TABLE 24.3** Causes of generalized peritonitis

- Perforation of viscus (e.g. appendix, diverticular disease)
- Mesenteric vascular occlusion leading to intestinal infarction
- Inflammatory conditions (most commonly appendicitis, cholecystitis (p. 406), diverticulitis, pancreatitis (p. 408))
- Late intestinal obstruction (most commonly due to large bowel tumor, adhesions, hernia or volvulus)

**TABLE 24.4** 'Medical' causes of acute abdominal pain

**Right upper quadrant**
- Pneumonia (p. 268)
- Hepatic congestion due to congestive heart failure
- Alcoholic hepatitis (p. 404)
- Viral hepatitis
- Acute gonococcal perihepatitis (Fitz–Hugh–Curtis syndrome)

*Continued*

**Epigastric**
- Acute myocardial infarction (p. 158)
- Pericarditis (p. 212)
- Pancreatitis (p. 408)

**Left upper quadrant**
- Pneumonia

**Central**
- Mesenteric ischemia/infarction
- Diabetic ketoacidosis (p. 429)
- Aortic dissection (p. 181)
- Acute intermittent porphyria
- Vaso-occlusive crisis of sickle cell disease (p. 514)
- Henoch–Schonlein purpura
- Typhoid (p. 549)
- Malaria (p. 546)
- Retroperitoneal hemorrhage (complicating heparin or warfarin therapy, or due to a bleeding disorder, leaking abdominal aortic aneurysm or vertebral fracture)

## Further reading

Humes DJ, Simpson J. Acute appendicitis. *BMJ* 2006; 333: 530–4.

Janes SEJ, et al. Management of diverticulitis. *BMJ* 2006; 332: 271–5.

Kauppinen R. Porphyrias. *Lancet* 2005; 365: 241–52.

Ng CS, et al. Evaluation of early abdominopelvic computed tomography in patients with acute abdominal pain of unknown cause: prospective randomised study. *BMJ* 2002; 325: 1387–9.

Sreenarasimhaiah J. Diagnosis and management of intestinal ischaemic disorders. *BMJ* 2003; 326: 1372–6.

# Specific Problems

# Cardiovascular

# 25 Acute coronary syndrome with persisting ST elevation or new left bundle branch block

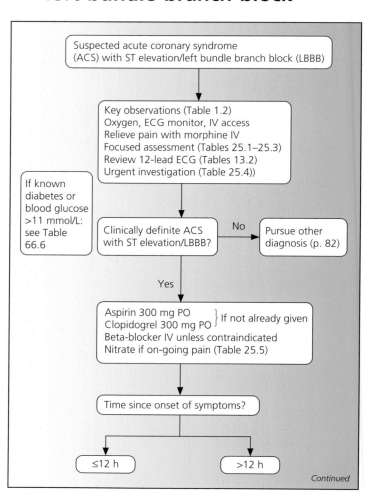

Suspected acute coronary syndrome (ACS) with ST elevation/left bundle branch block (LBBB)

Key observations (Table 1.2)
Oxygen, ECG monitor, IV access
Relieve pain with morphine IV
Focused assessment (Tables 25.1–25.3)
Review 12-lead ECG (Tables 13.2)
Urgent investigation (Table 25.4))

If known diabetes or blood glucose >11 mmol/L: see Table 66.6

Clinically definite ACS with ST elevation/LBBB?

No → Pursue other diagnosis (p. 82)

Yes

Aspirin 300 mg PO
Clopidogrel 300 mg PO } If not already given
Beta-blocker IV unless contraindicated
Nitrate if on-going pain (Table 25.5)

Time since onset of symptoms?

≤12 h

>12 h

*Continued*

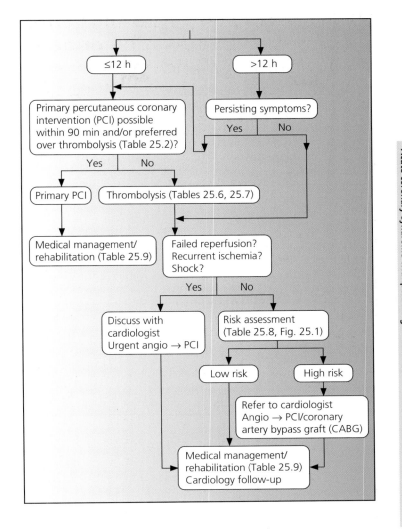

Acute coronary syndrome with persisting ST elevation or new left bundle branch block

**TABLE 25.1** Focused assessment in ST elevation acute coronary syndrome

- Time since onset of symptoms
- Are symptoms consistent with myocardial ischemia/infarction?
- Does ECG show persistent ST segment elevation consistent with acute coronary syndrome or left bundle branch block not known to be old?
- Are there signs of heart failure or shock?
- Which reperfusion strategy: primary percutaneous coronary intervention or fibrinolysis (Table 25.2)?

**TABLE 25.2** Factors favoring primary percutaneous coronary intervention (PCI) over fibrinolysis in ST elevation acute coronary syndrome

- Ability to implement primary PCI within 90 min from presentation
- Q waves on initial ECG
- Time to presentation >3 h
- Cardiogenic shock
- Severe heart failure and/or pulmonary edema
- Contraindications to fibrinolysis (Table 25.3)
- Diagnosis of ST elevation acute coronary syndrome in doubt

**TABLE 25.3** Contraindications and cautions for use of fibrinolysis in acute coronary syndrome with persistent ST elevation or new left bundle branch block

**Absolute contraindications**
- Prior intracranial hemorrhage
- Known structural cerebrovascular lesion (e.g. arteriovenous malformation)
- Known malignant intracranial neoplasm (primary or metastatic)
- Ischemic stroke within 3 months (except acute ischemic stroke within 3 h)
- Suspected aortic dissection
- Active bleeding or bleeding tendency (excluding menses)
- Significant closed head trauma or facial trauma within 3 months

**Relative contraindications and cautions**
- History of chronic, severe, poorly controlled hypertension
- Severe uncontrolled hypertension on presentation (systolic BP >180 mmHg or diastolic BP >110 mmHg) (could be an absolute contraindication in low risk patient)
- History of prior ischemic stroke >3 months, dementia or known intracranial pathology not covered in absolute contraindications
- Traumatic or prolonged (>10 min) cardiopulmonary resuscitation or major surgery within 3 weeks
- Recent (within 2–4 weeks) internal bleeding
- Non-compressible vascular punctures
- For streptokinase/anistreplase: prior exposure (>5 days ago) or prior allergic reaction to these agents
- Pregnancy
- Active peptic ulcer
- Current use of anticoagulants: the higher the INR, the higher the risk of bleeding

INR, international normalized ratio.

**TABLE 25.4** Investigation in ST elevation acute coronary syndrome

**Needed urgently**
- ECG (repeat 60 and 90 min after fibrinolysis to assess reperfusion; a reduction in ST elevation by more than 70% in the leads with maximal elevation is associated with the most favorable outcomes)
- Chest X-ray
- Echocardiography if:
  - There is cardiogenic shock (p. 174)
  - The diagnosis is in doubt and chest pain still present (to establish whether or not there is a left ventricular regional wall motion abnormality consistent with acute coronary syndrome)
- Blood glucose (see p. 428 for management of diabetes in acute coronary syndrome)
- Sodium, potassium and creatinine (recheck potassium if significant arrhythmia occurs or after large diuresis)
- Plasma markers of myocardial necrosis (p. 89)

**For later analysis**
- Full blood count
- Cholesterol (value is representative if checked within 24 h of acute coronary syndrome)

**TABLE 25.5** Initial drug therapy in ST elevation acute coronary syndrome

| Drug | Comment |
|---|---|
| **Morphine** | 5–10 mg IV, with additional doses of 2.5 mg IV at 5–10 min intervals until pain-free. Metoclopramide 10 mg IV can be given if needed for nausea/vomiting |
| **Aspirin** | 300 mg PO stat (chewed), 75 mg PO daily thereafter |
| **Clopidogrel** | 300 mg PO stat, 75 mg PO daily for one month |

*Continued*

| Drug | Comment |
|------|---------|
| **Beta-blocker** | If not contraindicated (by bradycardia, hypotension, heart failure, severe asthma), give metoprolol 5 mg IV over 5 min, repeated as needed up to total dose of 15 mg, target heart rate 60 bpm, followed by oral beta-blocker |
| **ACE inhibitor** | Started on the morning after admission unless contraindicated by hypotension |
| **Nitrate** | Indicated for on-going chest pain/pulmonary edema<br>• IV nitrate *or*<br>• Buccal nitrate 2–5 mg 8-hourly |

ACE, angiotension-converting enzyme.

**TABLE 25.6** Fibrinolytic regimens

| Fibrinolytic | Dose (IV) | Antithrombin co-therapy |
|--------------|-----------|-------------------------|
| **Streptokinase** | 1.5 MU in 100 ml of 5% glucose or normal saline over 30–60 min | None or IV heparin for 24–48 h (see below) |
| **Alteplase** | 15 mg bolus 0.75 mg/kg over 30 min Then 0.5 mg/kg over 60 min Total dose not to exceed 100 mg | After alteplase, reteplase and tenecteplase, give IV heparin for 24–48 h:<br>• Bolus 60 units/kg to a maximum of 4000 units<br>• Infusion 12 units/kg/h to a maximum of 1000 units/h<br>• Check APTT 3, 6, 12 and 24 h after starting treatment<br>Target APTT 50–70 s |
| **Reteplase** | 10 units bolus followed by further 10 units bolus at 30 min | |
| **Tenecteplase** | Single bolus:<br>• 30 mg if <60 kg<br>• 35 mg if 60–69 kg<br>• 40 mg if 70–79 kg<br>• 45 mg if 80–89 kg<br>• 50 mg if 90 kg or above | |

APTT, activated partial thromboplastin time.

Acute coronary syndrome with persisting ST elevation or new left bundle branch block

---

**TABLE 25.7** Fibrinolytic therapy: problems

**Hypotension during streptokinase infusion**
- Usually reversed by elevating the foot of the bed or slowing the infusion

**Allergic reaction to streptokinase**
- Give chlorphenamine 10 mg IV and hydrocortisone 100 mg IV (prophylactic treatment not needed)

**Vascular access after thrombolysis**
- If venepuncture is necessary, use a 22 G (blue) needle and compress the puncture site for 10 min
- Central venous lines should be inserted via a femoral vein (p. 589)
- For arterial puncture, use a 23 G (orange) needle in the radial or brachial artery and compress the puncture site for at least 10 min

**Uncontrollable bleeding**
- Stop the infusion of thrombolytic
- Transfuse whole fresh blood if available or fresh frozen plasma
- As a last resort, give tranexamic acid 1 g (10 mg/kg) IV over 10 min

**Symptomatic bradycardia unresponsive to atropine**
- If temporary pacing is required within 24 h of thrombolytic therapy, the lead should be placed via the femoral vein (p. 600)

**TABLE 25.8** Risk assessment after ST elevation acute coronary syndrome (ACS)*

| | High risk | Low risk |
|---|---|---|
| **Assess clinical criteria and LV systolic function (e.g. by echocardiography):** | | |
| Clinical | Hypotension<br>Heart failure<br>Major arrhythmia<br>Angina occurring spontaneously or on mobilization after ACS | No hypotension<br>No heart failure<br>No arrhythmia<br>No angina after ACS |
| LV ejection fraction | Less than 50% | 50% or greater |
| **Assess inducible ischemia†** | | |
| By stress echocardiography or myocardial perfusion imaging | Extensive hibernation or inducible ischemia affecting 20% or more of non-infarcted myocardium | Limited or mild inducible ischemia affecting <20% of non-infarcted myocardium, particularly if the ischemia is in the infarct zone rather than remote |
| By exercise ECG | Evidence of myocardial ischemia (angina/ST depression) in first or second stages of Bruce protocol | Able to complete three stages of Bruce protocol without evidence of myocardial ischemia |

LV, left ventricular.
* Based on clinical criteria, assessment of LV systolic function and the presence of inducible myocardial ischemia (European Society of Cardiology guidelines 2003). See also GRACE (Global Registry of Acute Coronary Events) prediction model (Fig. 25.1).
† Patients at low risk based on clinical/LV systolic function criteria, should have assessment of inducible ischemia (by stress echocardiography, myocardial perfusion imaging or exercise ECG).

**TABLE 25.9** Medical management/rehabilitation after acute coronary syndrome (ACS)

| Element | Comment |
|---|---|
| **Antiplatelet therapy** | Aspirin 75 mg daily continued indefinitely<br>Clopidogrel 75 mg daily for at least 1 month after ST elevation ACS and 1 year after non-ST elevation ACS |
| **Beta-blocker** | Continued indefinitely, especially in patients with LV ejection fraction <40% |
| **Statin** | Continued indefinitely<br>Target total cholesterol <4 mmol/L, LDL-C <2 mmol/L |
| **ACE inhibitor** | Continued indefinitely, especially in patients who have had heart failure or LV ejection fraction <40%<br>Use angiotensin-receptor blocker if there is a cough |
| **Eplerenone** | Indicated for patients with heart failure |
| **Implantable cardioverter-defibrillator** | Indicated for primary prevention in patients who are more than four weeks after myocardial infarction and in NYHA functional class 1 to 3 and have *either*:<br>• LV ejection fraction <35% and non-sustained VT on 24 h ECG monitoring and inducible VT on electrophysiological testing<br>*or*<br>• LV ejection fraction <30% and QRS duration 120 ms or more (NICE 2006) |
| **Rehabilitation/ exercise training** | Indicated for all patients, including those with heart failure |
| **Smoking cessation** | Stopping smoking has a major beneficial effect on prognosis. Smokers should be advised to stop and be referred if needed to a smoking cessation program |
| **Blood pressure control** | Target BP <130/85 mmHg |
| **Diabetes** | See p. 428 |

ACE, angiotensin-converting enzyme; LDL-C, low density lipoprotein C; LV, left ventricle; NICE, National Institute for Health and Clinical Excellence; NYHA, New York Heart Association; VT, ventricular tachycardia.

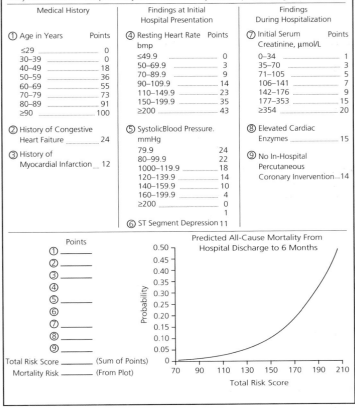

Risk Calculator for 6-Month Postdischarge Mortality
After Hospitalization for Acute Coronary Syndrome

Record the points for each variable at the bottom left and sum the points to calculate the total risk score. Find the total score on the x-axis of the nomogram plot. The corresponding probability on the y-axis is the estimated probability of all-cause mortality from hospital discharge to 6 months.

| Medical History | Findings at Initial Hospital Presentation | Findings During Hospitalization |
| --- | --- | --- |

① Age in Years    Points

| | |
| --- | --- |
| ≤29 | 0 |
| 30–39 | 0 |
| 40–49 | 18 |
| 50–59 | 36 |
| 60–69 | 55 |
| 70–79 | 73 |
| 80–89 | 91 |
| ≥90 | 100 |

② History of Congestive Heart Faiture    24

③ History of Myocardial Infarction    12

④ Resting Heart Rate    Points
bmp

| | |
| --- | --- |
| ≤49.9 | 0 |
| 50–69.9 | 3 |
| 70–89.9 | 9 |
| 90–109.9 | 14 |
| 110–149.9 | 23 |
| 150–199.9 | 35 |
| ≥200 | 43 |

⑤ SystolicBlood Pressure. mmHg

| | |
| --- | --- |
| 79.9 | 24 |
| 80–99.9 | 22 |
| 1000–119.9 | 18 |
| 120–139.9 | 14 |
| 140–159.9 | 10 |
| 160–199.9 | 4 |
| ≥200 | 0 |
| | 1 |

⑥ ST Segment Depression 11

⑦ Initial Serum    Points
Creatinine, μmol/L

| | |
| --- | --- |
| 0–34 | 1 |
| 35–70 | 3 |
| 71–105 | 5 |
| 106–141 | 7 |
| 142–176 | 9 |
| 177–353 | 15 |
| ≥354 | 20 |

⑧ Elevated Cardiac Enzymes    15

⑨ No In-Hospital Percutaneous Coronary Invervention    14

Points
① _____
② _____
③ _____
④ _____
⑤ _____
⑥ _____
⑦ _____
⑧ _____
⑨ _____

Total Risk Score _____ (Sum of Points)
Mortality Risk _____ (From Plot)

Predicted All-Cause Mortality From Hospital Discharge to 6 Months

**FIGURE 25.1** GRACE (Global Registry of Acute Coronary Events) prediction score card and nomogram for all-cause mortality from discharge to six months after acute coronary syndrome. (From Eagle, K. et al. *JAMA* 2004; **291**: 2727.)

Acute coronary syndrome with persisting ST elevation or new left bundle branch block

## Further reading

American College of Cardiology and American Heart Association. Guidelines for the management of patients with ST-elevation myocardial infarction (2004). American College of Cardiology website (http://www.acc.org/qualityandscience/clinical/statements.htm).

Boersma E, et al. Acute myocardial infarction. *Lancet* 2003; 361: 847–58.

Eagle KA, et al. A validated prediction model for all forms of acute coronary syndrome: estimating the risk of 6-month post-discharge death in an international registry. *JAMA* 2004; 291: 2727–33.

European Society of Cardiology. Guidelines for the management of patients with ST-elevation myocardial infarction (2003). European Society of Cardiology website (http://www.escardio.org/knowledge/guidelines/Guidelines_list.htm?hit=quick).

Keeley EC, Hillis LD. Primary PCI for myocardial infarction with ST-segment elevation. *N Engl J Med* 2007; 356: 47–54.

Ting HH, et al. Narrative review: reperfusion strategies for ST-segment elevation myocardial infarction. *Ann Intern Med* 2006; 145: 610–17.

Zimetbaum PJ, Josephson ME. Use of the electrocardiogram in acute myocardial infarction. *N Engl J Med* 2003; 348: 933–40.

Acute coronary syndrome with persisting ST elevation or new left bundle branch block

# 26 Acute coronary syndrome without persisting ST elevation

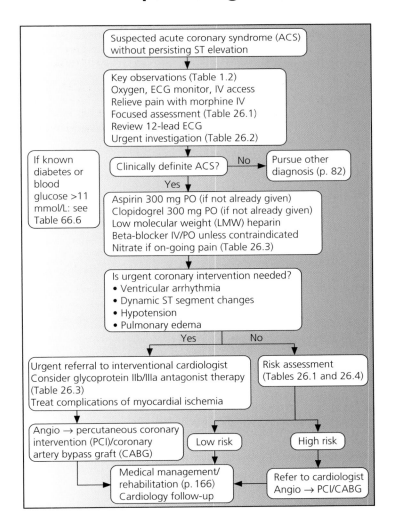

Suspected acute coronary syndrome (ACS) without persisting ST elevation

Key observations (Table 1.2)
Oxygen, ECG monitor, IV access
Relieve pain with morphine IV
Focused assessment (Table 26.1)
Review 12-lead ECG
Urgent investigation (Table 26.2)

Clinically definite ACS? — No → Pursue other diagnosis (p. 82)

If known diabetes or blood glucose >11 mmol/L: see Table 66.6

Yes ↓

Aspirin 300 mg PO (if not already given)
Clopidogrel 300 mg PO (if not already given)
Low molecular weight (LMW) heparin
Beta-blocker IV/PO unless contraindicated
Nitrate if on-going pain (Table 26.3)

Is urgent coronary intervention needed?
• Ventricular arrhythmia
• Dynamic ST segment changes
• Hypotension
• Pulmonary edema

Yes | No

Urgent referral to interventional cardiologist
Consider glycoprotein IIb/IIIa antagonist therapy (Table 26.3)
Treat complications of myocardial ischemia

Risk assessment (Tables 26.1 and 26.4)

Angio → percutaneous coronary intervention (PCI)/coronary artery bypass graft (CABG)

Low risk | High risk

Medical management/ rehabilitation (p. 166) Cardiology follow-up

Refer to cardiologist Angio → PCI/CABG

**TABLE 26.1** Focused assessment in non-ST elevation acute coronary syndrome (ACS)

**1 Is chest pain due to myocardial ischemia?**
This judgement is based on the typicality of symptoms, the likelihood of coronary disease (based on analysis of risk factors in patients not known to have coronary disease), and the presence of ECG changes during pain

**2 High or low risk?**

| Feature | High risk (any of these features present) | Low risk (all of these features present) |
|---|---|---|
| **Chest pain** | On-going<br>Recurrent | Resolved<br>No recurrence during observation |
| **Background** | Recent ACS<br>Known coronary disease (angiogram, previous ACS, PCI or CABG)<br>Diabetes<br>Renal impairment | No previously documented coronary disease<br>No diabetes or renal impairment |
| **Examination** | Hypotension<br>Pulmonary edema | Normal blood pressure<br>No signs of heart failure |
| **12-lead ECG** | Dynamic or fixed ST depression<br>Transient ST elevation<br>Deep anterior T wave inversion<br>ECG pattern (e.g. LBBB or paced rhythm) which precludes assessment of ST segment | Normal ECG or minor T wave changes only |
| **ECG monitoring** | Ventricular arrhythmia | No arrhythmia |
| **Plasma troponin** | Positive | Negative |

CABG, coronary artery bypass graft; LBBB, left bundle branch block; PCI, percutaneous coronary intervention.

**ALERT**
A normal ECG at presentation does not exclude an acute coronary syndrome.

---

**TABLE 26.2** Investigation in non-ST elevation acute coronary syndrome

**Needed urgently**
- ECG (repeat 60, 90 and 120 min, and if pain recurs)
- Chest X-ray
- Echocardiography:
  - If there is cardiogenic shock (p. 174)
  - If the diagnosis in doubt and chest pain still present (to establish whether or not there is a left ventricular regional wall motion abnormality consistent with acute coronary syndrome)
- Blood glucose (see p. 428 for management of diabetes in acute coronary syndrome)
- Sodium, potassium and creatinine (recheck potassium if significant arrhythmia occurs or after large diuresis)
- Plasma troponin (at presentation and measured 12 h after onset of chest pain)

**For later analysis**
- Full blood count
- Cholesterol (value is representative if checked within 24 h of acute coronary syndrome)

Acute coronary syndrome without persisting ST elevation

**TABLE 26.3** Drug therapy in unstable angina/non-ST elevation acute coronary syndrome

| Drug | Comments |
|------|----------|
| **Aspirin** | 300 mg PO (chewed) stat, 75 mg daily thereafter |
| **Clopidogrel** | 300 mg PO stat, 75 mg daily thereafter for 12 months |
| **Heparin (unfractionated or low molecular weight)** | Low molecular weight heparins have the advantages of subcutaneous administration and no requirement for monitoring of the activated partial thromboplastin time:<br>• Enoxaparin 100 units/kg 12-hourly SC for at least 48 h *or*<br>• Dalteparin 120 units/kg 12-hourly SC (maximum 10,000 units 12-hourly) for at least 48 h *or*<br>• Unfractionated heparin by IV infusion: see p. 507 |
| **Platelet glycoprotein IIb/IIIa receptor inhibitor** | Indicated in high risk patients being considered for urgent coronary intervention; discuss with interventional cardiologist first<br>• Tirofiban IV *or*<br>• Eptifibatide IV |
| **Beta-blocker** | If not contraindicated (by bradycardia, hypotension, heart failure, severe asthma):<br>• Metoprolol 5 mg IV over 5 min, repeated as needed up to total dose of 15 mg, target heart rate 60 bpm<br>• Continue beta-blocker PO (metoprolol or atenolol) |
| **Calcium antagonist** | Diltiazem or verapamil should be used if beta-blocker contraindicated:<br>• Diltiazem 90–180 mg 12-hourly PO *or*<br>• Verapamil 40–120 mg 8-hourly PO |
| **Nitrate** | Indicated for on-going chest pain/pulmonary edema:<br>• IV nitrate *or*<br>• Buccal nitrate 2–5 mg 8-hourly |

**TABLE 26.4** Risk assessment after non-ST elevation acute coronary syndrome*

- Initial risk assessment is based on clinical, ECG and troponin criteria (Table 26.1)
- Patients at high risk on these criteria should be referred to a cardiologist for coronary angiography
- Patients at low risk on these criteria should have a predischarge assessment of LV systolic function (e.g. by echocardiography) and of inducible myocardial ischemia (by stress echocardiography, myocardial perfusion imaging or exercise ECG) (see Table 25.8)
- Patients with impaired LV systolic function (ejection fraction <50%) and/or inducible myocardial ischemia should be referred to a cardiologist for coronary angiography

LV, left ventricular.
* See also GRACE (Global Registry of Acute Coronary Events) prediction model (Fig. 25.1).

Acute coronary syndrome without persisting ST elevation

## Further reading

American College of Cardiology and American Heart Association. Guideline update for the management of patients with unstable angina and non-ST-segment elevation myocardial infarction (2002). American College of Cardiology website (http://www.acc.org/qualityandscience/clinical/statements.htm).

Eagle KA, et al. A validated prediction model for all forms of acute coronary syndrome: estimating the risk of 6-month postdischarge death in an international registry. *JAMA* 2004; 291: 2727–33.

European Society of Cardiology. Guidelines for the management of patients with acute coronary syndromes without persisting ST-segment elevation (2002). European Society of Cardiology website (http://www.escardio.org/knowledge/guidelines/Guidelines_list.htm?hit=quick). Updated June 2007.

Peters RJG et al. Acute coronary syndromes without ST segment elevation. *BMJ* 2007; 334: 1265–9.

# 27 Cardiogenic shock

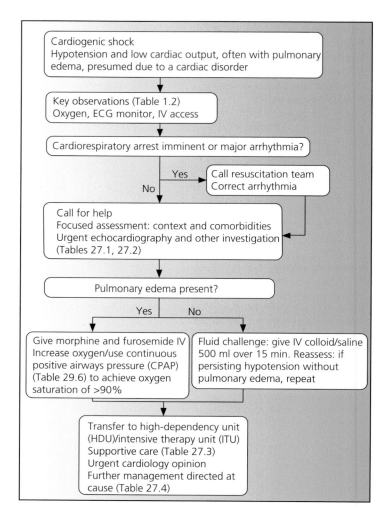

Cardiogenic shock
Hypotension and low cardiac output, often with pulmonary edema, presumed due to a cardiac disorder

Key observations (Table 1.2)
Oxygen, ECG monitor, IV access

Cardiorespiratory arrest imminent or major arrhythmia?

Yes → Call resuscitation team
Correct arrhythmia

No

Call for help
Focused assessment: context and comorbidities
Urgent echocardiography and other investigation
(Tables 27.1, 27.2)

Pulmonary edema present?

Yes

No

Give morphine and furosemide IV
Increase oxygen/use continuous positive airways pressure (CPAP) (Table 29.6) to achieve oxygen saturation of >90%

Fluid challenge: give IV colloid/saline 500 ml over 15 min. Reassess: if persisting hypotension without pulmonary edema, repeat

Transfer to high-dependency unit (HDU)/intensive therapy unit (ITU)
Supportive care (Table 27.3)
Urgent cardiology opinion
Further management directed at cause (Table 27.4)

**TABLE 27.1** Urgent investigation in cardiogenic shock

- ECG
- Chest X-ray
- Echocardiography
- Arterial blood gases and pH
- Blood glucose
- Sodium, potassium and creatinine
- Cardiac biomarkers (for later analysis)
- Full blood count
- Blood culture

**ALERT**

If cardiac output is low but the left ventricle is hyperdynamic on echo consider acute ventricular septal rupture or acute aortic or mitral regurgitation.

**ALERT**

The prognosis of cardiogenic shock is poor, especially in patients over 80 years with major comorbidities, and in such patients palliative care may be preferable to transfer for invasive investigation.

Cardiogenic shock

Cardiogenic shock

**TABLE 27.2** Echocardiographic findings in cardiogenic shock

| Cause of cardiogenic shock | Echocardiographic findings | | | |
| --- | --- | --- | --- | --- |
| | IVC | Right ventricle | Left ventricle | Other features |
| LV dysfunction due to ischemia/ infarction | Normal or dilated | Normal size and contraction (unless associated RV infarction) | Reduced contraction, regionally or globally | |
| Ventricular septal rupture complicating myocardial infarction | Dilated | Dilated with reduced contraction | Regional wall motion abnormality elsewhere hyperdynamic | Septal rupture with left to right shunt |
| Papillary muscle rupture complicating myocardial infarction | Normal or dilated | Normal size and contraction | | Severe mitral regurgitation Flail mitral valve Tip of papillary muscle may be seen |
| RV infarction | Dilated | Dilated with reduced contraction | Reduced contraction if associated inferior infarction | |
| Acute mitral or aortic regurgitation (pp. 196, 200) | Normal or dilated | Normal size and contraction | Non-dilated, hyperdynamic | Severe valve regurgitation and |

*Continued*

**Cardiogenic shock**

**Echocardiographic findings**

| Cause of cardiogenic shock | IVC | Right ventricle | Left ventricle | Other features |
|---|---|---|---|---|
| | | | | causative pathology (e.g. vegetations) |
| **Critical mitral stenosis (p. 199)** | Dilated | Dilated with reduced contraction (due to pulmonary hypertension) | Normal or small size and normal contraction | Calcified/fibrotic mitral valve with small orifice |
| **Critical aortic stenosis (p. 197)** | Normal or dilated | Normal or reduced (if associated severe pulmonary hypertension) | Normal or increased size with reduced activity | Calcified aortic valve with little or no movement |
| **Acute major pulmonary embolism (p. 231)** | Dilated | Dilated with reduced contraction | Normal or small size with normal or increased activity | (see p. 235) |
| **Cardiac tamponade (p. 216)** | Dilated | Diastolic collapse of free wall of right ventricle | | Pericardial effusion (see p. 218) |

IVC, inferior vena cava; LV, left ventricular; RV, right ventricular.

**TABLE 27.3** Cardiogenic shock: supportive care

| Element | Comment |
| --- | --- |
| **Airway and breathing** | Maintain patent airway (see Table 1.3)<br>Treat pulmonary edema (p. 185)<br>Increase inspired oxygen concentration to achieve arterial oxygen saturation >90%<br>Ventilatory support (CPAP) or endotracheal intubation and mechanical ventilation if appropriate (see Table 16.5) |
| **Circulation** | Correct major arrhythmia (p. 18)<br>Put in a central line to monitor CVP and for drug administration<br>Put in an arterial line<br>Start inotropic vasopressor agent if there is pulmonary edema (see Table 9.5)<br>Diagnose cause (ECG/echocardiography) and arrange definitive management if appropriate |
| **Renal function** | Put in bladder catheter to monitor urine output |
| **Blood glucose** | Use insulin infusion to control blood glucose in patients with diabetes or blood glucose >11 mmol/L (p. 428) |
| **Symptom control/ palliative care** | Use morphine to relieve distress/ breathlessness<br>Consider syringe driver (p. 583) |

CPAP, continuous positive airways pressure; CVP, central venous pressure.

**TABLE 27.4** Cardiogenic shock: definitive management

| Cause of cardiogenic shock | Definitive management |
|---|---|
| **Acute coronary syndrome (ACS)** | Coronary reperfusion by percutaneous coronary intervention (PCI) or coronary artery bypass grafting (CABG)<br>Thrombolysis for ST elevation ACS if PCI/CABG unavailable or contraindicated<br>Support with intra-aortic balloon pump prior to revascularization |
| **Ventricular septal rupture complicating acute coronary syndrome** | Surgical repair of septal rupture combined with CABG if indicated<br>Support with intra-aortic balloon pump prior to surgery |
| **Papillary muscle rupture complicating acute coronary syndrome** | Surgical repair/replacement of mitral valve combined with CABG if indicated<br>Support with intra-aortic balloon pump prior to surgery |
| **Right ventricular infarction** | Coronary reperfusion by PCI or thrombolysis |
| **Acute mitral or aortic regurgitation** | Valve surgery<br>Treat infective endocarditis (p. 203) if this is the cause |
| **Critical mitral stenosis** | Valve surgery or mitral balloon valvuloplasty |
| **Critical aortic stenosis** | Valve surgery |
| **Cardiac tamponade** | Pericardiocentesis (p. 609)<br>Treat cause of pericardial effusion (p. 217) |
| **Acute major pulmonary embolism** | Thrombolysis or thrombectomy (p. 231) |

Cardiogenic shock

## Further reading

Hasdai D, et al. Cardiogenic shock complicating acute coronary syndromes. *Lancet* 2000; 356: 749–56.

Menon V, Hochman JS. Management of cardiogenic shock complicating acute myocardial infarction. *Heart* 2002; 88: 531–37.

Murday A. Optimal management of acute ventricular septal rupture. *Heart* 2003; 89: 1462–66.

Trost JC, Hillis LD. Intra-aortic balloon counterpulsation. *Am J Cardiol* 2006; 97: 1391–98.

# 28 Aortic dissection

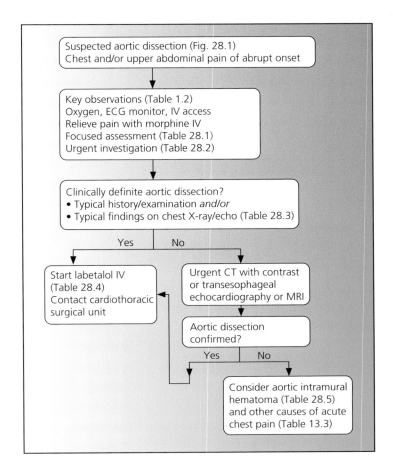

Suspected aortic dissection (Fig. 28.1)
Chest and/or upper abdominal pain of abrupt onset

Key observations (Table 1.2)
Oxygen, ECG monitor, IV access
Relieve pain with morphine IV
Focused assessment (Table 28.1)
Urgent investigation (Table 28.2)

Clinically definite aortic dissection?
• Typical history/examination *and/or*
• Typical findings on chest X-ray/echo (Table 28.3)

Yes          No

Start labetalol IV
(Table 28.4)
Contact cardiothoracic
surgical unit

Urgent CT with contrast
or transesophageal
echocardiography or MRI

Aortic dissection
confirmed?

Yes          No

Consider aortic intramural
hematoma (Table 28.5)
and other causes of acute
chest pain (Table 13.3)

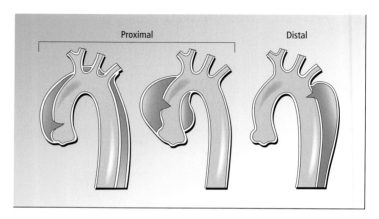

**FIGURE 28.1** Classification of aortic dissection.

---

**TABLE 28.1** Focused assessment in suspected aortic dissection

**History**
- Severe chest pain of abrupt onset, often tearing or ripping in quality
- Radiation of pain along the course of the aorta (e.g. anterior–posterior, chest–abdomen) or its major branches
- Associated neurological symptoms

**Background**
- Risk factors for aortic dissection: hypertension, Marfan syndrome, aortic root dilatation, bicuspid aortic valve or pregnancy

**Examination**
- Asymmetric or absent peripheral pulses (systolic blood pressure difference of >15 mmHg between the arms)?
- Signs of cardiac tamponade (raised jugular venous pressure, pulsus paradoxus, p. 217)?
- Aortic regurgitation (due to distortion or dilatation of the aortic root)?
- Signs of other complications of aortic dissection (e.g. stroke, paraparesis/paraplegia, mesenteric ischemia)?

---

**ALERT**
Pulse abnormalities are found in <20% of patients: their absence does not rule out aortic dissection.

---

**TABLE 28.2** Urgent investigation in suspected aortic dissection

- ECG
- Chest X-ray
- Arterial blood gases and pH
- Full blood count
- Blood glucose
- Sodium, potassium and creatinine
- Transthoracic echocardiogram

---

**TABLE 28.3** Chest X-ray and transthoracic echocardiographic findings in aortic dissection

**Chest X-ray**
- Widened mediastinum
- Double shadow on aortic knuckle
- Small left pleural effusion

**Transthoracic echocardiogram**
- Aortic dissection flap
- Dilated aorta
- Aortic regurgitation
- Pericardial effusion

---

**ALERT**
The chest X-ray and transthoracic echocardiogram may be normal in aortic dissection.

Aortic dissection

---

**TABLE 28.4** Hypotensive therapy with IV labetalol in acute aortic dissection

---

- Make up a solution of 1 mg/ml by diluting the contents of 2 × 100 mg ampoules to 200 ml with normal saline or glucose 5%
- Start the infusion at 15 ml/h and increase it every 15 min as necessary
- Put in a bladder catheter to monitor urine output
- Aim to reduce systolic blood pressure to <120 mmHg, providing the urine output remains >30 ml/h
- A nitrate infusion can be added if needed for blood pressure control

---

**TABLE 28.5** Aortic intramural hematoma

---

- The clinical picture of aortic dissection may be due to aortic intramural hematoma (without an intimal flap) in 15% of cases, which may be missed on CT
- Transesophageal echocardiography shows:
  - Aortic wall >4 mm thick
  - Echolucencies caused by blood in the aortic wall
  - Fascial planes in the aortic wall which 'shear' during systole
- Management of aortic intramural hematoma is the same as for dissection
- Continue hypotensive therapy and discuss further management with a cardiothoracic surgeon

## Further reading

Hagan PG, et al. The international registry of acute aortic dissection (IRAD): new insights into an old disease. *JAMA* 2000; 283: 897–903.

Klompas M. Does this patient have aortic dissection? *JAMA* 2002; 287: 2862–72.

Nienaber CA, Eagle KA. Aortic dissection: new frontiers in diagnosis and management. Part I: From etiology to diagnostic strategies. *Circulation* 2003; 108: 628–35. Part II: Therapeutic management and follow-up. *Circulation* 2003; 108: 772–78.

Tsai TT, et al. Acute aortic syndromes. *Circulation* 2005; 112: 3802–13.

# 29 Acute pulmonary edema

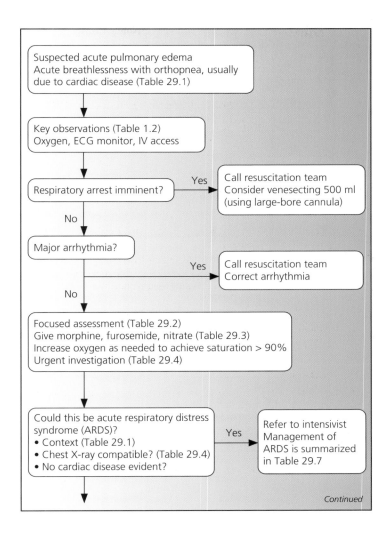

Suspected acute pulmonary edema
Acute breathlessness with orthopnea, usually
due to cardiac disease (Table 29.1)

Key observations (Table 1.2)
Oxygen, ECG monitor, IV access

Respiratory arrest imminent? → Yes → Call resuscitation team
Consider venesecting 500 ml
(using large-bore cannula)

No

Major arrhythmia? → Yes → Call resuscitation team
Correct arrhythmia

No

Focused assessment (Table 29.2)
Give morphine, furosemide, nitrate (Table 29.3)
Increase oxygen as needed to achieve saturation > 90%
Urgent investigation (Table 29.4)

Could this be acute respiratory distress
syndrome (ARDS)?
• Context (Table 29.1)
• Chest X-ray compatible? (Table 29.4)
• No cardiac disease evident?
→ Yes → Refer to intensivist
Management of
ARDS is summarized
in Table 29.7

*Continued*

Acute pulmonary edema

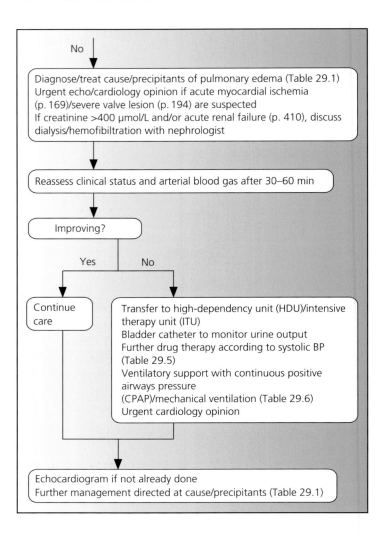

No

Diagnose/treat cause/precipitants of pulmonary edema (Table 29.1)
Urgent echo/cardiology opinion if acute myocardial ischemia
(p. 169)/severe valve lesion (p. 194) are suspected
If creatinine >400 µmol/L and/or acute renal failure (p. 410), discuss
dialysis/hemofibiltration with nephrologist

Reassess clinical status and arterial blood gas after 30–60 min

Improving?

Yes          No

Continue
care

Transfer to high-dependency unit (HDU)/intensive
therapy unit (ITU)
Bladder catheter to monitor urine output
Further drug therapy according to systolic BP
(Table 29.5)
Ventilatory support with continuous positive
airways pressure
(CPAP)/mechanical ventilation (Table 29.6)
Urgent cardiology opinion

Echocardiogram if not already done
Further management directed at cause/precipitants (Table 29.1)

**TABLE 29.1** Causes of acute pulmonary edema

## Causes due to elevated pressure in the pulmonary capillaries

- Cardiac disease: new presentation
  - Acute myocardial infarction or severe myocardial ischemia
  - Severe aortic stenosis
  - Acute myocarditis
  - Acute aortic regurgitation (aortic dissection, infective endocarditis, chest trauma)
  - Acute mitral regurgitation (infective endocarditis, ruptured chordae or papillary muscle, chest trauma)
  - Ventricular septal rupture after myocardial infarction
  - Severe mitral stenosis
  - Left atrial myxoma
- Precipitants of pulmonary edema in patients with previously stable valve or left ventricular disease
  - Acute myocardial infarction or myocardial ischemia
  - Arrhythmia
  - Poor compliance with diuretic therapy
  - Drugs causing fluid retention (e.g. NSAIDs, steroids)
  - Iatrogenic fluid overload
  - Endocarditis
  - Progression of disease
  - Intercurrent illness, e.g. pneumonia, anemia
- Renal disease
  - Acute or chronic renal failure
  - Renal artery stenosis (p. 223)
- Iatrogenic fluid overload
- Acute central nervous system disease
  - Subarachnoid hemorrhage
- Negative-pressure pulmonary edema (Table 29.8)

## Causes due to increased pulmonary capillary permeability (acute lung injury/ARDS); for management see Table 29.7

| Direct lung injury | Indirect lung injury |
|---|---|
| **Common causes** | |
| Pneumonia (viral or bacterial) | Sepsis |
| Aspiration of gastric contents | Severe trauma with shock and multiple transfusions |

*Continued*

**Less common causes**

| | |
|---|---|
| Pulmonary contusion | Cardiopulmonary bypass |
| Fat emboli | Drug overdose |
| Drowning | Acute pancreatitis |
| Inhalational injury | Transfusions of blood |
| Reperfusion pulmonary edema | products |
| after lung transplantation or | |
| pulmonary embolectomy | |

ARDS, acute respiratory distress syndrome; NSAIDs, non-steroidal anti-inflammatory drugs.

**TABLE 29.2** Focused assessment in acute pulmonary edema

**What is the cause of the pulmonary edema?**
- Usually cardiac disease (Table 29.1), less often acute renal failure
- Pulmonary edema developing in hospital is often due to fluid overload in patients with pre-existing cardiac or renal disease
- Consider acute respiratory distress syndrome in patients without evidence of cardiac disease (Table 29.1)
- In postoperative patients, negative-pressure pulmonary edema is occasionally seen (Table 29.8)
- Neurogenic pulmonary edema may complicate subarachnoid hemorrhage (p. 321)

**Acute pulmonary edema**

**TABLE 29.3** Initial drug therapy in acute pulmonary edema

| Drug | Comment |
|------|---------|
| **Oxygen** | Give oxygen 60–100% |
| | Pulse oximetry may be unreliable due to peripheral vasoconstriction |
| | Check arterial blood gases if the patient is hypotensive or there is no improvement within 30 min |
| | Target oxygen saturation >92%, $PaO_2 > 8$ kPa |
| **Morphine** | Give morphine 5–10 mg by slow IV injection to relieve breathlessness/distress. |
| **Furosemide** | Give furosemide 40 mg IV if plasma creatinine is <150 µmol/L and 80 mg if 150–200 µmol/L |
| | In patients with plasma creatinine >200 µmol/L, standard doses of furosemide are often ineffective. Try a furosemide infusion (100 mg IV over 60 min by syringe pump) |
| **Nitrate** | Give nitrate (sublingual, buccal or IV infusion) |

**TABLE 29.4** Urgent investigation in acute pulmonary edema

- ECG (Arrhythmia? Evidence of acute myocardial infarction or ischemia? Evidence of other cardiac disease, e.g. left ventricular hypertrophy, left bundle branch block?)
- Chest X-ray (to confirm the clinical diagnosis and exclude other causes of breathlessness). With non-cardiogenic pulmonary edema, the heart size is usually normal; septal lines and pleural effusions are usually absent; and air bronchograms are usually present
- Arterial blood gases and pH
- Blood glucose
- Creatinine, sodium and potassium
- Full blood count
- Erythrocyte sedimentation rate (ESR) or C-reactive protein
- Transthoracic echocardiography, especially if acute valve lesion or ventricular septal rupture is suspected, or distinction between cardiogenic/non-cardiogenic pulmonary edema is uncertain (in other patients, echocardiography should be done within 48 h)
- Cardiac biomarkers: plasma troponin and brain natriuretic peptide

**TABLE 29.5** Further drug therapy of acute cardiogenic pulmonary edema

| Systolic blood pressure | Action |
|---|---|
| **>110 mmHg** | Give another dose of furosemide 40–80 mg IV<br>Start a nitrate infusion |
| **90–110 mmHg** | Start a dobutamine infusion at 5 µg/kg/min; this can be given via a peripheral line<br>Increase the dose by 2.5 µg/kg/min every 10 min until systolic BP is >110 mmHg or a maximum dose of 20 µg/kg/min has been reached<br>A nitrate infusion can be added if systolic BP is maintained at >110 mmHg |
| **80–90 mmHg** | Start a dopamine infusion at 10 µg/kg/min; this must be given via a central line<br>Increase the dose by 5 µg/kg/min every 10 min until systolic BP is >110 mmHg<br>If systolic BP remains <90 mmHg despite dopamine 20 µg/kg/min, use norepinephrine instead<br>A nitrate infusion can be added if systolic BP is maintained at >110 mmHg |
| **<80 mmHg** | Start a norepinephrine infusion at 2.5 µg/kg/min; this must be given via a central line<br>Increase the dose by 2.5 µg/kg/min every 10 min until systolic BP is >110 mmHg<br>A nitrate infusion can be added if systolic BP is maintained at >110 mmHg |

Acute pulmonary edema

**TABLE 29.6** Ventilatory support for respiratory failure due to cardiogenic pulmonary edema

| Mode of ventilation | Indications | Contraindications | Disadvantages and complications |
|---|---|---|---|
| **Non-invasive ventilatory support with continuous positive airways pressure (CPAP)** | Oxygenation failure: oxygen saturation <92% despite $FiO_2 > 40\%$<br>Ventilatory failure: mild to moderate respiratory acidosis, arterial pH 7.25–7.35 | Recent facial, upper airway or upper gastrointestinal tract surgery<br>Vomiting or bowel obstruction<br>Copious secretions<br>Hemodynamic instability<br>Impaired consciousness, confusion or agitation | Discomfort from tightly fitting facemask<br>Discourages coughing and clearing of secretions |
| **Endotracheal intubation and mechanical ventilation** | Upper airway obstruction<br>Impending respiratory arrest<br>Airway at risk because of neurological disease or coma (GCS 8 or lower)<br>Oxygenation failure: $PaO_2$ <7.5–8 kPa despite supplemental oxygen/NIV<br>Ventilatory failure: moderate to severe respiratory acidosis, arterial pH < 7.25 | Severely impaired functional capacity and/or severe comorbidity<br>Cardiac disorder not remediable<br>Patient has expressed wish not to be ventilated | Adverse hemodynamic effects<br>Pharyngeal, laryngeal and tracheal injury<br>Pneumonia<br>Ventilator-induced lung injury (e.g. pneumothorax)<br>Complications of sedation and neuromuscular blockade |

GCS, Glasgow Coma Scale.

**Acute pulmonary edema**

**TABLE 29.7** Management of acute respiratory distress syndrome (ARDS)

| Element | Comment |
| --- | --- |
| **Transfer to ITU** | ARDS is usually part of multiorgan failure |
| **Oxygenation** | Increase inspired oxygen, target $PaO_2$ >8 kPa<br>Ventilation will be needed if $PaO_2$ is <8 kPa despite $FiO_2$ 60%<br>Ventilation in the prone position improves oxygenation<br>Hemoglobin should be kept around 10 g/dl (to give the optimum balance between oxygen-carrying capacity and blood viscosity) |
| **Fluid balance** | Renal failure is commonly associated with ARDS<br>Consider early hemofiltration |
| **Prevention and treatment of sepsis sepsis** | Sepsis is a common cause and complication of ARDS<br>Culture blood, tracheobronchial aspirate and urine daily<br>Treat presumed infection with broad-spectrum antibiotic therapy |
| **Nutrition** | Enteral feeding if possible, via nasogastric tube if ventilation needed |
| **DVT prophylaxis** | Give DVT prophylaxis with stockings and LMW heparin |
| **Prophylaxis against gastric stress ulceration** | Give proton pump inhibitor |

DVT, deep vein thrombosis; ITU, intensive therapy unit; LMW, low molecular weight.

Acute pulmonary edema

---

**TABLE 29.8** Negative-pressure pulmonary edema

- Seen in the early postoperative period
- Due to forced inspiration in the presence of upper airway obstruction (e.g. from laryngospasm after extubation)
- After relief of laryngospasm, patients develop clinical and radiological features of pulmonary edema
- Typically resolves over the course of a few hours with supportive care
- Cardiogenic pulmonary edema should be excluded by clinical assessment, ECG and echocardiography

---

## Further reading

European Society of Cardiology. Guidelines on the diagnosis and treatment of acute heart failure (2005). European Society of Cardiology website (http://www.escardio.org/knowledge/guidelines/Guidelines_list.htm?hit=quick).

McMurray JJV, Pfeffer MA. Heart failure. *Lancet* 2005; 365: 1877–89.

Peter JV, et al. Effect of non-invasive positive pressure ventilation (NIPPV) on mortality in patients with acute cardiogenic pulmonary oedema: a meta-analysis. *Lancet* 2006; 367: 1155–63.

Ware LB, Matthay MA. The acute respiratory distress syndrome. *N Engl J Med* 2000; 342: 1334–49.

Ware LB, Matthay MA. Acute pulmonary edema. *N Engl J Med* 2005; 353: 2788–96.

Acute pulmonary edema

# 30 Cardiac valve disease and prosthetic heart valves

Suspected valve disease:
- Unexplained hypotension/pulmonary edema (murmur may not be audible)
- Exertional syncope with ejection systolic murmur
- Fever with evidence of infective endocarditis
- Incidental finding of murmur

↓

Key observations (Table 1.2)
Urgent echocardiography and other investigation if acute illness (Tables 30.1, 30.2, 30.3)

↓

Further management directed by cause and severity of valve lesion, and clinical setting (Tables 30.4–30.6)

## ALERT
In severe aortic stenosis with a low cardiac output, the transvalve gradient will fall and the aortic stenosis may be erroneously graded as moderate.

## ALERT
If mitral regurgitation reported as 'mild' or 'moderate' is associated with a hyperdynamic left ventricle in a patient with shock, the likely diagnosis is critical regurgitation.

**TABLE 30.1** Urgent investigation in suspected valve disease

- ECG
- Chest X-ray
- Echocardiogram if pulmonary edema, unexplained hypotension, likely endocarditis, thromboembolism
- Full blood count and film
- Erythrocyte sedimentation rate (ESR) and C-reactive protein
- Blood culture (three sets) if infective endocarditis is suspected
- Blood glucose
- Sodium, potassium and creatinine
- Liver function tests
- Urine stick test and microscopy

**TABLE 30.2** Echocardiography in valve disease: key information

- Valve(s) affected and grade of stenosis or regurgitation
- Left ventricular size and function
- If there is acute severe aortic regurgitation, evidence of raised left ventricular end-diastolic pressure (early closure of the mitral valve and E deceleration time <150 ms)
- Evidence for etiology, e.g. infective endocarditis (p. 203), ruptured chord
- Pulmonary artery pressure and right ventricular function
- Ascending aortic diameter and evidence of abscess or dissection

## Further reading

American College of Cardiology and American Heart Association. Guidelines for the management of patients with valvular heart disease (2006). American College of Cardiology website (http://www.acc.org/qualityandscience/clinical/topic/topic.htm).

Butchart EC et al. Recommendation for the management of patients after heart valve surgery. *Eur Heart J* 2005; 26: 2463–71.

European Society of Cardiology. Guidelines on the management of valvular heart disease (2007). European Society of Cardiology website (http://www.escardio.org/knowledge/guidelines/Guidelines_list.htm?hit=quick).

Seiler C. Management and follow up of prosthetic heart valves. *Heart* 2004; 90: 818–24.

**TABLE 30.3** Causes of acute pulmonary edema in native and prosthetic valve disease

| Setting | Causes |
|---|---|
| **Acute native valve regurgitation** | Acute aortic regurgitation:<br>• Endocarditis<br>• Aortic dissection<br>• Deceleration injury, e.g. RTA<br>Acute mitral regurgitation:<br>• Myocardial infarction giving papillary muscle rupture or dysfunction<br>• Endocarditis<br>• Ruptured chord in floppy mitral valve<br>• Deceleration injury e.g. RTA |
| **Prosthetic valve** | Dehiscence (early, caused by surgical technique or friable tissue; or late, usually caused by endocarditis)<br>Thrombosis causing a stuck mechanical leaflet. Rare in biological valves<br>Primary failure causing either obstruction (as a result of calcification) or regurgitation (as a result of a tear in a biological cusp). Rarely occurs before 5 years in the mitral position or 7 years in the aortic position unless the patient is aged <45 years<br>Endocarditis |
| **Chronic native valve disease or prosthetic valve** | Acute myocardial infarction or myocardial ischemia<br>Arrhythmia<br>Poor compliance with diuretic therapy<br>Drugs causing fluid retention (e.g. NSAIDs, steroids)<br>Iatrogenic fluid overload<br>Endocarditis<br>Progression of disease |

NSAIDs, non-steroidal anti-inflammatory drugs; RTA, road traffic accident.

**TABLE 30.4** Aortic valve disease

| Valve lesion | Setting | Management |
|---|---|---|
| **Severe aortic stenosis** | Presenting with heart failure | Start a loop diuretic<br>If hypotensive, start dobutamine (p. 190)<br>The only definitive treatment is valve replacement<br>A low left ventricular ejection fraction may be reversible and is not a contraindication to aortic valve replacement |
| | Noted incidentally/ needing non-cardiac surgery | Severe aortic stenosis is a contraindication to all but life-saving non-cardiac surgery. Otherwise requires cardiac referral and consideration of aortic valve replacement before proceeding with original management plan<br>Avoid epidural anesthetics<br>Avoid vasodilators, e.g. angiotensin-converting enzyme inhibitors which should only be used under specialist guidance<br>Avoid drugs with negative inotropic effect<br>Moderate aortic stenosis may also cause symptoms and be associated with sudden death and should prompt cardiac referral |

*Continued*

Cardiac valve disease and prosthetic heart valves

Cardiac valve disease and prosthetic heart valves

| Valve lesion | Setting | Management |
|---|---|---|
| **Severe aortic regurgitation** | Presenting with heart failure | Consider infective endocarditis<br><br>Request urgent cardiac opinion if there are signs of a high LV end-diastolic pressure since these patients can deteriorate rapidly<br><br>Critical aortic regurgitation can lead to vasoconstriction with normalization of the diastolic pressure (usually <70 mmHg and often 30 or 40 mmHg in severe regurgitation)<br><br>Give a loop diuretic<br><br>If systolic BP <100 mmHg, start dobutamine<br><br>If oxygen saturation <92% despite 60% oxygen and patient tiring, discuss mechanical ventilation<br><br>Discuss urgent specialist investigation and surgery with a cardiologist |
| | Noted incidentally/ needing non-cardiac surgery | Refer for a cardiology opinion especially if there are indications for surgery:<br>• Exertional breathlessness<br>• LV systolic diameter >5.0 cm<br>• Aortic root dilatation<br>Patients with LV compensation usually tolerate non-cardiac surgery well |

BSA, body surface area; LV, left ventricular.

**ALERT**
In severe valve disease, a murmur may not be obvious if the cardiac output is low and/or breath sounds loud.

**ALERT**
Severe aortic stenosis is frequently associated with systemic hypertension rather than hypotension and narrow pulse pressure.

**TABLE 30.5** Mitral valve disease

| Valve lesion | Setting | Management |
|---|---|---|
| **Severe mitral stenosis** | Presenting with pulmonary edema | Give a loop diuretic<br>Left atrial pressure is highly dependent on heart rate. Treat atrial fibrillation with digoxin and if the ventricular rate is >100 bpm, add verapamil or a beta-blocker. If there is sinus tachycardia give a beta-blocker, e.g. metoprolol 25 mg 12-hourly PO<br>Avoid mechanical ventilation unless essential because of the risks of circulatory collapse. Maintain peripheral vascular resistance with norepinephrine<br>Discuss mitral valve replacement or balloon valvotomy with a cardiologist<br>*Continued* |

Cardiac valve disease and prosthetic heart valves

| Valve lesion | Setting | Management |
|---|---|---|
| | Noted incidentally /needing non-cardiac surgery | Indications for intervention are:<br>• Symptoms<br>• High pulmonary artery pressure<br>Patients with critical mitral stenosis tolerate non-cardiac surgery badly unless the rate is controlled pharmacologically. Also consider urgent balloon valvotomy |
| **Severe mitral regurgitation** | Presenting with heart failure | Start a loop diuretic<br>Start dobutamine if systolic BP <100 mmHg or norepinephrine if systolic BP <90 mmHg<br>Discuss with a cardiologist the insertion of a balloon pump preparatory to surgery |
| | Noted incidentally/ needing non-cardiac surgery | Refer for a cardiology opinion especially if there are indications for surgery:<br>• Exertional breathlessness<br>• LV systolic diameter >4.0 cm (in non-ischemic regurgitation)<br>Patients with LV compensation usually tolerate non-cardiac surgery well |

LV, left ventricular.

| TABLE 30.6 Prosthetic heart valves | |
|---|---|
| **Complication** | **Management** |
| **Heart failure or hypotension** | *Obstruction:* <br>• Recognized by reduced or absent opening of cusps or mechanical leaflet associated with high pressure drop across the valve on Doppler <br>• Requires emergency cardiac referral <br>• Transesophageal echocardiography is usually needed to determine the cause (thrombosis, pannus overgrowth, vegetations, mechanical obstruction) <br>• Surgery is the definitive treatment for left-sided obstruction; thrombolysis for right-sided thrombosis <br><br>*Regurgitation:* <br>• Recognized by rocking of the prosthesis associated with a large regurgitant color jet or the combination of highly active left ventricle and low cardiac output <br>• Requires emergency cardiac referral for consideration of redo surgery |
| **Thromboembolism** (arrange transthoracic echocardiogram) | The risk of thromboembolism is most closely related to non-prosthetic factors, e.g. atrial fibrillation, large left atrium, impaired left ventricle <br><br>Check that there are no signs of prosthetic dysfunction (breathlessness, abnormal murmur, muffled closure sound) or signs of infective endocarditis (p. 203) <br><br>Look at anticoagulation record and check INR, full blood count, CRP and blood culture (three sets) if white cell count or CRP raised <br><br>If INR low (<3 for a mechanical valve) and there is no evidence of endocarditis, increase warfarin dose aiming for a range of 3–4. |

*Continued*

Cardiac valve disease and prosthetic heart valves

| Complication | Management |
|---|---|
| | Arrange an early appointment with the anticoagulation clinic<br>If thromboembolism persists discuss with a cardiologist and consider transesophageal echocardiography looking for thrombus or pannus formation |
| **Bleeding** | See p. 512 |
| **Fever** | Always consider infective endocarditis but do not forget non-cardiac causes<br>Send three sets of blood cultures before starting antibiotic therapy.<br>The sensitivity of transthoracic echo for vegetations is much lower than for native valves, about 15%, and transesophageal echocardiography is usually necessary to confirm the diagnosis<br>Surgery is more likely to be necessary than for native valves |
| **Anemia** | Investigate as for any anemia, not forgetting the possibility of endocarditis<br>Virtually all mechanical valves produce minor hemolysis (disrupted cells on the film, high LDH and bilirubin, low haptoglobin) caused by normal transprosthetic regurgitation. Usually the hemoglobin remains normal<br>Hemolytic anemia suggests leakage usually around the valve (paraprosthetic regurgitation), which is often small and only detectable on transesophageal echocardiography<br>Refer for a cardiac opinion |

CRP, C-reactive protein; INR, international normalized ratio; LDH, lactate dehydrogenase.

# 31 Infective endocarditis

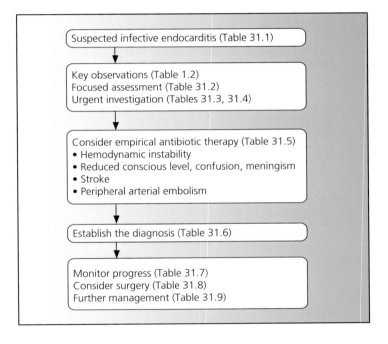

Suspected infective endocarditis (Table 31.1)

Key observations (Table 1.2)
Focused assessment (Table 31.2)
Urgent investigation (Tables 31.3, 31.4)

Consider empirical antibiotic therapy (Table 31.5)
• Hemodynamic instability
• Reduced conscious level, confusion, meningism
• Stroke
• Peripheral arterial embolism

Establish the diagnosis (Table 31.6)

Monitor progress (Table 31.7)
Consider surgery (Table 31.8)
Further management (Table 31.9)

**TABLE 31.1** Could this be infective endocarditis?

Consider infective endocarditis in the following clinical settings:
- Multisystem illness, especially with fever (see Table 76.1, p. 479)
- Stroke + fever, especially in a young patient
- Arterial embolism + fever
- Prosthetic heart valve + fever
- IV drug use + fever
- IV drug use + 'pneumonia' (septic pulmonary emboli from tricuspid valve endocarditis)
- Central venous catheter + fever
- *Streptococcus viridans* bacteremia
- *Staphyloccus aureus* bacteremia (incidence of infective endocarditis in patients with *Staph. aureus* bacteraemia is ~10%, and ~40% in those with prosthetic heart valve)
- Community-acquired *Enterococcus* bacteremia
- Acute aortic or mitral regurgitation (typically presents with acute pulmonary edema)

**TABLE 31.2** Focused assessment of the patient with suspected infective endocarditis

**History**
- Major symptoms and time course
- Symptoms of systemic embolism (transient ischemic attack, stroke, abdominal pain, limb ischemia) or pulmonary embolism (with right-sided valve endocarditis, typically seen with IV drug use)?
- Previous endocarditis or other known high risk cardiac lesion (congenital heart disease other than atrial septal defect, acquired native valve disease or prosthetic heart valve, hypertrophic cardiomyopathy)?
- Antibiotic history (prior antibiotic therapy may render blood cultures negative)
- Dental history
- IV drug use?

**Examination**
- Key observations (see Table 1.2) and systematic examination (see Table 1.9)
- Careful examination of the skin, nails, conjunctival and oral mucosae and fundi, looking for stigmata of infective endocarditis (petechiae, splinter hemorrhages, and rarely Janeway lesions, Osler nodes and Roth spots)
- Alternative source of sepsis?

**TABLE 31.3** Initial investigation in suspected infective endocarditis

- Blood culture (three sets drawn 1 h apart; unless critically ill in which case take two sets, one from each arm)
- Full blood count
- Erythrocyte sedimentation rate (ESR) and C-reactive protein
- Blood glucose
- Sodium, potassium, creatinine and liver function tests
- Urine stick test, microscopy and culture
- ECG
- Chest X-ray
- Echocardiography (Table 31.4)

**TABLE 31.4** Indications for transthoracic echocardiography in suspected infective endocarditis

**Urgent**
- Arterial embolism (stroke or peripheral)
- Hypotension or pulmonary edema
- Clinically severe aortic or mitral regurgitation (rapid deterioration may occur)
- Suspicion of an abscess (ill patient, long PR interval, *Staphylococcus aureus*)

**As soon as possible**
- Positive blood culture with organism associated with endocarditis, e.g. *Streptococcus viridans*, *Strep. bovis*, *Staph. aureus*
- Intravenous drug use
- Prosthetic heart valve
- Central venous catheter-related sepsis persisting for >72 h after antibiotic therapy
- New regurgitant murmur (endocarditis rarely causes new obstruction)

**Not indicated**
- Low clinical suspicion of endocarditis (e.g. fever with ejection systolic flow murmur, Table 31.6)

**TABLE 31.5** Empirical antibiotic therapy in suspected infective endocarditis*

**Suspected infective endocarditis in patients with prosthetic heart valves, penicillin allergy, suspected MRSA:**
- Vancomycin 1 g 12-hourly IV *plus*
- Gentamicin 80 mg 8-hourly IV *plus*
- Rifampicin 450 mg 12-hourly PO

**Suspected infective endocarditis of native heart valve in other patients – acute presentation:**
- Flucloxacillin 2 g 4-hourly IV *plus*
- Gentamicin 80 mg 8-hourly IV

**Suspected infective endocarditis of native heart valve in other patients – subacute presentation:**
- Benzylpenicillin 1.2 g 4-hourly IV *plus*
- Gentamicin 80 mg 8-hourly IV

MRSA, meticillin-resistant *Staphylococcus aureus*.

* These are regimens for when therapy has to be started before blood culture results are available. Contact a microbiologist for advice, particularly in patients with penicillin allergy.

**TABLE 31.6** Modified Duke criteria for the diagnosis of infective endocarditis (IE)

**Pathological criteria**
- Positive histology or microbiology of pathological material obtained at removal of a peripheral embolus (as well as at autopsy or cardiac surgery)

**Major criteria: microbiology**
- Two or more positive blood cultures with typical organisms, e.g. *Streptococcus viridans*, *Strep. bovis*, or
- Persistent bacteremia with a less specific organism, e.g. *Staphylococcus aureus*, *Staph. epidermidis*, or
- Positive serology for *Coxiella burnetti*

**Major criteria: echocardiography**
- Typical vegetation, *or*
- Intracardiac abscess or fistula, *or*
- Valve destruction causing new regurgitation, *or*
- New partial detachment of a prosthetic valve

**Minor criteria: clinical**
- Predisposing cardiac lesion or IV drug use
- Fever >38°C
- Vascular phenomena such as systemic arterial embolism and septic pulmonary embolism
- Immunological phenomena such as glomerulonephritis, Osler nodes, Roth spots
- Microbiological evidence consistent with IE but not meeting major criterion

**Diagnosis of infective endocarditis**
*Definite IE*:
- Pathological criteria positive, *or*
- Two major criteria, *or*
- One major and three minor criteria, *or*
- Five minor criteria

*Possible IE*:
- One major and one minor criterion, *or*
- Three minor criteria

*Rejected diagnosis of IE*:
- Firm alternative diagnosis, *or*
- Resolution of syndrome after 4 days or less of antibiotic therapy, *or*
- Does not meet above criteria

---

**TABLE 31.7** Monitoring in infective endocarditis

- Record blood results on a flow chart
- Check creatinine and electrolytes initially daily (Table 31.9)
- Check C-reactive protein and white cell count initially every other day
- Check vancomycin/gentamicin levels as directed by microbiology department
- With aortic valve endocarditis, record an ECG daily while fever persists (prolongation of PR interval is a sign of abscess formation: arrange transesophageal echocardiography)
- Repeat transthoracic echocardiography if there is a change in clinical status and before discharge (to provide baseline against which to compare grade of regurgitation and size of left ventricle on outpatient studies)

---

**ALERT**
Care in infective endocarditis should be shared between a cardiologist and microbiologist. Seek early advice from a cardiac surgeon if there is severe valve regurgitation, suspected endocarditis of a prosthetic heart valve, or fungal/*Coxiella* endocarditis.

**ALERT**
Surgery is usually needed if sepsis is uncontrolled after 1 week of antibiotic therapy.

**TABLE 31.8** Indications for surgery in infective endocarditis

**Absolute**
- Heart failure due to severe valve regurgitation
- Failure of sepsis to resolve with the correct antibiotic at the correct dose (including development of intracardiac abscesses or fistulae due to perivalvular spread of infection)
- Recurrent emboli despite adequate antibiotic therapy

**Relative**
- Endocarditis due to *Staphylococcu aureus*, *Coxiella burnetti*, *Brucella* species or fungi
- Prosthetic valve endocarditis (harder to sterilize than native valves)
- Large (>10 mm) and mobile vegetations if associated with another criterion for surgery

---

**TABLE 31.9** Infective endocarditis (IE): further management

- Correct anemia with transfusion if hemoglobin is <9 g/dl
- If creatinine rises:
  - Consider the possible causes: prerenal failure; glomerulonephritis related to IE; interstitial nephritis related to antibiotic; vancomycin or gentamicin nephrotoxicity; other causes, e.g. bladder outflow obstruction
  - Check urine stick test and microscopy and ultrasound of urinary tract
  - Reduce antibiotic doses as necessary
  - Discuss management with a cardiac surgeon if renal failure is due to severe valve regurgitation or uncontrolled sepsis
  - Seek advice from a nephrologist if glomerulonephritis/interstitial nephritis suspected
- Seek an opinion from a maxillofacial surgeon if endocarditis is due to *Streptococcus viridans* or other oral commensals
- Arrange investigation of colon if endocarditis is due to *Strep. bovis* (associated with colonic polyps (~50%) and colonic cancer (~20%)) but do not delay cardiac surgery if indicated

## Further reading

European Society of Cardiology. Guidelines on prevention, diagnosis and treatment of infective endocarditis (2004). European Society of Cardiology website (http://www.escardio.org/knowledge/guidelines/Guidelines_list.htm?hit=quick).

Moreillon P, Que Y-A. Infective endocarditis. *Lancet* 2004; 363: 139–49.

Moss R, Munt B. Injection drug use and right sided endocarditis. *Heart* 2003; 89: 577–81.

Piper C, et al. Prosthetic valve endocarditis. *Heart* 2001; 85: 590–93.

Infective endocarditis

# 32 Acute pericarditis

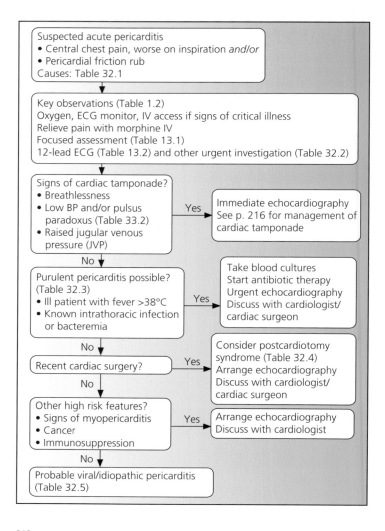

---

**TABLE 32.1** Causes of acute pericarditis (estimated incidence)

- Idiopathic (85–90%)
- Infectious diseases (viral, bacterial, fungal, tuberculous) (7%)
- Acute myocardial infarction (pericarditis occurs in 5–10% of patients with myocardial infarction)
- Malignancy (7%)
- Rheumatic diseases, e.g. systemic lupus erythematosus (3–5%)
- Aortic dissection (<1%)
- Advanced renal failure (pericarditis occurs in 5% of patients before renal replacement therapy)
- Pericardial surgery or trauma (Dressler/postcardiotomy syndrome) (<1%)
- Adverse drug reaction (<1%)

---

**TABLE 32.2** Urgent investigation in suspected pericarditis

- Chest X-ray
- ECG (see Table 13.2)
- Plasma markers of myocardial necrosis (see Table 13.5)
- Blood glucose
- Sodium, potassium and creatinine
- Full blood count
- Erythrocyte sedimentation rate (ESR) and C-reactive protein
- Echocardiogram if clinical evidence of myocarditis or pericardial effusion (large cardiac silhouette or pulmonary edema on chest X-ray, raised jugular venous pressure, hypotension)
- Blood for viral serology (for later analysis)
- Blood culture (if suspected bacterial infection)
- Autoantibody screen (for later analysis)

---

**TABLE 32.3** Purulent pericarditis

---

- Purulent pericarditis is usually due to spread of intrathoracic infection, e.g. following thoracic surgery or trauma, or complicating bacterial pneumonia
- Start antibiotic therapy with flucloxacillin (vancomycin or teicoplanin if penicillin allergy) and gentamicin IV after taking blood cultures
- Obtain an echocardiogram to look for an effusion or evidence of endocarditis
- Perform pericardiocentesis (p. 609) if there is an effusion large enough to be drained safely (echo-free space >2 cm). Send fluid for Gram stain and culture. Consider tuberculous or fungal infection if the effusion is purulent but no organisms are seen on Gram stain
- Discuss further management with a cardiologist or cardiothoracic surgeon

---

**TABLE 32.4** Postcardiotomy (Dressler) syndrome

---

- Occurs 2–4 weeks after open heart surgery
- Recognized but rare complication of acute myocardial infarction
- Acute self-limiting illness with fever, pericarditis and pleuritis
- ECG usually shows only non-specific ST/T abnormalities
- Chest X-ray shows:
  - Large cardiac silhouette (due to pericardial effusion)
  - Pleural effusions
  - Transient pulmonary infiltrates (occasionally seen)
- White cell count and ESR raised (often >70 mm/h)
- Treat with NSAID or colchicine

---

ESR, erythrocyte sedimentation rate; NSAID, non-steroidal anti-inflammatory drug.

**TABLE 32.5** Idiopathic pericarditis

- Likely diagnosis in young and otherwise healthy adults with acute pericarditis
- May be preceded by a flu-like illness
- Usually a self-limiting disorder lasting 1–3 weeks
- Echocardiography is not indicated unless the jugular venous pressure is raised or the chest X-ray shows a large cardiac silhouette
- Treat with NSAID (e.g. ibuprofen 1600–2400 mg daily) until the pain has resolved
- Recurrent pericarditis occurs in 15–40% of patients, and can be treated with colchicine

NSAID, non-steroidal anti-inflammatory drug.

## Further reading

European Society of Cardiology. Guidelines on the diagnosis and management of pericardial diseases (2004). European Society of Cardiology website (http://www.escardio.org/knowledge/guidelines/Guidelines_list.htm?hit=quick).

Goodman LJ. Purulent pericarditis. *Curr Treatment Options Cardiovasc Med* 2000; 2: 343–50.

Lange RA, Hillis LD. Acute pericarditis. *N Engl J Med* 2004; 351: 2195–202.

Spodick DH. Acute pericarditis: current concepts and practice. *JAMA* 2003; 289: 1150–3.

Troughton RW, et al. Pericarditis. *Lancet* 2004; 363: 717–27.

# 33 Cardiac tamponade

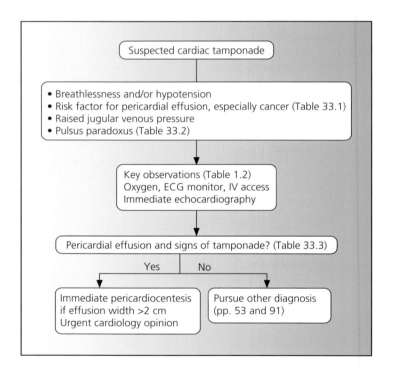

Suspected cardiac tamponade

- Breathlessness and/or hypotension
- Risk factor for pericardial effusion, especially cancer (Table 33.1)
- Raised jugular venous pressure
- Pulsus paradoxus (Table 33.2)

Key observations (Table 1.2)
Oxygen, ECG monitor, IV access
Immediate echocardiography

Pericardial effusion and signs of tamponade? (Table 33.3)

Yes     No

Immediate pericardiocentesis
if effusion width >2 cm
Urgent cardiology opinion

Pursue other diagnosis
(pp. 53 and 91)

**ALERT**
Once the decision to drain an effusion is made, do not delay.

---

**TABLE 33.1** Causes of cardiac tamponade

**Bleeding into pericardial space**
- Penetrating and blunt chest trauma including external cardiac compression
- Bleeding from cardiac chamber or coronary artery caused by perforation/laceration as a complication of cardiac catheterization, percutaneous coronary intervention, pacemaker insertion, pericardiocentesis or central venous cannulation
- Bleeding after cardiac surgery
- Cardiac rupture after myocardial infarction
- Aortic dissection with retrograde extension into pericardial space
- Anticoagulant therapy or thrombolytic therapy given (inappropriately) for pericarditis

**Serous or sero-sanguinous pericardial effusion**
- Neoplastic involvement of pericardium (most commonly in carcinoma of breast or bronchus, or lymphoma)
- Pericarditis complicating connective tissue diseases (e.g. systemic lupus erythematosus, rheumatoid arthritis)
- Postcardiotomy syndrome pericarditis
- Tuberculous and viral pericarditis
- Uremic pericarditis
- Idiopathic pericarditis (tamponade is a rare complication)

**Purulent pericarditis**
- Pyogenic bacterial infection

---

**TABLE 33.2** Pulsus paradoxus

**1 What is it?**
- An exaggeration of the normal inspiratory fall in systolic blood pressure to >10 mmHg
- Pulsus paradoxus may be palpable in the radial artery, with the pulse disappearing on inspiration

*Continued*

**2 When does it happen?**
- Typically in cardiac tamponade, but it may not always occur (e.g. if there is an atrial septal defect or severe aortic regurgitation)
- Pulsus paradoxus may occur in other conditions (e.g. acute severe asthma, right ventricular infarction)

**3 How is it measured?**
- Inflate the blood pressure cuff above systolic BP
- Slowly deflate the cuff, watching the chest, and note the pressure at which sounds are first heard in expiration alone
- Continue deflating the cuff and note the pressure at which sounds are heard thoughout expiration and inspiration
- The difference in these systolic pressures is the degree of pulsus paradoxus

**TABLE 33.3** What to look for on echocardiography in suspected cardiac tamponade

- Presence, size and distribution (circumferential or loculated) of pericardial fluid
- Signs of tamponade:
  - Diastolic collapse of the free wall of the right ventricle
  - A fall in mitral inflow velocity or aortic velocity by >25% on inspiration
  - Engorgement of the inferior vena cava with no respiratory variation
- Best approach for pericardiocentesis: subcostal or anterior. Choose the approach with the larger width of effusion (which should be 2 cm or greater), and decide on the optimum needle trajectory, avoiding the liver or lung (p. 609)

## Further reading

Bilchick KC, Wise RA. Paradoxical physical findings described by Kussmaul: pulsus paradoxus and Kussmaul's sign. *Lancet* 2002; 359: 1940–2.
Spodick DH. Acute cardiac tamponade. *N Engl J Med* 2003; 349: 684–90.

# 34 Severe hypertension

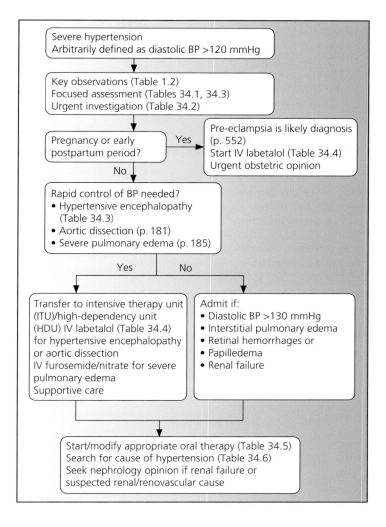

Severe hypertension
Arbitrarily defined as diastolic BP >120 mmHg

Key observations (Table 1.2)
Focused assessment (Tables 34.1, 34.3)
Urgent investigation (Table 34.2)

Pregnancy or early postpartum period? — Yes → Pre-eclampsia is likely diagnosis (p. 552)
Start IV labetalol (Table 34.4)
Urgent obstetric opinion

No

Rapid control of BP needed?
• Hypertensive encephalopathy (Table 34.3)
• Aortic dissection (p. 181)
• Severe pulmonary edema (p. 185)

Yes                No

Transfer to intensive therapy unit (ITU)/high-dependency unit (HDU) IV labetalol (Table 34.4) for hypertensive encephalopathy or aortic dissection
IV furosemide/nitrate for severe pulmonary edema
Supportive care

Admit if:
• Diastolic BP >130 mmHg
• Interstitial pulmonary edema
• Retinal hemorrhages or
• Papilledema
• Renal failure

Start/modify appropriate oral therapy (Table 34.5)
Search for cause of hypertension (Table 34.6)
Seek nephrology opinion if renal failure or suspected renal/renovascular cause

---

**TABLE 34.1** Focused assessment in severe hypertension

**History**
- Previous treatment and compliance
- Previous investigations
- Known cardiac or renal disease?
- Recent stroke or subarachnoid hemorrhage? (Lowering the blood pressure may worsen the neurological deficit: discuss management with a neurologist)
- Features of hypertensive encephalopathy (Table 34.3)?

**Examination**
- Blood pressure in both arms
- Presence and symmetry of the major pulses, check for radiofemoral delay
- Carotid, abdominal and femoral bruits
- Check for signs of heart failure and aortic regurgitation
- Abdominal mass (e.g. palpable kidneys or abdominal aortic aneurysm)
- Fundi: retinal hemorrhages, exudates or papilledema (not due to other causes) define accelerated phase or 'malignant' hypertension; hypertension is associated with microvascular damage, present in all organs but visualized in the retina

---

**TABLE 34.2** Urgent investigation in severe hypertension

- Blood glucose
- Sodium, potassium and creatinine (check daily)
- Full blood count
- Plasma renin/aldosterone (for later analysis)
- Urine stick test and microscopy
- Ultrasound of kidneys and urinary tract
- Urinary catecholamine excretion
- Urinary free cortisol excretion if suspected Cushing syndrome (Table 34.6)
- Chest X-ray
- ECG

---

**TABLE 34.3** Clinical features of hypertensive encephalopathy*

**Early**
- Headache
- Nausea and vomiting
- Confusional state
- Retinal hemorrhages, exudates or papilledema

**Late**
- Focal neurological signs
- Fits
- Coma

---

* Hypertensive encephalopathy is due to cerebral edema resulting from hyperperfusion as a consequence of severe hypertension with failure of cerebral autoregulation. It may be difficult to distinguish between hypertensive encephalopathy, subarachnoid hemorrhage (p. 321) and stroke. Hypertensive encephalopathy is favored by the gradual onset of symptoms and the absence (or late appearance) of focal neurological signs. If there is diagnostic doubt, a CT scan should be obtained to exclude cerebral or subarachnoid hemorrhage before starting IV therapy.

---

**TABLE 34.4** Intravenous labetalol for aortic dissection and hypertensive encephalopathy

- Make up a solution of 1 mg/ml by diluting the contents of 2 × 100 mg ampoules to 200 ml with normal saline or glucose 5%
- Start the infusion at 15 ml/h and increase it every 15 min as necessary
- Put in a bladder catheter to monitor urine output
- In aortic dissection, aim to reduce systolic blood pressure to <120 mmHg, providing the urine output remains >30 ml/h
- In hypertensive encephalopathy, aim to reduce BP to ~160–170/100–110 mmHg over 4–6 h
- A nitrate infusion can be added if needed for blood pressure control.

**TABLE 34.5** Initial oral therapy for severe hypertension

| Clinical features | Initial drug therapy |
| --- | --- |
| **Pheochromocytoma suspected** | Labetalol 100–200 mg 12-hourly PO |
| **Renal artery stenosis suspected** | Amlodipine 5–10 mg daily PO *plus* Bisoprolol 2.5–5 mg daily PO |
| **Other patients** | Amlodipine 5–10 mg daily *plus* Bisoprolol 2.5–5 mg daily PO |
| **If there is pulmonary edema or other signs of fluid retention** | Add furosemide 20–40 mg daily PO to one of the above regimens |

**TABLE 34.6** Causes of secondary hypertension

| Cause | Clues/investigation |
| --- | --- |
| **Intrinsic renal disease** | Family history of heritable renal disease (e.g. polycystic kidney disease) Abnormal urine stick test and microscopy Raised creatinine Abnormal kidneys on ultrasound Discuss further investigation with nephrologist if intrinsic renal disease suspected |
| **Primary hyperaldosteronism** | Low plasma potassium High plasma aldosterone with suppressed plasma renin |
| **Cushing syndrome** | Truncal obesity, thin skin with purple abdominal striae, proximal myopathy (unable to rise from chair without using arms) Increased urinary free cortisol excretion |
| **Pheochromocytoma** | Paroxysmal headache, sweating or palpitation Hypertensive crisis following anesthesia or administration of contrast Family history of pheochromocytoma Increased urinary catecholamine excretion |

*Continued*

| Cause | Clues/investigation |
| --- | --- |
| **Coarctation of aorta** | Radiofemoral delay<br>Coarctation demonstrated by echocardiography/MRI |
| **Renal artery stenosis** | May be due to fibromuscular dysplasia (age <50 with no family history of hypertension) or, more commonly, to atherosclerosis (age >50 with other atherosclerotic arterial disease)<br>Refractory hypertension<br>Deteriorating blood pressure control in compliant, long-standing hypertensive patients<br>Rise in creatinine on treatment with ACE inhibitor<br>Renal impairment with minimal proteinuria<br>Low plasma sodium and potassium (due to secondary hyperaldosteronism)<br>Difference in kidney size >1.5 cm on ultrasound |
| **Other causes** | Many causes including drugs, obstructive sleep apnea, acromegaly |

ACE, angiotension-converting enzyme.

Severe hypertension

## Further reading

Lenders JWM, et al. Phaeochromocytoma. *Lancet* 2005; 366: 665–75.

Moser M, Setaro JF. Resistant or difficult-to-control hypertension. *N Engl J Med* 2006; 355: 385–92.

Newell-Price J, et al. Cushing's syndrome. *Lancet* 2006; 367: 1605–17.

Safian RD, Textor SC. Renal-artery stenosis. *N Engl J Med* 2001; 344: 431–42.

Vidt DG. Hypertensive emergencies. *J Clin Hypertension* 2004; 6: 520–5.

Wong T, Mitchell P. The eye in hypertension. *Lancet* 2007; 369: 425–35.

Young WF Jr. Minireview. Primary aldosteronism – changing concepts in diagnosis and treatment. *Endocrinology* 2002; 144: 208–13.

# 35 Deep vein thrombosis

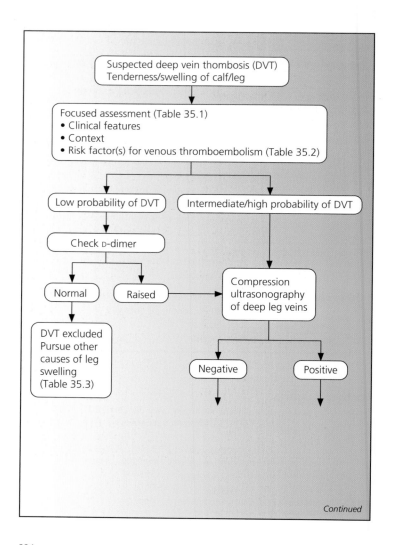

Suspected deep vein thombosis (DVT)
Tenderness/swelling of calf/leg

Focused assessment (Table 35.1)
• Clinical features
• Context
• Risk factor(s) for venous thromboembolism (Table 35.2)

Low probability of DVT

Intermediate/high probability of DVT

Check D-dimer

Normal

Raised

Compression ultrasonography of deep leg veins

DVT excluded
Pursue other causes of leg swelling
(Table 35.3)

Negative

Positive

*Continued*

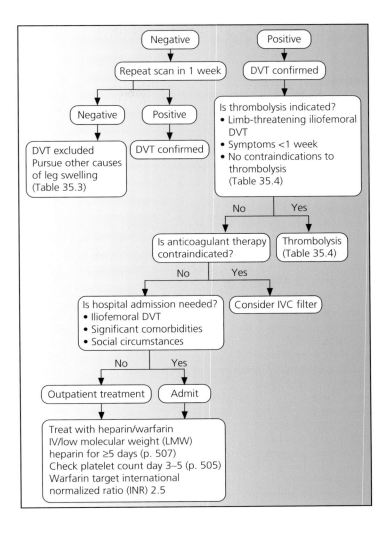

Deep vein thrombosis

**TABLE 35.1** Focused assessment in suspected deep vein thrombosis (DVT)

| Variable | Points |
|---|---|
| **History** | |
| Active cancer (treatment on-going, or within previous 6 months, or palliative) | 1 |
| Paralysis, paresis or recent plaster immobilization of the legs | 1 |
| Recently bed-ridden for more than 3 days, or major surgery within 4 weeks | 1 |
| **Examination** | |
| Entire leg swollen | 1 |
| Calf swelling by >3 cm when compared with asymptomatic leg (measured 10 cm below tibial tuberosity) | 1 |
| Pitting edema (greater in the symptomatic leg) | 1 |
| Localized tenderness along the distribution of the deep venous system | 1 |
| Collateral superficial veins (non-varicose) | 1 |
| **Alternative diagnosis** | |
| Alternative diagnosis as likely or more likely than DVT (Table 35.3)? | −2 |

| Clinical probability (prevalence of DVT) | Score |
|---|---|
| Low (<5%) | 0 or less |
| Intermediate | 1–2 |
| High (>60%) | >3 |

From Wells, P.S. et al. Value of assessment of pretest probability of deep-vein thrombosis in clinical management. *Lancet* 1997; **350**: 1795–8.

**TABLE 35.2** Risk factors for venous thromboembolism

| Risk factor | Comment |
|---|---|
| **Increasing age** | DVT/pulmonary embolism is rare in patients under 50 with no risk factors: if found, screen for thrombophilic disorder (see below) |
| **Previous DVT or PE** | Risk of recurrence after first spontaneous DVT is ~25% at 4 years |
| **Surgery** | Especially major abdominal or pelvic surgery, or hip/knee replacement |
| **Cancer** | Especially metastatic or abdominal/pelvic cancer |
| **Acute medical illness** | E.g. heart failure, respiratory failure, pneumonia |
| **Immobility** | Prolonged travel<br>Prolonged bed rest<br>Stroke |
| **Pregnancy and puerperium** | Associated with a two-fold and 14-fold increased risk for first DVT |
| **Trauma** | Especially spinal injuries, pelvic fractures or leg fractures |
| **Oral contraceptive (OC) and HRT** | Risk in OC and HRT users is approximately three times that in non-users |
| **Hematological disorders** | Deficiency of antithrombin, protein C or protein S<br>Resistance to activated protein C<br>Factor V Leiden<br>Prothrombin G20210A mutation<br>High level of factor VIII, factor IX or factor XI<br>Polycythemia rubra vera<br>Thrombocytosis<br>Heparin-induced thrombocytopenia<br>Paroxysmal nocturnal hemoglobinuria |

*Continued*

Deep vein thrombosis

| Risk factor | Comment |
|---|---|
| **Other disorders** | Antiphospholipid syndrome |
| | Behçet syndrome |
| | Nephrotic syndrome |
| | Hyperhomocysteinemia |
| | Ulcerative colitis |
| | Presence of central venous cannula, pacing leads or IVC filter |
| | Severe obesity |
| | IV drug abuse |

DVT, deep vein thrombosis; HRT, hormone replacement therapy; IVC, inferior vena cava; PE, pulmonary embolism.

---

**TABLE 35.3** Causes of leg swelling

**Venous/lymphatic**
- Deep vein thrombosis
- Superficial thrombophlebitis
- Inferior vena cava (IVC) obstruction (e.g. by tumor)
- Varicose veins with chronic venous hypertension
- Postphlebitic syndrome
- Congenital lymphedema
- After vein harvesting for coronary bypass grafting
- Dependent edema (e.g. in paralysed limb)
- Severe obesity with compression of iliofemoral veins by abdominal fat

**Musculoskeletal**
- Calf hematoma
- Ruptured Baker (popliteal) cyst (which may complicate rheumatoid arthritis or osteoarthritis of the knee)
- Muscle tear

*Continued*

---

**Skin**
- Cellulitis (recognized by tenderness, erythema and induration of the skin; p. 469)

**Systemic** (edema is bilateral, but may be asymmetric)
- Congestive heart failure
- Liver failure
- Renal failure
- Nephrotic syndrome
- Hypoalbuminemia
- Chronic respiratory failure
- Pregnancy
- Idiopathic edema of women
- Calcium antagonists
- Drugs causing salt/water retention (e.g. NSAIDs)

---

NSAIDs, non-steroidal anti-inflammatory drugs.

---

**Deep vein thrombosis**

**ALERT**
Deep vein thrombosis is common (incidence about one per 1000 per year) but leg swelling is usually due to other causes.

---

**TABLE 35.4** Thrombolysis in venous thromboembolism (limb-threatening iliofemoral deep vein thrombosis or acute major pulmonary embolism with persisting hypotension/shock)

**Absolute contraindications**
- History of hemorrhagic stroke
- Active intracranial neoplasm
- Recent (<2 months) intracranial surgery or trauma
- Active or recent internal bleeding in previous 6 months

**Relative contraindications**
- Bleeding disorder
- Uncontrolled severe hypertension (systolic BP > 200 mmHg or diastolic BP > 110 mmHg)
- Ischemic stroke within previous 2 months
- Surgery within previous 10 days
- Thrombocytopenia (<100 × $10^9$/L)

**Regimen**
- Give alteplase 100 mg IV over 2 h
- Then check the activated partial thromboplastin time (APTT)
- Unfractionated heparin should be given by IV infusion (p. 507) (without a loading dose) when the APTT is less than twice the upper limit of normal. If the APTT is above this value, recheck it every 4 h

---

## Further reading

Goodacre S, et al. Meta-analysis: the value of clinical assessment in the diagnosis of deep venous thrombosis. *Ann Intern Med* 2005; 143: 129–39.

Hirsh J, Bates SM. Clinical trials that have influenced the treatment of venous thrombo-embolism: a historical perspective. *Ann Intern Med* 2001; 134: 409–17.

Joffe HV, Goldhaber SZ. Upper-extremity deep vein thrombosis. *Circulation* 2002: 106: 1874–80.

Kyrle PA, Eichinger S. Deep vein thrombosis. *Lancet* 2005; 365: 1163–74.

Wells PS, et al. Does this patient have a deep vein thrombosis? *JAMA* 2006; 295; 199–207.

# 36 Pulmonary embolism

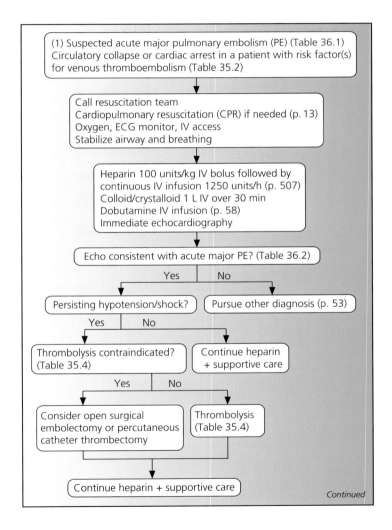

(1) Suspected acute major pulmonary embolism (PE) (Table 36.1)
Circulatory collapse or cardiac arrest in a patient with risk factor(s)
for venous thromboembolism (Table 35.2)

Call resuscitation team
Cardiopulmonary resuscitation (CPR) if needed (p. 13)
Oxygen, ECG monitor, IV access
Stabilize airway and breathing

Heparin 100 units/kg IV bolus followed by
continuous IV infusion 1250 units/h (p. 507)
Colloid/crystalloid 1 L IV over 30 min
Dobutamine IV infusion (p. 58)
Immediate echocardiography

Echo consistent with acute major PE? (Table 36.2)

Yes — No

Persisting hypotension/shock? | Pursue other diagnosis (p. 53)

Yes — No

Thrombolysis contraindicated? (Table 35.4) | Continue heparin + supportive care

Yes — No

Consider open surgical embolectomy or percutaneous catheter thrombectomy | Thrombolysis (Table 35.4)

Continue heparin + supportive care

*Continued*

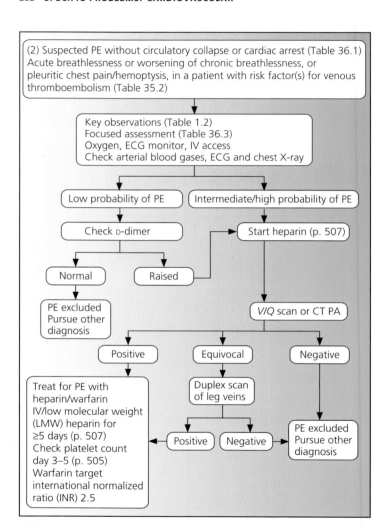

(2) Suspected PE without circulatory collapse or cardiac arrest (Table 36.1)
Acute breathlessness or worsening of chronic breathlessness, or
pleuritic chest pain/hemoptysis, in a patient with risk factor(s) for venous
thromboembolism (Table 35.2)

Key observations (Table 1.2)
Focused assessment (Table 36.3)
Oxygen, ECG monitor, IV access
Check arterial blood gases, ECG and chest X-ray

Low probability of PE

Intermediate/high probability of PE

Check D-dimer

Start heparin (p. 507)

Normal

Raised

PE excluded
Pursue other
diagnosis

V/Q scan or CT PA

Positive

Equivocal

Negative

Treat for PE with
heparin/warfarin
IV/low molecular weight
(LMW) heparin for
≥5 days (p. 507)
Check platelet count
day 3–5 (p. 505)
Warfarin target
international normalized
ratio (INR) 2.5

Duplex scan
of leg veins

Positive

Negative

PE excluded
Pursue other
diagnosis

**Pulmonary embolism**

**ALERT**

One or more risk factors for venous thromboembolism (Table
35.1) are present in ~85% of patients with pulmonary embolism.

**TABLE 36.1** Main clinical presentations of pulmonary embolism

| Variable | Circulatory collapse, previously well | Circulatory collapse, with underlying CPD | Pulmonary infarction | Isolated dyspnea |
|---|---|---|---|---|
| Frequency | 5% | 10% | 60% | 25% |
| Pulmonary arterial occlusion | Extensive | Small/moderate | Small/moderate | Moderate/large |
| Examination | Hypotension<br>Raised JVP | Hypotension<br>May have raised JVP<br>Signs of underlying CPD | Focal lung signs | Tachypnea (>20/min) |
| Chest X-ray | Usually normal | May reflect underlying CPD | Often focal shadowing | Usually normal |
| ECG | Often acute RV strain (RAD, RBBB) | Unhelpful, because abnormalities are mainly due to underlying CPD | Normal | Non-specific abnormalities |
| Arterial blood gases | Markedly abnormal | Unhelpful, because abnormalities are mainly due to underlying CPD | May be normal | Usually abnormal |

CPD, cardiopulmonary disease; JVP, jugular venous pressure; RAD, right axis deviation; RBBB, right bundle branch block; RV, right ventricular.
From British Thoracic Society, Standards of Care Committee. Suspected pulmonary embolism: a practical approach. *Thorax* 1997; **52** (Suppl. 4).

**Pulmonary embolism**

**TABLE 36.2** Assessing the likelihood of pulmonary embolism: Wells and Revised Geneva Scores

**Wells Score** (*Thromb Haemost* 2000; **83**: 416–20)

| Variable | Points |
|---|---|
| **History** | |
| Previous DVT/PE | 1.5 |
| Surgery under general anesthesia or fracture of lower limbs within previous month or immobilization | 1.5 |
| Cancer (receiving treatment, treated in past 6 months or palliative care) | 1 |
| Hemoptysis | 1 |
| **Examination** | |
| Clinical features of DVT | 3 |
| Heart rate >100 bpm | 1.5 |
| **Alternative diagnosis** | |
| No alternative diagnosis evident | 3 |

| Clinical probability of pulmonary embolism | Score |
|---|---|
| Low | <2 |
| Intermediate | 2–6 |
| High | >6 |

**Revised Geneva Score** (*Ann Intern Med* 2006; **144**: 165–71)

| Variable | Points |
|---|---|
| **History** | |
| Age >65 years | 1 |
| Previous DVT/PE | 3 |
| Surgery under general anesthesia or fracture of lower limbs within previous month | 2 |
| Active malignancy within previous year | 2 |
| Unilateral lower limb pain | 3 |
| Hemoptysis | 2 |

*Continued*

| Examination | |
|---|---|
| Heart rate 75–94 bpm | 3 |
| Heart rate 95 bpm or faster | 5 |
| Pain on lower limb deep venous palpation and unilateral edema | 4 |

| Clinical probability of pulmonary embolism | Score |
|---|---|
| Low | 0–3 |
| Intermediate | 4–10 |
| High | 11 or more |

**TABLE 36.3** Echocardiographic features of acute major pulmonary embolism

- Dilated right ventricle and right atrium
- Hypokinetic right ventricle with systolic septal flattening (best seen in the parasternal short axis view)
- Moderate or severe tricuspid regurgitation
- Dilated inferior vena cava with little or no change with respiration
- Elevated pulmonary artery pressure (peak velocity of tricuspid regurgitant jet <4.0 m/sec)
- Absence of significant left heart abnormalities that can cause pulmonary hypertension
- Free-floating thrombi may be seen in the right heart
- Time to peak pulmonary artery velocity short (<60 msec)

## Further reading

British Thoracic Society. Guidelines for the management of suspected acute pulmonary embolism. *Thorax* 2003; 58: 470–84.

Fedullo PF, Tapson VF. The evaluation of suspected pulmonary embolism. *N Engl J Med* 2003; 349: 1247–56.

Goldhaber SZ. Echocardiography in the management of pulmonary embolism. *Ann Intern Med* 2002; 136: 691–700.

Goldhaber SZ. Pulmonary embolism. *Lancet* 2004; 363: 1295–305.

Kucher N, Goldhaber SZ. Management of massive pulmonary embolism. *Circulation* 2005; 112: e28–e32.

Le Gal G, et al. Prediction of pulmonary embolism in the emergency department: the revised Geneva score. *Ann Intern Med* 2006; 144: 165–71.

Wells PS, et al. Derivation of a simple clinical model to categorize patients' probability of pulmonary embolism: increasing the model's utility with the simplified D-dimer. *Thromb Haemost* 2000; 83: 416–20.

# 37 Problems with pacemakers and implantable cardioverter-defibrillators

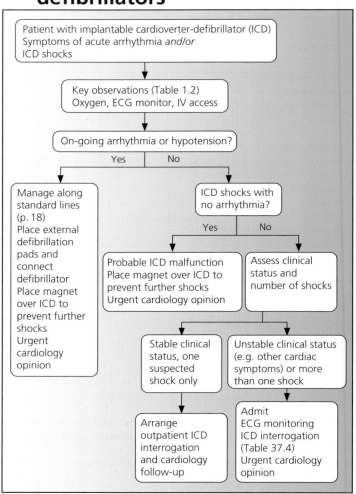

Patient with implantable cardioverter-defibrillator (ICD)
Symptoms of acute arrhythmia *and/or*
ICD shocks

↓

Key observations (Table 1.2)
Oxygen, ECG monitor, IV access

↓

On-going arrhythmia or hypotension?

Yes — No

**Yes:**
Manage along standard lines (p. 18)
Place external defibrillation pads and connect defibrillator
Place magnet over ICD to prevent further shocks
Urgent cardiology opinion

**No:**
ICD shocks with no arrhythmia?

Yes — No

**Yes:**
Probable ICD malfunction
Place magnet over ICD to prevent further shocks
Urgent cardiology opinion

**No:**
Assess clinical status and number of shocks

→ Stable clinical status, one suspected shock only
→ Arrange outpatient ICD interrogation and cardiology follow-up

→ Unstable clinical status (e.g. other cardiac symptoms) or more than one shock
→ Admit
ECG monitoring
ICD interrogation (Table 37.4)
Urgent cardiology opinion

**TABLE 37.1** Pacemaker and implantable cardioverter-defibrillator (ICD) functions

### 1 Pacemaker functions

| Pacemaker type/ indications | Pacemaker code | Comment |
| --- | --- | --- |
| **Single lead atrial pacemaker**<br>Indication: sinoatrial disorder (sinus bradycardia/pauses) with normal AV conduction | AAI or AAIR | Pacemaker senses and paces right atrium<br>If no intrinsic activity is sensed within right atrium, the pacemaker paces at its preprogramed rate<br>AAIR indicates rate-adaptive capability: the pacemaker increases the atrial pacing rate in response to stimuli such as movement |
| **Single lead ventricular pacemaker**<br>Indications: AV block with atrial fibrillation, intermittent AV block | VVI or VVIR | Pacemaker senses and paces right ventricle<br>If atrial electrical activity is conducted through the AV node/bundle of His and depolarizes the ventricles, the pacemaker is inhibited<br>If no intrinsic activity is sensed within right ventricle, the pacemaker paces at its preprogramed rate<br>VVIR indicates rate-adaptive capability: the pacemaker increases the pacing rate in response to stimuli such as movement |

*Continued*

| Pacemaker type/ indications | Pacemaker code | Comment |
|---|---|---|
| **Dual lead atrial and ventricular pacemaker**<br>Indications: AV block with sinus rhythm, sinoatrial disorder with impaired AV conduction | DDD or DDDR (Fig. 37.1) | Pacemaker senses and paces both the right atrium and the right ventricle<br>If no intrinsic activity is sensed in right atrium, the pacemaker paces at its preprogramed rate<br>If intrinsic activity or paced atrial activity is not conducted to the ventricles within a preprogramed interval, the pacemaker paces the right ventricle<br>DDDR indicates rate-adaptive capability: the pacemaker increases the pacing rate in response to stimuli such as movement |
| **Cardiac resynchronization therapy (CRT) (biventricular pacing)**<br>Indications: heart failure NYHA class 3 or 4, LVEF <35%, QRS duration >120 ms | CRT or CRT-D | Pacing both right and left ventricle to correct dyssynchronous contraction of the left ventricle and improve ejection<br>CRT may be combined with defibrillation capability (CRT-D) (see below)<br>Pacing leads are placed in the right atrium, right ventricle and in a venous branch over the free wall of the left ventricle (via the coronary sinus) |

*Continued*

| 2 ICD functions | |
| --- | --- |
| **ICD function** | **Comment** |
| **Sensing** | Recognition of atrial and ventricular electrogram signals |
| **Detection** | Classification of sensed signals according to programable heart rate zones |
| **Provision of therapy to terminate ventricular fibrillation (VF) or ventricular tachycardia (VT)** | VF is terminated by high energy (up to 30 J) unsynchronized shocks delivered between coil electrode in right ventricle and ICD casing and/or another electrode<br>VT is managed in one of four ways:<br>• Observation with no action<br>• Antitachycardia pacing (burst pacing at a rate faster than the VT rate)<br>• Low energy (<5 J) synchronized shock<br>• High energy unsynchronized shock<br>Placement of a magnet over the ICD suspends VT/VF detection (but not pacing for bradycardia) |
| **Pacing for bradycardia** | As provided by a pacemaker (see above) |

AV, atrioventricular; LVEF, left ventricular ejection fraction; NYHA, New York Heart Association.

Problems with pacemakers and implantable cardioverter-defibrillators

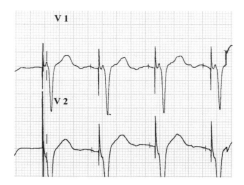

**FIGURE 37.1** ECG showing dual chamber pacing. The small atrial and larger ventricular pacing spikes can be seen, preceding the P waves and QRS complexes, respectively.

**TABLE 37.2** Complications of pacemakers and implantable cardioverter-defibrillators (ICDs)

### At implantation/shortly after implantation
- Pneumothorax
- Air embolism
- Pulse generator pocket hematoma
- Malposition of lead
- Displacement of lead
- Perforation of great vessels or myocardium by lead causing pericardial effusion/tamponade
- Diaphragmatic stimulation
- Thrombosis of subclavian vein

### Later
- Lead malfunction (insulation failure, conduction fracture)
- Pulse generator malfunction
- Infection of lead
- Infection of pulse generator pocket
- Erosion of pulse generator pocket
- Thrombosis of subclavian and central veins

**TABLE 37.3** Assessment of suspected pacemaker malfunction

- Check the details of the pacemaker: is it a single or dual chamber system (Table 37.1) and what is the pacing mode? Contact the hospital where the system was implanted to obtain further details
- Record a 12-lead ECG, a long rhythm strip and a penetrated chest X-ray for the postion of the leads
- Does the ECG show no pacing spikes, spikes without capture or spikes without sensing? Interpretation is given below
- Contact the cardiology department to arrange a check of the pacemaker and discuss management with a cardiologist (including need for temporary pacing)

| ECG | Causes |
| --- | --- |
| **No spikes** | Normal sensing<br>Malfunction of pulse generator<br>Spike buried in QRS complex<br>Electromagnetic interference |
| **Spikes without capture (failure to capture)** | High threshold:<br>• Lead fracture<br>• Lead displacement<br>• Myocardial fibrosis<br>• Myocardial perforation<br>Lead not properly connected to pulse generator<br>Depletion of battery of pulse generator<br>Spike in ventricular refractory period |
| **Spikes without sensing (failure to sense)** | Lead displacement<br>Low intrinsic P/R wave (i.e. not at sensing threshold) |

Problems with pacemakers and implantable cardioverter-defibrillators

**TABLE 37.4** Findings on interrogation of an implantable cardioverter-defibrillator (ICD) after the patient reports a shock

| Finding | Action |
| --- | --- |
| **VT/VF with appropriate termination by shock** | Assess potential causes: <br> • Myocardial ischemia <br> • Non-compliance with drug therapy <br> • Electrolyte disorder <br> • Intercurrent illness <br> Consider starting/modifying drug therapy to prevent recurrence. <br> Refer to cardiologist |
| **Inappropriate shock due to missensing of SVT/AF** | Assess causes and treat <br> Refer to cardiologist |
| **Inappropriate shock due to missensing of electrical noise** | Environmental noise: avoid exposure <br> Electrical noise from ICD malfunction: <br> • Program VT/VF detection off <br> • Admit for further management <br> • Refer to cardiologist |
| **No shock or arrhythmia** | Phantom shock. Reassure |

AF, atrial fibrillation; SVT, supraventricular tachycardia.
From Stevenson, W.G. et al. *Circulation* 2004; **110**: 3866–9.

## Further reading

Sohail MR, et al. Management and outcome of permanent pacemaker and implantable cardioverter-defibrillator infections. *J Am Coll Cardiol* 2007; 49: 1851–9.

Stevenson WG, et al. Clinical assessment and management of patients with implanted cardioverter-defibrillators presenting to nonelectrophsiologists. *Circulation* 2004; 110: 3866–9.

Trohman RG, et al. Cardiac pacing: the state of the art. *Lancet* 2004; 364: 1701–19.

Problems with pacemakers and implantable cardioverter-defibrillators

# Respiratory

# 38 Airway management and upper airway obstruction

**TABLE 38.1** Methods of airway management

| Procedure/ airway | Indications and comments | Technique | Contraindications and potential complications |
|---|---|---|---|
| **Head tilt/ chin lift/jaw thrust** (Figs 38.1, 38.2) | Reduced conscious level with airway obstruction by tongue and other soft tissues Jaw thrust is indicated if the patient may have a cervical spine injury | *Head tilt/chin lift*: Place one hand on the patient's forehead and gently tilt it back; using the fingers of the other hand, gently lift the chin *Jaw thrust*: Keep the patient's head and neck in neutral alignment. Grasp the jaw on both sides and lift it forward | Potential worsening of cervical spine injury: if such injury is suspected, combine maneuver with manual in-line stabilization of head and neck |
| **Manual clearing of the airway** | Reduced conscious level with persistent airway obstruction despite above | Use finger sweep to remove foreign body Remove broken or displaced dentures but | May provoke vomiting if the gag reflex is intact |

*Continued*

| Procedure/ airway | Indications and comments | Technique | Contraindications and potential complications |
|---|---|---|---|
| | maneuvers or to confirm patent airway in unconscious patient | leave well-fitting dentures in place | |
| **Suctioning of upper airway** | Liquid in upper airway (secretions, blood, gastric contents) or to confirm patent airway in unconscious patient<br><br>If there is no reflex response (gagging or coughing) to suctioning, an ETT should be placed to protect the airway | Use wide-bore rigid sucker (Yankauer) attached to suction device | May provoke vomiting if the gag reflex is intact |
| **Oropharyn-geal airway** (Fig. 38.3) | Reduced conscious level | Use size 2, 3 and 4 for small, medium and large adults, respectively | May provoke laryngospasm or vomiting<br>May become obstructed by soft tissues or fall out |

*Continued*

| Procedure/ airway | Indications and comments | Technique | Contraindications and potential complications |
|---|---|---|---|
| **Nasopharyn-geal airway** | Reduced conscious level<br>Use if oropharyngeal airway not tolerated or if there is oral trauma | Use size 6 or 7 mm (internal diameter) for adults | May cause bleeding from nasal mucosa<br>If tube is too long, it may provoke laryngospasm or vomiting |
| **Bag-mask device**<br>(Fig. 38.4) | Hypoventilation/ apnea | Attach oxygen supply to bag, flow rate 10 L/min<br>Easier to do with two people: one holds the mask in place and lifts the jaw, while the other squeezes the bag<br>Deliver 10 breaths/ min, each breath over 1 s, with sufficient volume to produce visible chest rise (tidal volume of 500–600 ml) | May cause gastric distension, resulting in regurgitation, aspiration, splinting of diaphragm |

*Continued*

Airway management and upper airway obstruction

| Procedure/ airway | Indications and comments | Technique | Contraindications and potential complications |
|---|---|---|---|
| **Laryngeal mask airway (LMA)** | Reduced conscious level, requiring ventilation<br><br>Easier to insert than ETT | Place only if trained to do so | Does not protect airway as reliably as ETT against aspiration |
| **Endotracheal tube** | Reduced conscious level, requiring ventilation and/or if airway needs protection | Place only if trained to do so | Unrecognized esophageal intubation may occur if operator is inexperienced |

ETT, endotracheal tube.

Airway management and upper airway obstruction

**TABLE 38.2** Clinical features of upper airway obstruction

**Acute**
- Acute respiratory distress (dyspnea, tachypnea, ability to speak only in short sentences or single words, agitation, sweating)
- Inspiratory stridor (indicates obstruction at level of larynx or above)
- Coughing and choking
- Suprasternal retraction
- Gurgling due to liquid or semisolid material in major airways
- Grunting and snoring (indicates pharynx partially obstructed by soft palate or epiglottis)
- Acute respiratory failure with increased $PaCO_2$
- Respiratory arrest

**Subacute/chronic**
- Dyspnea (typically misdiagnosed as an exacerbation of chronic obstructive pulmonary disease)
- Inspiratory stridor
- Increased respiratory rate
- Abnormal voice
- Respiratory failure with increased $PaCO_2$
- Respiratory arrest

Airway management and upper airway obstruction

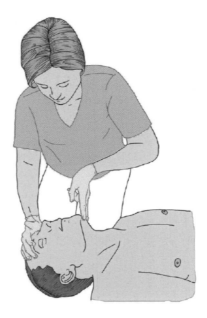

**FIGURE 38.1** Head tilt and chin lift. (Redrawn from European Resuscitation Council Guidelines for Resuscitation 2005.)

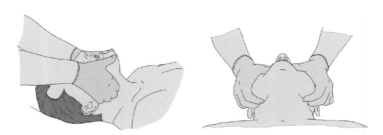

**FIGURE 38.2** Jaw thrust. (Redrawn from European Resuscitation Council Guidelines for Resuscitation 2005.)

Airway management and upper airway obstruction

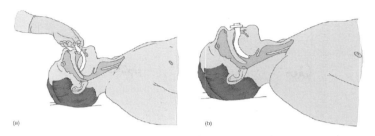

(a)                                    (b)

**FIGURE 38.3** Insertion of oropharyngeal airway during (a) and after (b) procedure. (Reproduced from European Resuscitation Council Guidelines for Resuscitation 2005.)

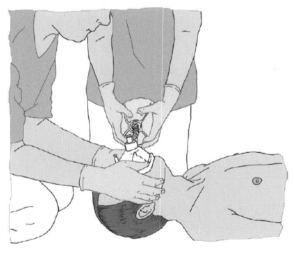

**FIGURE 38.4** Two-person technique for bag-mask ventilation. (Redrawn from European Resuscitation Council Guidelines for Resuscitation 2005.)

Airway management and upper airway obstruction

> **TABLE 38.3** Causes of upper airway obstruction
>
> **Conscious patient**
> - Anaphylaxis (tongue/laryngeal edema)
> - Angioedema (tongue/laryngeal edema)
> - Foreign body
> - Carcinoma of the larynx
> - Laryngeal trauma
> - Vocal cord paralysis
> - Neck hematoma (e.g. from attempted central vein cannulation)
>
> **Unconscious patient**
> - Any of the above causes
> - Tongue and soft tissues of oropharynx
> - Inhalation of foreign body, secretions, vomitus or blood

## Further reading

Erns A, et al. Central airway obstruction. *Am J Resp Crit Care Med* 2004; 169: 1278–97.

Walz JM, et al. Airway management in critical illness. *Chest* 2007; 131: 608–20.

# 39 Acute asthma

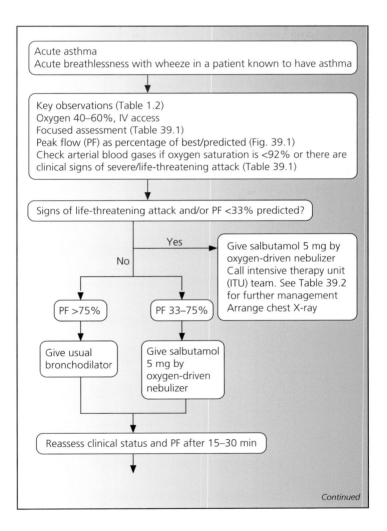

Acute asthma
Acute breathlessness with wheeze in a patient known to have asthma

↓

Key observations (Table 1.2)
Oxygen 40–60%, IV access
Focused assessment (Table 39.1)
Peak flow (PF) as percentage of best/predicted (Fig. 39.1)
Check arterial blood gases if oxygen saturation is <92% or there are clinical signs of severe/life-threatening attack (Table 39.1)

↓

Signs of life-threatening attack and/or PF <33% predicted?

Yes →

Give salbutamol 5 mg by oxygen-driven nebulizer
Call intensive therapy unit (ITU) team. See Table 39.2 for further management
Arrange chest X-ray

No

PF >75%        PF 33–75%

Give usual bronchodilator

Give salbutamol 5 mg by oxygen-driven nebulizer

↓

Reassess clinical status and PF after 15–30 min

↓

*Continued*

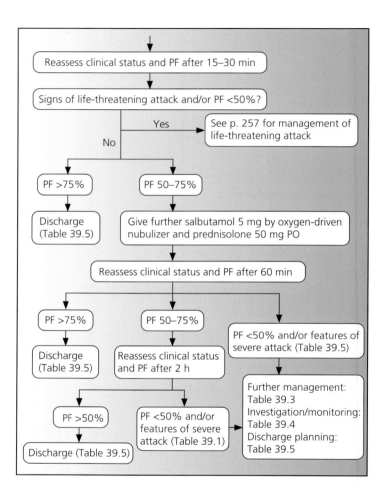

Acute asthma

---

**TABLE 39.1** Focused assessment in acute asthma

**1 Is this acute asthma?**
- Acute breathlessness and wheeze with reduced peak flow
- Known asthma? Regular treatment? Usual peak flow?
- Previous similar episodes responding to bronchodilator therapy (?previous hospital/intensive therapy unit admissions)
- Diurnal and seasonal variation in symptoms
- Symptoms provoked by allergen exposure or exercise
- Sleep disturbance by breathlessness and wheeze

**2 How severe is the attack?**
- Fully conscious?
- Able to talk in complete sentences or just gasped words?
- Check respiratory rate, tidal volume, arterial oxygen saturation, peak flow, heart rate and blood pressure. Listen over the lungs

**3 Signs of a life-threatening asthma attack**
- Silent chest, cyanosis, feeble respiratory effort
- Bradycardia or hypotension
- Exhaustion, confusion or coma
- Peak flow <33% of predicted (Fig. 39.1) or previous best
- Arterial oxygen saturation <92%

**4 Signs of a severe asthma attack**
- Unable to complete sentences
- Respiratory rate >25/min
- Peak flow 33–50% of predicted (Fig. 39.1) or previous best
- Heart rate >110 bpm

Acute asthma

---

**ALERT**
Asthma is the commonest cause of acute breathlessness with wheeze, but other diagnoses (p. 93) should be considered especially in older patients or if the response to treatment is poor.

Acute asthma

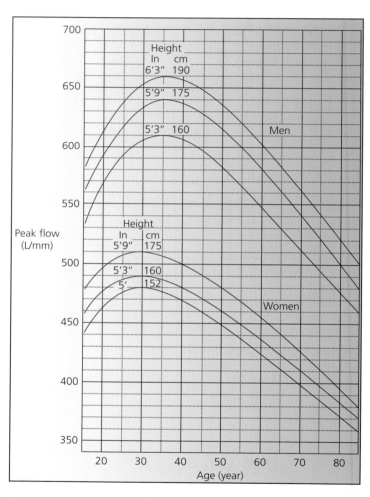

**FIGURE 39.1** Normal peak flow. (From Gregg, I. and Nunn, A.J. *BMJ* 1989; **298**: 1068–70.)

**TABLE 39.2** Immediate management of life-threatening asthma attack

| Element | Comment |
| --- | --- |
| **Obtain help** | Call for help from a chest physician or senior colleague in medicine, and an anesthetist in case urgent endotracheal intubation/ ventilation is needed |
| **Oxygen** | Give oxygen 60–100% |
| **Nebulized bronchodilator** | Give salbutamol 5 mg plus ipratropium 500 µg by oxygen-driven nebulizer, repeated every 15–30 min |
| **Corticosteroid** | Give prednisolone 50 mg PO and hydrocortisone 100 mg IV |
| *If not improving after 15–30 min, consider adding:* | |
| **IV bronchodilator** | Aminophylline 250 mg IV over 20 min (not if the patient is already taking an oral theophylline) *or* Salbutamol 250 µg IV over 10 min followed by an infusion Monitor ECG if IV bronchodilator given |
| **Magnesium** | Magnesium sulfate 1.2–2 g IV over 20 min |

*Acute asthma*

## Further reading

British Thoracic Society and Scottish Intercollegiate Guidelines Network. British guideline on the management of asthma. *Thorax* 2003; 58 (suppl I): i1–i94.

Holgate ST, Polosa R. The mechanisms, diagnosis, and management of severe asthma in adults. *Lancet* 2006; 368: 80–93.

| **TABLE 39.3** Further management of acute severe asthma | |
|---|---|
| **Element** | **Comment** |
| **Oxygen** | Give humidified oxygen 40–60% to maintain $SaO_2$ >92% |
| **Bronchodilator** | Give salbutamol 5 mg plus ipratropium 500 μg by oxygen-driven nebulizer, every 30 min to 6-hourly as required<br>Switch from nebulized to inhaled bronchodilator therapy when peak flow (PF) is >75% of predicted/best |
| **Corticosteroid** | Continue prednisolone 40–50 mg PO daily or hydrocortisone 100 mg 6-hourly IV<br>Oral prednisolone should be given until the acute attack has completely resolved (no sleep disturbance, normal effort tolerance, and PF >80% of predicted/best)<br>As a rule of thumb, oral prednisolone should be continued for double the length of time it takes for PF to return to this level, to a maximum of 21 days<br>Start inhaled steroid at least 24 h before discharge and check inhaler technique |
| **Antibiotic therapy** | Only a minority of asthma attacks are provoked by bacterial infection and antibiotics are not routinely required<br>Give antibiotic therapy as for pneumonia (p. 272) if there is focal shadowing on the chest X-ray or fever or purulent sputum |
| **Supportive care** | Ensure a fluid intake of 2–3 L/day<br>Check electrolytes the day after admission |

*Continued*

| Element | Comment |
|---|---|
| | Salbutamol and steroid may result in significant hypokalemia. Give potassium supplement if the plasma level is <3.5 mmol/L |
| **Monitoring** | Continuous monitoring of arterial oxygen saturation while needing supplemental oxygen |
| | Recheck arterial blood gases if $SaO_2$ <92% or there is clinical deterioration |
| | Check PF before and after inhaled bronchodilator (and at least four times daily during admission) |
| | Discharge when PF is stable at >75% predicted/best, with <25% diurnal variation in the 24 h before discharge, on the same medication that will be taken at home |

**Acute asthma**

**TABLE 39.4** Investigation and monitoring in acute asthma

**Arterial blood gases**
- Check arterial blood gases if there are clinical signs of a severe or life-threatening attack (Table 39.1) or if arterial oxygen saturation by oximetry is <92%
- Recheck arterial blood gases within 2 h of starting treatment if:
  - Initial $PaO_2$ is <8 kPa unless oxygen saturation by oximetry is >92%
  - Initial $PaCO_2$ is normal or raised
  - There is clinical deterioration
- Check arterial blood gases again if the patient's condition has not improved after 4–6 h

*Continued*

**Chest X-ray**
- Arrange a chest X-ray for:
  - Life-threatening attack
  - Poor response to treatment
  - If ventilation is needed
  - Suspected pneumomediastinum or pneumothorax
  - Suspected pneumonia

**Blood tests**
- Check electrolytes, creatinine, glucose and full blood count if admission is needed
- Check serum theophylline level if aminophylline infusion is needed for >24h (target level 55–110 μmol/L)

**Peak flow**
- Check and record peak flow 15–30 min after starting treatment and thereafter according to the response
- Check and record peak flow nebulized and inhaled bronchodilator (at least four times daily) during hospital stay and until controlled after discharge

From British guidelines on the management of asthma. *Thorax* 2003; **58**: Suppl I.

---

**TABLE 39.5** Checklist before discharge after acute asthma

- Stable on discharge medication for 24h
- Inhaler technique checked and recorded
- Peak flow >75% of predicted/best and diurnal variation <25%
- Oral and inhaled steroid prescribed
- Inhaler technique checked
- Own peak flow meter and written asthma action plan
- General practitioner follow-up arranged within two working days
- Follow-up appointment in asthma clinic within 4 weeks

# 40 Acute exacerbation of chronic obstructive pulmonary disease

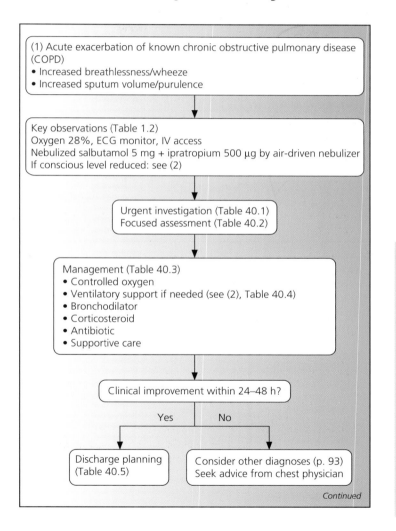

(1) Acute exacerbation of known chronic obstructive pulmonary disease (COPD)
- Increased breathlessness/wheeze
- Increased sputum volume/purulence

Key observations (Table 1.2)
Oxygen 28%, ECG monitor, IV access
Nebulized salbutamol 5 mg + ipratropium 500 µg by air-driven nebulizer
If conscious level reduced: see (2)

Urgent investigation (Table 40.1)
Focused assessment (Table 40.2)

Management (Table 40.3)
- Controlled oxygen
- Ventilatory support if needed (see (2), Table 40.4)
- Bronchodilator
- Corticosteroid
- Antibiotic
- Supportive care

Clinical improvement within 24–48 h?

Yes → Discharge planning (Table 40.5)

No → Consider other diagnoses (p. 93)
Seek advice from chest physician

*Continued*

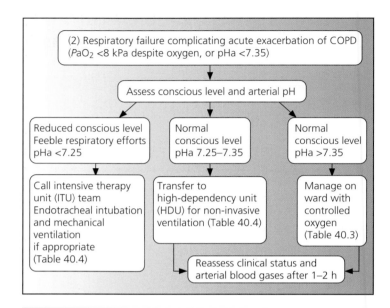

(2) Respiratory failure complicating acute exacerbation of COPD
($PaO_2$ <8 kPa despite oxygen, or pHa <7.35)

Assess conscious level and arterial pH

Reduced conscious level
Feeble respiratory efforts
pHa <7.25

Normal
conscious level
pHa 7.25–7.35

Normal
conscious level
pHa >7.35

Call intensive therapy
unit (ITU) team
Endotracheal intubation
and mechanical
ventilation
if appropriate
(Table 40.4)

Transfer to
high-dependency unit
(HDU) for non-invasive
ventilation (Table 40.4)

Manage on
ward with
controlled
oxygen
(Table 40.3)

Reassess clinical status and
arterial blood gases after 1–2 h

**TABLE 40.1** Urgent investigation in acute exacerbation of chronic
obstructive pulmonary disease (COPD)

- Chest X-ray (check for focal shadowing indicative of pneumonia, or
  pneumothorax)
- Arterial blood gases and pH
- ECG
- Echocardiography if there are clinical signs of congestive heart failure,
  raised plasma brain natriuretic peptide or if the diagnosis is uncertain
- Plasma brain natriuretic peptide (if normal, effectively excludes
  associated left ventricular dysfunction)
- Sputum culture if purulent sputum or focal shadowing on chest X-ray
- Blood culture if febrile or focal shadowing on chest X-ray
- Blood glucose
- Sodium, potassium and creatinine
- Plasma theophylline level (if taking theophylline)
- Full blood count
- C-reactive protein

Acute exacerbation of chronic obstructive pulmonary disease

**TABLE 40.2** Focused assessment in suspected acute exacerbation of chronic obstructive pulmonary disease (COPD)

**History**
- Breathlessness: usual and recent change
- Wheeze: usual and recent change
- Sputum: usual volume/purulence and recent change
- Effort tolerance: usual (e.g. ability to cope with activities of daily living unaided; distance walked on the flat; number of stairs climbed without stopping) and recent change
- Previous acute exacerbations requiring hospital admission/ventilation
- Previous lung function tests and arterial blood gases (from the notes): an $FEV_1$ 50–80% of predicted signifies mild COPD; 30–50%, moderate COPD; less than 30%, severe COPD
- Requirement for home nebulized bronchodilator and/or oxygen therapy
- Concurrent illness, especially cardiac

**Examination**
- Conscious level
- Respiratory rate
- Arterial oxygen saturation
- Use of accessory muscles of respiration
- Paradoxical abdominal breathing
- Lung signs
- Peak flow
- Heart rate, blood pressure, jugular venous pressure
- Peripheral edema

$FEV_1$, forced expiratory volume in 1 s.

## Further reading

Calverley PMA, Walker P. Chronic obstructive pulmonary disease. *Lancet* 2003; 362: 1051–61.

Keenan SP. Which patients with acute exacerbations of chronic obstructive pulmonary disease benefit from noninvasive positive-pressure ventilation? A systematic review of the literature. *Ann Intern Med* 2003; 138: 861–70.

National clinical guideline on management of chronic obstructive pulmonary disease in adults in primary and secondary care. *Thorax* 2004; 59 (suppl I): i1–i232.

Acute exacerbation of chronic obstructive pulmonary disease

**TABLE 40.3** Management of acute exacerbation of chronic obstructive pulmonary disease (COPD)

| Element | Comment |
|---------|---------|
| **Oxygen** | Give oxygen if $SaO_2$ on air is <92%/$PaO_2$ <8 kPa ($SaO_2$ <88%, $PaO_2$ <7.5 kPa if known chronic respiratory failure) |
| | Start with an inspired oxygen of 28% (or 2 L/min by nasal prongs) |
| | Check arterial gases and pH 1 h after starting oxygen |
| | Increase inspired oxygen to 35% if $PaO_2$ is <7.5 kPa (<6.5 kPa if known chronic respiratory failure) |
| | If this oxygen level cannot be attained, or arterial pH falls below 7.35, consider ventilatory support (flow diagram 2, Table 40.4): ask advice from a chest physician |
| | Supplemental oxygen should be continued until arterial oxygen saturation is >90% breathing air |
| **Ventilatory support** | See flow diagram 2 and Table 40.4 |
| **Bronchodilator** | Give salbutamol 2.5–5.0 mg by nebulizer up to 4-hourly *and/or* |
| | Ipratropium 500 µg by nebulizer up to 4-hourly |
| | Switch from nebulized to inhaled bronchodilator therapy when the patient no longer needs supplemental oxygen |
| | If the patient is severely ill and does not respond to nebulized salbutamol and ipratropium:<br>• Give aminophylline 250 mg IV over 20 min (not if the patient is already taking a theophylline)<br>• Follow this with an infusion of aminophylline 750–1500 mg over 24 h, according to body size |
| **Corticosteroid** | Give prednisolone 30 mg daily for 7–14 days |
| | Consider osteoporosis prophylaxis in patients needing frequent courses of corticosteroid |

*Continued*

| Element | Comment |
| --- | --- |
| **Antibiotic therapy** | Indicated if there is evidence of infection, as shown by fever, or increased sputum volume and purulence<br>Initial therapy is with amoxycillin 500 mg 8-hourly PO<br>If the patient is allergic to penicillin or has received a penicillin in the previous month, use trimethoprim 200 mg 12-hourly PO or doxycycline 200 mg daily PO<br>Modify therapy in light of sputum and blood culture results. Give a 7-day course<br>If there is no response to amoxycillin, consider using co-amoxiclav or ciprofloxacin. In ill patients, use cefuroxime or cefotaxime IV |
| **Supportive care** | Ensure a fluid intake of 2–3 L/day<br>Check electrolytes the day after admission. Salbutamol and steroids may result in significant hypokalemia. Give potassium supplement if the plasma level is <3.5 mmol/L<br>Physiotherapy is of little value unless sputum is copious (>25 ml/day) or there is mucus plugging with lobar atelectasis<br>DVT prophylaxis with stockings/LMW heparin<br>Assess/treat comorbidities, e.g. atrial fibrillation, congestive heart failure |
| **Monitoring** | Continuous monitoring of arterial oxygen saturation while needing supplemental oxygen<br>Monitoring of arterial blood gases as required in patients receiving ventilatory support |

DVT, deep vein thrombosis; LMW, low molecular weight.

Acute exacerbation of chronic obstructive pulmonary disease

**Acute exacerbation of chronic obstructive pulmonary disease**

TABLE 40.4 Ventilatory support in acute exacerbation of chronic obstructive pulmonary disease (COPD)

| Method | Indications | Contraindications | Comments |
|---|---|---|---|
| **NIV with bilevel positive airways pressure (BiPAP)** | $PaO_2$ <7.5–8 kPa despite supplemental oxygen<br>Arterial pH <7.35 | Decreased conscious level<br>Respiratory rate <12/min<br>Arterial pH <7.25<br>Copious secretions<br>Orofacial abnormalities which prevent fitting of the mask | Around 20% of patients cannot tolerate NIV<br>If arterial pH is <7.3, admit to ITU<br>Consider mechanical ventilation if no improvement in arterial pH and other variables within 1–2 h of starting NIV |
| **Endotracheal intubation and mechanical ventilation** | Impending respiratory arrest<br>Deteriorating conscious level<br>$PaO_2$ <7.5–8 kPa despite supplemental oxygen/NIV<br>Arterial pH <7.25<br>Inability to protect airway or to clear copious secretions | Known severe COPD with severely impaired functional capacity and/or severe comorbidity<br>Patient has expressed wish not to be ventilated | Potential complications of barotraumas and infection, and inability to wean some patients from the ventilator |
| **Doxapram** | $PaO_2$ <7.5–8 kPa despite supplemental oxygen<br>Arterial pH <7.35<br>NIV not available and mechanical ventilation not appropriate | Respiratory rate >20/min | Has not been proven to improve survival or reduce the need for mechanical ventilation |

ITU, intensive therapy unit; NIV, non-invasive positive pressure ventilation.

**TABLE 40.5** Checklist before discharge after acute exacerbation of chronic obstructive pulmonary disease (COPD)

- Clinically stable off IV therapy for >24 h
- Bronchodilator therapy needed no more than 6-hourly, with the patient on same medication (nebulized or inhaled) that will be taken at home
- Inhaler technique checked
- Spirometry checked/arranged
- Able to walk at least short distances unaided
- Social support at home organized
- Advice on smoking cessation given if needed
- General practitioner follow-up arranged within 1 week
- Follow-up appointment in chest clinic within 4–6 weeks

Acute exacerbation of chronic obstructive pulmonary disease

# 41 Pneumonia (1): community-acquired pneumonia

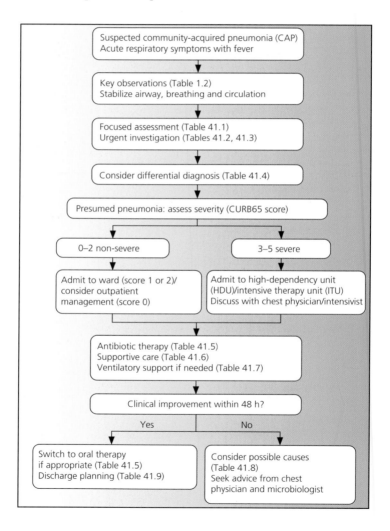

**TABLE 41.1** Focused assessment in suspected community-acquired pneumonia (CAP)

**1 Is this pneumonia?**
- Suspect pneumonia if there are acute respiratory symptoms (cough, purulent sputum, pleuritic chest pain or breathlessness) and fever
- Associated non-respiratory symptoms (e.g. confusion, upper abdominal pain, diarrhea) are common and may dominate the picture
- Examination shows abnormal chest signs in 80% of patients with pneumonia (most often an increased respiratory rate (>20/min) and focal crackles)
- Other diagnoses to consider, especially in patients with atypical features or who fail to respond to antibiotic therapy, are given in Table 41.4

**2 How severe is the pneumonia?**
- Severe pneumonia is indicated by a CURB65 score of 3 or more, and moderate pneumonia by a score of 2, scoring one point each for:
  - New confusion (C)
  - Plasma urea >7 mmol/L (U)
  - Respiratory rate >30/min (R)
  - Systolic BP <90 mmHg or diastolic BP <60 mmHg (B)
  - Age over 65 years
- If the CURB65 score is 4 or 5, discuss admission to ITU with an intensive care physician or chest physician: this decision will also take into account arterial blood gases, chest X-ray findings and comorbidities. Other patients with severe pneumonia should be admitted to HDU

HDU, high-dependency unit; ITU, intensive therapy unit.

**ALERT**
Pneumonia usually presents with acute respiratory symptoms, but should always be considered in patients with unexplained sepsis or confusional state. Examination of the chest may be normal, and if you suspect pneumonia, a chest X-ray is needed.

**TABLE 41.2** Urgent investigation in suspected community-acquired pneumonia (CAP)

- Chest X-ray (Table 41.3)
- Arterial blood gases and pH (if oxygen saturation is <92% or there are clinical features of severe pneumonia)
- Sputum culture (in CAP if severe, or if non-severe and no prior antibiotic therapy)
- Blood culture (×2)
- Full blood count
- C-reactive protein
- Blood glucose
- Sodium, potassium, creatinine and urea
- Liver function tests
- Urine stick test
- Urine for pneumococcal antigen in all severe CAP and in non-severe CAP if antibiotic therapy has been started before admission
- Urine for *Legionella* antigen in all severe CAP or if clinical suspicion of *Legionella* is high
- Blood for *Mycoplasma* serology in all severe CAP or if clinical suspicion of *Mycoplasma* is high (acute/convalescent samples needed)

**TABLE 41.3** Features to look for on the chest X-ray in suspected pneumonia

| Feature | Comment |
|---|---|
| **Focal shadowing** | Required to make the diagnosis of pneumonia, but may initially be absent in patients who are severely neutropenic or hypovolemic, and in early *Pneumocystis carinii* (*jiroveci*) pneumonia |

*Continued*

| Pleural effusion | If present, aspirate a sample and send for Gram stain and culture |
|---|---|
| Cavitation | Particularly associated with tuberculosis and *Staphylococcus aureus* infection, but may also occur in Gram-negative and anaerobic infections |
| Pneumothorax | May occur in cavitating pneumonias and is particularly associated with *P. carinii* (*jiroveci*) pneumonia (see Table 83.4) |

---

**TABLE 41.4** Differential diagnosis of suspected pneumonia

**Pulmonary vascular disorders**
- Pulmonary embolism
- Pulmonary edema

**Neoplastic disorders**
- Bronchial carcinoma
- Alveolar cell carcinoma
- Lymphoma

**Immune-mediated disorders**
- Wegener granulomatosis (p. 481)
- Diffuse alveolar hemorrhage in pulmonary–renal syndromes (pp. 400, 484)
- Systemic lupus erythematosus
- Sarcoidosis
- Acute interstitial pneumonia
- Eosinophilic pneumonia syndromes
- Bronchiolitis obliterans – organizing pneumonia

**Other disorders**
- Drug toxicity (e.g. amiodarone pneumonitis)
- Subdiaphragmatic abscess

**TABLE 41.5** Initial antibiotic therapy of community-acquired pneumonia (CAP)

| Setting | Initial antibiotic therapy Not allergic to penicillin | Penicillin allergy |
|---|---|---|
| **Non-severe CAP (oral)** | Amoxycillin + erythromycin PO *or* Amoxycillin + clarithromycin PO | Erythromycin *or* Clarithromycin or Doxycycline |
| **Severe CAP** Initial therapy IV, high dose | Co-amoxiclav *or* Cefuroxime *or* Cefotaxime *or* Ceftriaxone + erythromycin *or* Clarithromycin + rifampicin | Levofloxacin + erythromycin *or* Clarithromycin + rifampicin |
| Oral therapy *Switch to oral therapy when*: <br> • There is no microbiological evidence of *Legionella*, staphylococcal or Gram-negative enteric bacilli infection <br> • Clinically improving <br> • Able to swallow safely <br> • No vomiting/ileus | Substitute co-amoxiclav PO for IV cephalosporin Continue oral macrolide (+ rifampicin if indicated) | Continue oral levofloxacin and macrolide (+ rifampicin if indicated) |

**TABLE 41.6** Supportive care in pneumonia

| Element | Comment |
|---|---|
| **Oxygen** | Humidified oxygen should be continued until $PaO_2$ is >8 kPa (60 mmHg) with the patient breathing air, or arterial oxygen saturation is >92% |
| **Ventilatory support** | See Table 41.7 |
| **Fluid balance** | Insensible losses are greater than normal due to fever (allow 500 ml/day/°C) and tachypnea<br>Patients with severe pneumonia should receive IV fluids (2–3 L/day) with daily check of creatinine and electrolytes if abnormal on admission<br>Monitor central venous pressure and urine output if patient is oliguric or if plasma creatinine is >200 µmol/L |
| **DVT prophylaxis** | Give DVT prophylaxis with stockings and LMW heparin |
| **Pain relief** | Relieve pleuritic chest pain with paracetamol and/or NSAIDs |
| **Physiotherapy** | Indicated if patient is producing sputum, but having difficulty expectorating it, and in bronchiectasis<br>Nebulized normal saline may be helpful when sputum is thick and difficult to expectorate |
| **Bronchodilator therapy** | Nebulized Salbutamol or ipratropium should be given to patients with chronic obstructive pulmonary disease or asthma (p. 253) |

DVT, deep vein thrombosis; LMW, low molecular weight; NSAIDs, non-steroidal anti-inflammatory drugs.

Pneumonia (1): community-acquired pneumonia

**TABLE 41.7** Ventilatory support for respiratory failure due to pneumonia

| Mode of ventilation | Indications | Contraindications | Disadvantages and limitations |
|---|---|---|---|
| **NIV with bilevel positive airways pressure (BiPAP)** | Oxygenation failure: oxygen saturation <92% despite $FiO_2$ >40% Ventilatory failure: mild to moderate respiratory acidosis, arterial pH 7.25–7.35 | Recent facial, upper airway or upper gastrointestinal tract surgery Vomiting or bowel obstruction Copious secretions Hemodynamic instability Impaired consciousness, confusion or agitation | Discomfort from tightly fitting facemask Discourages coughing and clearing of secretions |
| **Endotracheal intubation and mechanical ventilation** | Upper airway obstruction Impending respiratory arrest Airway at risk because of neurological disease or coma (GCS score 8 or lower) Oxygenation failure: $PaO_2$ <7.5–8 kPa despite supplemental oxygen/NIV Ventilatory failure: moderate to severe respiratory acidosis, arterial pH <7.25 | Severely impaired functional capacity and/or severe comorbidity Cardiac disorder not remediable Patient has expressed wish not to be ventilated | Adverse hemodynamic effects Pharyngeal, laryngeal and tracheal injury Ventilator-induced lung injury (e.g. pneumothorax) Complications of sedation and neuro-muscular blockade |

GCS, Glasgow Coma Scale; NIV, non-invasive positive pressure ventilation.

**TABLE 41.8** Causes of failure to improve after 48h of antibiotic therapy

- Wrong diagnosis (Table 41.4)
- Slow response in elderly patient
- Endobronchial obstruction (e.g. bronchial carcinoma, foreign body)
- Unexpected pathogen or pathogen not covered by initial choice of antibiotic therapy
- Antibiotic ineffective or causing allergic reaction
- Overwhelming infection
- Impaired local or systemic defences (e.g. bronchiectasis, HIV, myeloma)
- Pulmonary (parapneumonic effusion, empyema, lung abscess, adult respiratory distress syndrome) or extrapulmonary (pericarditis, endocarditis, septic arthritis) complication

**TABLE 41.9** Checklist before discharge after pneumonia

- Clinically stable for >48h:
  - Normal mental state
  - Temperature <37.8°C
  - Respiratory rate <24/min
  - Arterial oxygen saturation breathing air >90%
  - Heart rate <100 bpm
  - Systolic BP >90 mmHg
- Able to walk at least short distances unaided (or close to preadmission functional status)
- Social support at home organized if needed
- Advice on smoking cessation given if needed
- General practitioner follow-up arranged within 1 week
- Follow-up appointment in chest clinic at 6 weeks, with chest X-ray taken before visit

## Further reading

Baudouin SV. The pulmonary physician in critical care. 3: Critical care management of community acquired pneumonia. *Thorax* 2002; 57: 267–71.

Hoare Z, Lim WS. Pneumonia: update on diagnosis and management. *BMJ* 2006; 332: 1077–9.

Macfarlane J, et al. British Thoracic Society guidelines for the management of community acquired pneumonia in adults – 2004 update. British Thoracic Society website (http://www.brit-thoracic.org.uk/guidelines.html).

# 42 Pneumonia (2): hospital-acquired pneumonia

**TABLE 42.1** Initial antibiotic therapy of hospital-acquired pneumonia (HAP)

| Setting | Initial antibiotic therapy Not allergic to penicillin | Penicillin allergy |
|---|---|---|
| **Non-severe HAP** | Co-amoxiclav | Clarithromycin |
| **Severe HAP** | Piperacillin + tazobactam + gentamicin *or* Ceftazidime + gentamicin Add clarithromycin if *Legionella* suspected Add vancomycin or teicoplanin if MRSA suspected | Meropenem + gentamicin |

MRSA, meticillin-resistant *Staphylococcus aureus*.

**ALERT**
Hospital-acquired pneumonia is overdiagnosed, and management is contentious. Seek advice from a microbiologist on antibiotic therapy for patients with severe hospital-acquired pneumonia.

Pneumonia (2): hospital-acquired pneumonia

**TABLE 42.2** Aspiration (inhalation) pneumonia

| Inoculum | Effects on airway and lungs | Clinical features | Management |
|---|---|---|---|
| **Acid** | Chemical pneumonitis | Acute dyspnea, tachypnea, possible cyanosis, bronchospasm, fever, pink frothy sputum, infiltrates in one or both lower lobes, hypoxemia | Positive-pressure breathing, IV fluids, tracheal suction |
| **Oropharyngeal bacteria** | Bacterial infection | Usually insidious onset; cough, fever, purulent sputum, infiltrate involving dependent pulmonary segment or lobe, with or without cavitation | Antibiotic therapy (Table 42.1) |
| **Inert fluids** | Mechanical obstruction, reflex airway closure | Acute dyspnea, cyanosis, pulmonary edema | Tracheal suction, intermittent positive-pressure breathing with oxygen, bronchodilator |
| **Particulate matter** | Mechanical obstruction | Dependent on level of obstruction, ranging from acute apnea to chronic cough with or without recurrent infections | Extraction of particulate matter, antibiotic therapy |

# Further reading

American Thoracic Society. Guidelines for the management of adults with hospital-acquired, ventilator-associated, and healthcare-associated pneumonia. *Am J Resp Crit Care Med* 2005; 171: 388–416.

# 43 Pneumothorax

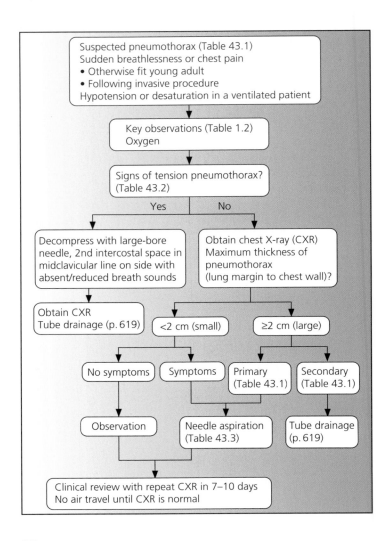

Suspected pneumothorax (Table 43.1)
Sudden breathlessness or chest pain
• Otherwise fit young adult
• Following invasive procedure
Hypotension or desaturation in a ventilated patient

↓

Key observations (Table 1.2)
Oxygen

↓

Signs of tension pneumothorax?
(Table 43.2)

Yes — No

**Yes:**
Decompress with large-bore needle, 2nd intercostal space in midclavicular line on side with absent/reduced breath sounds
↓
Obtain CXR
Tube drainage (p. 619)

**No:**
Obtain chest X-ray (CXR)
Maximum thickness of pneumothorax
(lung margin to chest wall)?

<2 cm (small) — ≥2 cm (large)

<2 cm (small):
No symptoms — Symptoms
↓
No symptoms → Observation
Symptoms → Needle aspiration (Table 43.3)

≥2 cm (large):
Primary (Table 43.1) — Secondary (Table 43.1)
Primary → Needle aspiration (Table 43.3)
Secondary → Tube drainage (p. 619)

↓

Clinical review with repeat CXR in 7–10 days
No air travel until CXR is normal

---

**TABLE 43.1** Classification and causes of pneumothorax

**Spontaneous pneumothorax**
*Primary*
- No clinical lung diseae
- Typically occurs in tall thin males aged 10–30 years
- Rare in patients over 40

*Secondary*
- Airways disease (COPD, cystic fibrosis, acute severe asthma)
- Infectious lung disease (*Pneumocystis carinii* (*jiroveci*) pneumonia; necrotizing pneumonia caused by anaerobic, Gram-negative bacteria or *Staphylococcus aureus*)
- Interstitial lung disease (e.g. sarcoidosis)
- Connective tissue disease (e.g. rheumatoid arthritis, Marfan syndrome)
- Malignancy (bronchial carcinoma or sarcoma)
- Thoracic endometriosis

**Traumatic pneumothorax** (due to penetrating or blunt chest trauma)

**Iatrogenic pneumothorax**
- Transthoracic needle aspiration
- Subclavian vein puncture
- Thoracentesis and pleural biopsy
- Pericardiocentesis
- Barotrauma related to mechanical ventilation

---

COPD, chronic obstructive pulmonary disease.

Pneumothorax

---

**TABLE 43.2** Signs of tension pneumothorax

- Pleuritic chest pain
- Respiratory distress (dyspnea, tachypnea, ability to speak only in short sentences or single words, agitation, sweating)
- Falling arterial oxygen saturation
- Ipsilateral hyperexpansion, hypomobility, hyperresonance with decreased breath sounds
- Tachycardia
- Hypotension (late sign)
- Tracheal deviation (inconsistent sign)
- Elevated jugular venous pressure (inconsistent sign)

---

**TABLE 43.3** Needle aspiration of pneumothorax

1 Identify the 3rd to 4th intercostal space in the midaxillary line
2 Infiltrate with lidocaine down to and around the pleura over the pneumothorax
3 Connect a 21 G (green) needle to a three-way tap and a 60 ml syringe
4 With the patient semirecumbent, insert the needle into the pleural space. Withdraw air and expel it via the three-way tap
5 Obtain a chest X-ray to confirm resolution of the pneumothorax

## Further reading

Baumann MH, et al. Management of spontaneous pneumothorax. An American College of Chest Physicians Delphi consensus statement. *Chest* 2001; 119: 590–602.

Henry M, et al. British Thoracic Society guidelines for the management of spontaneous pneumothorax. *Thorax* 2003; 58 (suppl II): ii39–ii52.

Leigh-Smith S, Harris T. Tension pneumothorax – time for a rethink? *Emerg Med J* 2005; 22: 8–16.

# 44 Pleural effusion

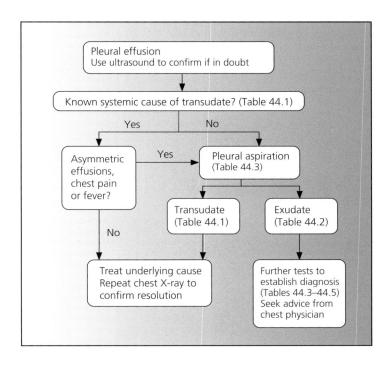

---

**TABLE 44.1** Transudative pleural effusions

- Congestive heart failure
- Cirrhosis
- Nephrotic syndrome
- Peritoneal dialysis
- Hypothyroidism
- Pulmonary embolism (in 10–20% of cases)
- Malignancy (in 5% of cases)

---

**ALERT**

Pleural effusion is distinguished from pulmonary consolidation on the chest X-ray by:

- shadowing higher laterally than medially
- shadowing does not conform to that of a lobe or segment
- no air bronchogram
- trachea and mediastinum maybe pushed to opposite side (if large effusion).

If in doubt, use ultrasound to confirm effusion and establish if loculated.

---

**TABLE 44.2** Exudative pleural effusions

- Parapneumonic effusion and empyema
- Malignancy
- Pulmonary embolism
- Congestive heart failure after diuretic therapy
- Mesothelioma
- Tuberculosis
- Rheumatoid arthritis and systemic lupus erythematosus
- Esophageal rupture
- Pancreatitis
- Postcardiotomy syndrome
- Drug-induced
- Chylothorax

**TABLE 44.3** Pleural fluid analysis (1)

| Test | Comment |
| --- | --- |
| **Visual inspection** | Blood-stained effusion (pleural fluid hematocrit 1–20% of peripheral hematocrit) is likely to be due to malignancy, pulmonary embolism or trauma<br>Purulent fluid signifies empyema |
| **Protein and lactate dehydrogenase (LDH)** | These are the only tests needed if the effusion is likely to be a transudate<br>Pleural fluid LDH correlates with the degree of pleural inflammation<br>Exudative pleural effusions have a protein concentration >30 g/L<br>If the pleural fluid protein is around 30 g/L, Light's criteria are helpful in distinguishing between a transudate and exudate. An exudate is identified by one or more of the following:<br>• Pleural fluid protein to serum protein ratio >0.5<br>• Pleural fluid LDH to serum LDH ratio >0.6<br>• Pleural fluid LDH more than two-thirds the upper limit of normal for serum LDH |

**Pleural effusion**

**TABLE 44.4** Pleural fluid analysis (2): additional tests for exudative pleural effusion

| Test | Comment |
|------|---------|
| **Pleural fluid pH and glucose** (check these if a parapneumonic or malignant pleural effusion is suspected. Send sample in heparinized syringe for measurement of pH in blood gas analyzer) | Low pH (<7.3)/low glucose (<3.3 mmol/L) pleural fluid may be seen in:<br>• Complicated parapneumonic effusion and empyema<br>• Malignancy<br>• Rheumatoid or lupus pleuritis<br>• Tuberculosis<br>• Esophageal rupture |
| **Cytology** (total and differential cell count; malignant cells) | Neutrophilia (>50% cells) indicate acute pleural disease<br>Lymphocytosis is seen in malignancy, tuberculous pleuritis and in pleural effusions after CABG<br>The yield of cytology is influenced by the histological type of malignancy: >70% positive in adenocarcinoma, 25–50% in lymphoma, 10% in mesothelioma |
| **Microbiology** (Gram stain and culture; markers of tuberculosis (TB)) | Send fluid for markers of TB if TB is suspected or there is a pleural fluid lymphocytosis |
| **Other tests depending on the clinical setting** (e.g. amylase, triglyceride) | Elevated pleural fluid amylase is seen in acute pancreatitis and esophageal rupture<br>Check triglyceride level if chylothorax is suspected (opaque white effusion); chylothorax (triglyceride >1.1 g/L) is due to disruption of the thoracic duct by trauma or lymphoma |

CABG, coronary artery bypass graft.

> **TABLE 44.5** Further investigation to establish cause of exudative pleural effusion
>
> - Contrast-enhanced CT of thorax and abdomen
> - Closed pleural biopsy (only if suspected tuberculosis)
> - Thoracoscopy and biopsy
> - CT pulmonary angiography if pulmonary embolism is suspected

**ALERT**
If pleural fluid cytology is negative in suspected malignancy, CT should be done before complete drainage of the effusion, as the presence of pleural fluid enhances the diagnostic accuracy of the scan.

## Further reading

Heffner JE, et al. A meta-analysis derivation of continuous likelihood ratios for diagnosing pleural fluid exudates. *Am J Resp Crit Care Med* 2003; 167: 1591–9.

Light RW. Pleural effusion. *N Engl J Med* 2002; 346: 1971–7.

Maskell NA, et al. British Thoracic Society guidelines for the investigation of a unilateral pleural effusion in adults. *Thorax* 2003; 58 (suppl II): ii8–ii17.

Rahman NM, et al. Investigating suspected malignant pleural effusion. *BMJ* 2007; 334: 206–7.

Thomsen TW, et al. Thoracentesis. *N Engl J Med* 2006; 355: e16.

# 45 Hemoptysis

**TABLE 45.1** Causes of hemoptyis

| Cause | Comment |
|---|---|
| **Carcinoma of bronchus** | Persistent blood-streaking of mucoid sputum; weight loss |
| **Tuberculosis** | Blood-streaking of purulent sputum; weight loss; fever |
| **Bronchiectasis** | Blood-streaking of copious purulent sputum; chronic sputum production; previous episodes of hemoptysis occurring over months or years |
| **Acute bronchitis** | Blood-streaking of mucopurulent sputum |
| **Pneumonia** | 'Rusty' sputum; acute illness with fever and breathlessness; signs of consolidation |
| **Lung abscess** | Blood-streaking of purulent sputum; fever; pleuritic chest pain |
| **Pulmonary infarction** | Gross blood not mixed with sputum; pleuritic chest pain and breathlessness; at risk of deep vein thrombosis |
| **Pulmonary edema** | Frothy blood-tinged sputum; severe breathlessness; associated cardiac disease |
| **Lung contusion** | Preceding chest trauma |
| **Mycetoma** | Fungal ball on chest X-ray; previous pulmonary tuberculosis |
| **Vascular malformation** | Recurrent hemoptysis; Osler–Weber–Rendu syndrome with multiple telangiectasia |
| **Bronchial adenoma** | Recurrent hemoptysis in an otherwise well woman |
| **Bleeding tendency** | Hemoptysis following persistent coughing; bleeding from other sites |
| **Pulmonary vasculitis** | Wegener granulomatosis (upper and lower respiratory tract involvement, |

*Continued*

| Cause | Comment |
|---|---|
| | antineutrophil cytoplasmic antibodies present); Goodpasture syndrome (pulmonary and renal involvement, antiglomerular basement membrane antibodies present) |
| **Eisenmenger syndrome** | Cyanosis and clubbing |
| **Other causes of pulmonary hypertension** | Mitral stenosis; primary pulmonary hypertension |

**TABLE 45.2** Management of massive hemoptysis (>1000 ml in 24 h)

- There is a risk of death from drowning or exsanguination
- Lie the patient head down (position with bleeding side down, if known) and give high-flow oxygen
- Call an anesthetist: endotracheal intubation may be needed to allow suctioning of the airway and adequate ventilation
- Put in a large-bore IV cannula and take blood for urgent cross-match and other investigation (Table 45.3)
- Restore circulating volume and correct coagulopathy (see Table 57.4)
- Contact a thoracic surgeon for advice on further management. Bleeding may occasionally be stopped through a rigid bronchoscope, but usually requires resection of the bleeding segment or lobe, or bronchial artery embolization

**ALERT**
Hemoptysis can be distinguished from hematemesis by its color and pH: hemoptysis is bright red and alkaline; hematemesis is brown and acid. Bleeding from the nasopharynx may be mistaken for hemoptysis: if in doubt, ask the advice of an ear, nose and throat surgeon.

Hemoptysis

**TABLE 45.3** Investigation in hemoptysis

**Massive hemoptysis**
- Full blood count
- Coagulation screen
- Cross-match 6 units
- Blood glucose
- Sodium, potassium and creatinine
- Arterial blood gases
- Chest X-ray when stable

**Other patients**
- Chest X-ray
- Arterial blood gases if there is pleuritic chest pain or breathlessness, or oxygen saturation <92%
- ECG
- Sputum for Gram and Ziehl–Neelsen stains, culture and cytology
- Full blood count
- Erythrocyte sedimentation rate and C-reactive protein
- Antineutrophil cytoplasmic antibodies and antiglomerular basement membrane antibodies (only if pulmonary vasculitis is suspected)
- Coagulation screen if bleeding tendency is suspected
- Blood glucose
- Sodium, potassium and creatinine
- Urine stick test and microscopy

**Further investigation**
- Bronchoscopy
- CT of thorax
- Echocardiography to look for evidence of pulmonary hypertension and its cause
- Bronchial angiography to identify site of bleeding; embolization may be indicated

## Further reading

Campbell IA, Bah-Sow O. Pulmonary tuberculosis: diagnosis and treatment. *BMJ* 2006; 332: 1194–7.

Hoffman PC, et al. Lung cancer. *Lancet* 2000; 355: 479–85.

Jackman DM, Johnson BE. Small-cell lung cancer. *Lancet* 2005; 366: 1385–96.

Lordan JL, et al. The pulmonary physician in critical care. Illustrative case 7: assessment and management of massive haemoptysis. *Thorax* 2003; 58: 814–19.

# Neurological

# 46 Examination of the nervous system in acute medicine

**TABLE 46.1** Screening examination of the nervous system in acute medicine

| Element | Comment |
|---|---|
| **Conscious level** | Assess conscious level by the simple four-point AVPU scale (alert; responsive to voice; responsive to pain; unresponsive) or by the Glasgow Coma Scale (Table 46.2) |
| **Mental state, speech and language** | If the patient is able to give a lucid and detailed history, with fluent speech in a normal voice, no further assessment of mental state and speech is needed |
| | If you suspect dysphasia, assess speech fluency and check naming, repetition and comprehension (one-, two- and three-stage commands) |
| | See Tables 46.3 and 46.4 for further assessment of mental state and language |
| **Skull and spine** | Check for signs of head injury |
| | Test for neck stiffness |
| | Check for spinal deformity or tenderness |
| **Cranial nerves** | Check as a minimum: |
| | • Visual fields |
| | • Pupils: size, symmetry and response to light |
| | • Eye movements |
| | • Facial strength |
| | • Hearing (finger rub) |

*Continued*

| Element | Comment |
| --- | --- |
| **Fundoscopy** | Check for spontaneous retinal vein pulsation (if present, excludes raised intracranial pressure), papilledema, retinal hemorrhages and exudates |
| **Motor system** | If the patient is unable to stand or walk because of systemic illness, check, as a minimum, limb tone and ability to lift arms and legs off the bed (Tables 46.5, 46.6). Check if there is lateralized weakness |
| **Reflexes** | Check biceps, triceps, knee and ankle reflexes (Table 46.7) |
| **Plantar responses** | Extensor plantar response usually indicates structural lesion in motor pathway (cortex, subcortex, brainstem or spinal cord) |
| **Sensation** | Test light touch sensation in the forearms/hands and lower legs/feet (Fig. 46.1). Test vibration sense over the first MTP joint |

MTP, metatarsophalangeal.

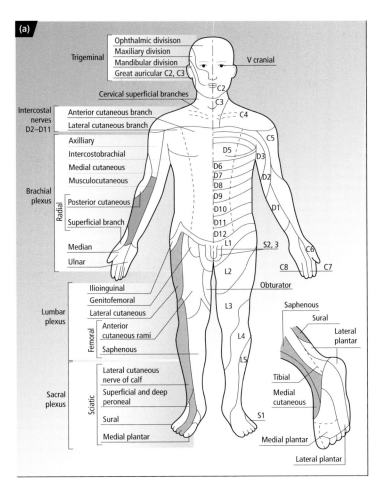

**FIGURE 46.1** Sensory innervation of the skin. Cutaneous areas of distribution of spinal segments and sensory fibers of the peripheral nerves: (a) anterior and (b) posterior views. (From Walton J, *Brain's Diseases of the Nervous System*, 10th edn. Oxford: Oxford University Press, 1993.)

Examination of the nervous system in acute medicine

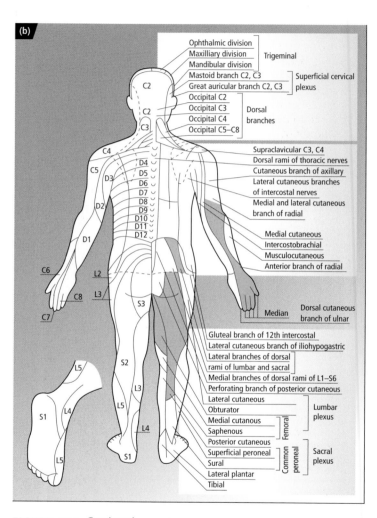

**(b)**

Ophthalmic division
Maxilliary division ⎤ Trigeminal
Mandibular division
Mastoid branch C2, C3 ⎤ Superficial cervical
Great auricular branch C2, C3 ⎦ plexus
Occipital C2
Occipital C3 ⎤ Dorsal
Occipital C4 ⎦ branches
Occipital C5–C8

Supraclavicular C3, C4
Dorsal rami of thoracic nerves
Cutaneous branch of axillary
Lateral cutaneous branches
of intercostal nerves
Medial and lateral cutaneous
branch of radial

Medial cutaneous
Intercostobrachial
Musculocutaneous
Anterior branch of radial

Dorsal cutaneous
Median   branch of ulnar

Gluteal branch of 12th intercostal
Lateral cutaneous branch of iliohypogastric
Lateral branches of dorsal
rami of lumbar and sacral
Medial branches of dorsal rami of L1–S6
Perforating branch of posterior cutaneous
Lateral cutaneous
Obturator ⎤ Lumbar
Medial cutanous ⎤ plexus
Saphenous ⎦ Femoral
Posterior cutaneous
Superficial peroneal ⎤ Sacral
Sural ⎤ plexus
Lateral plantar ⎦ Common peroneal
Tibial

**FIGURE 46.1** *Continued*

**TABLE 46.2** Assessment of conscious level using the Glasgow Coma Scale

- This is a scale based on the assessment of three clinical signs: eye opening, motor response and verbal response
- To assess the motor response, ask the patient to move the limb. If there is no response, apply firm pressure to the nailbed. Test and record for each of the limbs. Test for a localizing response by pressure on the supraorbital notch or sternal rub. For the purpose of assessment of conscious level, the best motor response is taken. Differences between the limbs will be important in identifying any focal neurological lesion
- The score for eye opening, motor response and verbal response is summed, although you should record the elements of the score as well, e.g. E2, M4, V2 (eye opening 2, motor response 4, verbal response 2)
- Coma is defined as a score of 8 or below, and a reduced conscious level as a score between 9 and 14

| Sign | Score |
|---|---|
| **Eye opening** | |
| None – the eyes remain closed | 1 |
| To pain – the eyes open in response to a painful stimulus applied to the trunk or limb (a painful stimulus to the head usually provokes closing of the eyes) | 2 |
| To voice | 3 |
| Spontaneous – the eyes are open with blinking | 4 |
| **Motor response** | |
| None | 1 |
| Extensor response | 2 |
| Abnormal flexor response | 3 |
| Withdrawal | 4 |
| Localizing – uses limb to locate or resist the painful stimulus | 5 |
| Voluntary – obeys commands | 6 |
| **Verbal response** | |
| None – no sound whatsoever is produced | 1 |
| Incomprehensible – mutters or groans only | 2 |
| Inappropriate – intelligible but isolated words | 3 |
| Confused speech | 4 |
| Oriented speech | 5 |
| **Total score** | 3–15 |

**TABLE 46.3** Abbreviated mental status examination of the elderly*

- Age
- Time (to nearest hour)
- Address for recall at end of test; this should be repeated by the patient to ensure it has been heard correctly: 42 West Street
- Year
- Name of hospital
- Recognition of two people (e.g. doctor, nurse)
- Date of birth (day and month is sufficient)
- Year of Second World War
- Name of present monarch
- Count backwards from 20 to 1

* Each correct answer scores 1 mark. The healthy elderly score is 8–10. From Qureshi, K.N. and Hodkinson, H.M. Evaluation of a ten-question mental test in the institutionalized elderly. *Age and Ageing* 1974; **3**: 152–7.

**TABLE 46.4** Mini mental state examination* (from Folstein M, et al. 1975)

| Assessment | Method | Score |
|---|---|---|
| Orientation for time | Day, date, month, season, year | 1 point for each. Total 5 |
| Orientation for place | Country, county, city/town, hospital, name of ward/unit | 1 point for each. Total 5 |
| Registration of three words | Repeat three words, e.g. ball, jar, fan | 1 point for each. Score first attempt only. Total 3 |
| Attention/ concentration | Repeat three words up to five times until they are learned Spell WORLD backwards | Count the number of letters to first mistake, e.g. DLORW counts 2. Total 5 |
| Short-term memory | Tell me the three items we named a few minutes ago | 1 point for each. Total 3 |
| Language | • Point to a pen and a wrist watch and ask the patient to name them | 1 point for each. Total 2 |
| | • Repeat the phrase, 'no ifs, ands or buts' | 1 point |
| | • Tell the patient to follow the instructions: 'Take this piece of paper in your right hand, fold it in half and put it on the floor' | 1 point for each. Total 3 |
| | • Show the patient a piece of paper with the words 'CLOSE YOUR EYES' written on it and ask him/her to follow the instructions | 1 point |
| | • Ask the patient to write a short sentence | 1 point for a complete sentence |
| Construction | Ask the patient to copy a diagram, e.g. two 5-sided shapes that intersect to create a 4-sided shape | 1 point |

* Maximum score 30. Scores of 24 or below indicate an acute confusional state or dementia.

**Examination of the nervous system in acute medicine**

| **TABLE 46.5** Grading of muscle power | |
| --- | --- |
| **Grade** | **Description** |
| 0 | No contraction |
| 1 | Flicker or trace of contraction |
| 2 | Active movement with gravity eliminated |
| 3 | Active movement against gravity |
| 4– | Active movement against gravity and slight resistance |
| 4 | Active movement against gravity and moderate resistance |
| 4+ | Active movement against gravity and strong resistance |
| 5 | Normal power |

**TABLE 46.6** Muscle groups: root and peripheral nerve supply

| Movement | Muscle group | Main roots | Peripheral nerve |
|---|---|---|---|
| **Shoulder abduction** | Deltoid | C5 | Axillary |
| **Shoulder adduction** | Latissimus dorsi | C7 | Brachial plexus |
| | Pectoralis major | C5–C7 | Brachial plexus |
| **Elbow flexion** | Biceps | C5, C6 | Musculocutaneous |
| | Brachioradialis | C6 | Radial |
| **Elbow extension** | Triceps | C7 | Radial |
| **Radial wrist extension** | Extensor carpi radialis longus | C6 | Radial |
| **Finger flexion** | Flexor digitorum profundus | C8 | Anterior interosseous/ulnar |
| **Finger extension** | Extensor digitorum communis | C7 | Posterior interosseous |
| **Finger abduction (index, middle, and ring fingers)** | Dorsal interossei | T1 | Ulnar |
| **Thumb abduction** | Abductor pollicis brevis | T1 | Median |
| **Hip flexion** | Iliopsoas | L1, L2 | Femoral |
| **Hip extension** | Gluteus maximus | L5–S1 | Inferior gluteal |
| **Hip adduction** | Adductors | L2, L3 | Obturator |
| **Knee flexion** | Hamstrings | S1 | Sciatic |
| **Knee extension** | Quadriceps | L3, L4 | Femoral |
| **Ankle dorsiflexion** | Tibialis anterior | L4 | Deep peroneal |
| **Ankle plantarflexion** | Gastrocnemius | S1, S2 | Tibial |
| | Soleus | S1, S2 | Tibial |
| **Ankle eversion** | Peroneus longus | L5–S1 | Superficial peroneal |
| **Great toe dorsiflexion** | Extensor hallucis longus | L5 | Deep peroneal |

**Examination of the nervous system in acute medicine**

**TABLE 46.7** Tendon reflexes: root and peripheral nerve supply

| Tendon reflex | Muscle | Main roots | Peripheral nerve |
|---|---|---|---|
| **Biceps** | Biceps | C5, C6 | Musculocutaneous |
| **Supinator** | Brachioradialis | C6 | Radial |
| **Triceps** | Triceps | C7 | Radial |
| **Finger** | Long finger flexors | C7, C8 | Median/ulnar |
| **Knee** | Quadriceps | L3, L4 | Femoral |
| **Ankle** | Gastrocnemius | S1, S2 | Sciatic (tibial) |

## Further reading

Folstein M, et al. 'Mini mental state': a practical method for grading the cognitive state of patients for the clinician. *J Psychiatr Res* 1975; 12: 189–98.

Rasvi SSM, Bone I. Neurological consultations in the medical intensive care unit. *J Neurol Neurosurg Psychiatry* 2003; 74 (suppl III): iii16–iii23.

Examination of the nervous system in acute medicine

# 47 Stroke

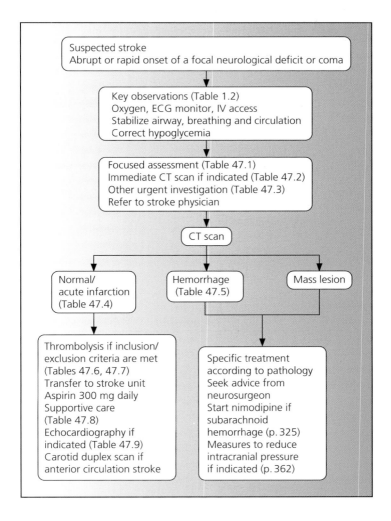

Suspected stroke
Abrupt or rapid onset of a focal neurological deficit or coma

↓

Key observations (Table 1.2)
Oxygen, ECG monitor, IV access
Stabilize airway, breathing and circulation
Correct hypoglycemia

↓

Focused assessment (Table 47.1)
Immediate CT scan if indicated (Table 47.2)
Other urgent investigation (Table 47.3)
Refer to stroke physician

↓

CT scan

↓

| Normal/ acute infarction (Table 47.4) | Hemorrhage (Table 47.5) | Mass lesion |

Thrombolysis if inclusion/ exclusion criteria are met (Tables 47.6, 47.7)
Transfer to stroke unit
Aspirin 300 mg daily
Supportive care (Table 47.8)
Echocardiography if indicated (Table 47.9)
Carotid duplex scan if anterior circulation stroke

Specific treatment according to pathology
Seek advice from neurosurgeon
Start nimodipine if subarachnoid hemorrhage (p. 325)
Measures to reduce intracranial pressure if indicated (p. 362)

Stroke

**TABLE 47.1** Focused assessment in suspected stroke

1 **Stabilize airway, breathing, circulation and blood glucose (p. 3)**

2 **Is this a stroke and not some other illness which may mimic stroke?**
- History of trauma or alcohol abuse (extradural or subdural hematoma)?
- Progressive onset over days (subdural hematoma, tumor)?
- Fever (brain abscess, meningitis, encephalitis, endocarditis, cerebral lupus, cerebral malaria)?
- Neck stiffness (meningitis, subarachnoid hemorrhage)?
- Severe hypertension (diastolic pressure >120 mmHg and papilledema with retinal hemorrhages and exudates) (hypertensive encephalopathy)?

3 **Does the stroke have a potentially treatable cause?**
*Important diagnoses to consider are*:
- Subarachnoid hemorrhage (p. 321)
- Embolism from the heart
- Carotid or vertebral artery dissection (preceding neck trauma or associated ipsilateral headache, Horner syndrome, pulsatile tinnitus)
- Cerebral venous sinus thrombosis (risk factors as for deep vein thrombosis, plus local infection and trauma)
- Vasoocclusive crisis of sickle cell disease
- Vasculitis (e.g. giant cell arteritis, systemic lupus erythematosus)

---

**TABLE 47.2** Indications for immediate CT scan in suspected stroke

---

- Thrombolysis is being considered (to rule out hemorrhage or early ischemic change, a marker for hemorrhagic transformation after thrombolysis) (see Table 47.6)
- Evidence of head injury (to rule out extradural or subdural hematoma)
- Patient taking warfarin or has a bleeding tendency (to rule out intracranial hemorrhage)
- Deteriorating conscious level (if so neurosurgical intervention to evacuate a hematoma or relieve obstructive hydrocephalus would be considered)
- Meningitis, encephalitis, subdural empyema or brain abscess are possible diagnoses
- Diagnosis of stroke is uncertain

Stroke

---

**TABLE 47.3** Urgent investigation in suspected stroke

---

- Full blood count
- ESR or C-reactive protein (if raised, consider vasculitis, endocarditis, myxoma)
- Coagulation screen (prothrombin time (INR if taking warfarin), activated partial thromboplastin time)
- Sickle solubility test if possible sickle cell disease (p. 514)
- Blood glucose
- Sodium, potassium, creatinine, lipids
- Urine stick test
- Blood culture (×2) if febrile or endocarditis is suspected
- ECG (?atrial fibrillation, left ventricular hypertrophy, myocardial infarction)
- Cranial CT (see Table 47.2 for indications for immediate CT; in other patients, CT should be done within 24 h)
- Chest X-ray
- Echocardiography if indicated (Table 47.9)

ESR, erythrocyte sedimentation rate; INR, international normalized ratio.

**TABLE 47.4** Causes of cerebral infarction

| Cause | Comment |
|---|---|
| **Atheromatous disease of the extracranial and large intracranial cerebral arteries** | Causes ~50% of ischemic strokes<br>May have carotid bruit<br>Stuttering progression of neurological deficit |
| **Embolism from the heart** | Causes ~20% of ischemic strokes<br>Sudden onset of neurological deficit, maximal at onset<br>Causes of embolism include:<br>• Atrial fibrillation (thrombus in left atrium)<br>• Prosthetic heart valve<br>• Rheumatic mitral valve disease<br>• Atrial myxoma |
| **Lacunar infarction** | Causes ~25% of ischemic strokes<br>Due to occlusion of a single perforating artery in the basal ganglia or pons by lipohyalinosis or microatheroma<br>Conscious level, higher cerebral functions and visual fields are not affected |
| **Other causes** | Cerebral venous sinus thrombosis (risk factors as for deep vein thrombosis (Table 35.2), plus local infection and trauma)<br>Embolism from aorta<br>Carotid or vertebral artery dissection (carotid dissection is the commonest cause of stroke in patients under 45 years)<br>Cerebral vasculitis<br>Aortic dissection with occlusion of carotid artery (p. 181)<br>CADASIL syndrome (cerebral autosomal dominant arteriopathy with subcortical infarcts and leukoencephalopathy)<br>MELAS syndrome (mitochondrial myopathy, encephalopathy, lactic acidosis, and stroke-like episodes) |

**TABLE 47.5** Causes of cerebral hemorrhage

| Cause | Comment |
|---|---|
| **Hypertension** | Hypertensive hemorrhages occur from microaneurysms on penetrator arteries that branch off major intracerebral arteries<br>Typically causes hemorrhage in the putamen, thalamus, pons and cerebellum |
| **Bleeding disorder** | Most often due to warfarin anticoagulation, with INR >5 |
| **Amyloid angiopathy** | Typically causes lobar hemorrhage (in cortex and subcortical white matter) in elderly patient |
| **Other causes** | Hemorrhagic transformation of cerebral infarction (commonly seen in infarction due to cerebral venous sinus thrombosis)<br>Reperfusion after carotid endarterectomy/angioplasty<br>Vascular malformation<br>Mycotic aneurysm |

INR, international normalized ratio.

**ALERT**
Approximately 80% of strokes are due to cerebral infarction, ~15% to primary intracerebral hemorrhage and ~5% to subarachnoid hemorrhage. Headache, vomiting and coma at onset are more common in hemorrhagic stroke, but accurate differentiation requires CT.

**TABLE 47.6** Inclusion/exclusion criteria for thrombolysis for acute ischemic stroke

### Inclusion criteria (yes to all before thrombolysis)

- Age 18–80?
- Clinical diagnosis of ischemic stroke with a measurable neurological deficit?
- Time of symptom onset (when patient was last seen normal) well established as <3h before treatment should begin?
- Hemorrhage excluded on CT

### Exclusion criteria (no to all before thrombolysis)

- Evidence of intracranial hemorrhage on pretreatment non-contrast head CT?
- Clinical presentation suggestive of subarachnoid hemorrhage even with normal CT?
- CT shows multilobar infarction (hypodensity greater than one-third cerebral hemisphere)?
- History of intracranial hemorrhage?
- Uncontrolled hypertension? At time treatment should begin, is systolic BP >185mmHg or diastolic BP >110mmHg on repeated measurements?
- Known arteriovenous malformation, neoplasm or aneurysm?
- Witnessed seizure at stroke onset?
- Active internal bleeding or acute trauma?
- Bleeding tendency, including but not limited to:
  - Platelet count <100 × $10^9$/L
  - Heparin received within 48h, resulting in an activated partial thromboplastin time (APTT) that is greater than upper limit of normal

  Current use of warfarin with INR >1.7 or prothromin time (PT) >15s
- Within 3 months of intracranial or intraspinal surgery, serious head trauma or previous stroke?
- Arterial puncture at a non-compressible site within past 7 days?

*Continued*

**Relative contraindications/precautions**
- Only minor or rapidly improving stroke symptoms (clearing spontaneously)
- Within 14 days of major surgery or serious trauma
- Recent gastrointestinal or urinary tract hemorrhage (within previous 21 days)
- Recent acute myocardial infarction (within previous 3 months)
- Postmyocardial infarction pericarditis
- Abnormal blood glucose level (<2.8 or >22.2 mmol/L)

INR, international normalized ratio.

**TABLE 47.7** Thrombolytic therapy for acute ischemic stroke

- Admit to HDU or acute stroke unit
- Give alteplase 0.9 mg/kg body weight, to a maximum dose of 90 mg: 10% of dose IV over 1 min and rest infused over 1 h
- Check neurological signs and general observations:
  - Every 15 min for 2 h, *then*
  - Every 30 min for 6 h, *then*
  - Every 60 min for 16 h
- Follow-up CT scan at 24 h
- Keep blood pressure at or below 180/105 mmHg for first 24 h
- Antiplatelet therapy, heparin and warfarin should not be given for at least 24 h after the alteplase infusion is completed

HDU, high-dependency unit.

Stroke

**TABLE 47.8** Supportive care after stroke

| Element | Comment |
|---|---|
| **Management on acute stroke unit** | Shown to improve the outcome of stroke<br>Start physiotherapy within 1–2 days to prevent contractures and pressure ulceration, and encourage recovery of function<br>Patients with language disorders should be referred for speech therapy |
| **Fluid and electrolyte balance** | Avoid dehydration (which may cause hemoconcentration and worsen cerebral blood flow) and fluid overload (possibly worsening cerebral edema)<br>If the patient is conscious, check if 50 ml of water can be swallowed safely with the patient sitting upright. If so, fluids can be given by mouth<br>If conscious level is depressed, if voluntary cough is weak or absent, or if water cannot be swallowed safely, oral fluids should not be given. Start an IV or SC infusion (usually 2 L in 24 h) or insert a fine-bore nasogastric tube<br>Use normal saline in the first 24 h. Glucose IV should be avoided as a high blood glucose level may worsen prognosis<br>Check electrolytes and creatinine, initially daily, and correct derangements of plasma sodium (p. 439) and potassium (p. 446) |
| **Feeding** | If the patient is unable to swallow safely after the stroke, consider placing a fine-bore nasogastric tube to allow feeding<br>If swallowing has not recovered by 2 weeks after the stroke, consider feeding via a percutaneous gastrostomy tube |

*Continued*

| Element | Comment |
|---|---|
| **Deep vein thrombosis (DVT) prophylaxis** | DVT is a common complication<br>The incidence can be reduced by early mobilization and graded compression stockings<br>Low-dose SC heparin may result in hemorrhagic transformation of a cerebral infarct and should not routinely be used<br>Patients with cerebral infarction who have had a previous DVT or pulmonary embolism, or who are severely obese (BMI >40) should be considered for prophylactic LMW heparin |
| **When to treat hypertension?** | Acute treatment (within the first week) is not indicated unless there is hypertensive encephalopathy, aortic dissection or intracerebral hemorrhage with severe hypertension (systolic pressure >230 mmHg or diastolic >140 mmHg)<br>If IV therapy is needed, use IV labetolol (p. 184) so that the dose can be titrated carefully<br>If the patient has been taking antihypertensive therapy, this should be continued |
| **Blood glucose** | Hyperglycemia is an adverse risk factor but the threshold for and benefits of treatment are not established<br>Use an insulin sliding scale if the blood glucose is >15 mmol/L (p. 427) |
| **Fever** | In patients febrile at presentation, consider brain abscess, meningitis and infective endocarditis<br>Fever beginning 12–48 h after presentation may be due to the stroke itself, aspiration pneumonia (in patients with a reduced |

*Stroke*

*Continued*

| Element | Comment |
| --- | --- |
| | conscious level or disordered swallowing; p. 278), urinary tract infection or venous thromboembolism. Examine the patient, send blood and urine for culture, check full blood count and C-reactive protein, and obtain a chest X-ray |
| | If you suspect aspiration pneumonia, options for initial treatment (before culture results are known) are co-amoxiclav or a fluoroquinolone plus clindamycin or metronidazole |
| | Measures to reduce body temperature (paracetamol, fan) may help reduce neuronal damage |
| **Bladder function** | Urinary incontinence is common but often temporary, and is best managed without bladder catheterization |
| | Exclude fecal impaction and urinary tract infection |

BMI, body mass index; LMW, low molecular weight.

> **TABLE 47.9** Echocardiography after stroke or transient ischemic attack
>
> **Urgent transthoracic or transesophageal echocardiography**
> - Possible infective endocarditis (p. 206)
> - Possible aortic dissection (p. 183)
> - Possible atrial myxoma (systemic symptoms; signs of mitral valve disease; high ESR)
>
> **Routine transthoracic echocardiography**
> - Pansystolic murmur
> - Any diastolic murmur
> - Atrial fibrillation (to determine cause of AF)
> - Other major ECG abnormality (e.g. Q waves indicative of previous myocardial infarction, LV hypertrophy with strain pattern (?hypertrophic cardiomyopathy), complete left bundle branch block (?dilated cardiomyopathy))
> - Significant cardiac enlargement on chest X-ray (e.g. CTR >0.6)
>
> **Routine transesophageal echocardiography**
> - Possible infective endocarditis but normal transthoracic study
> - Mechanical heart valve prosthesis (to exclude thrombus and vegetations)
> - Age <50 with unexplained stroke (may be indicated in patients >50 with unexplained stroke: discuss with a neurologist or stroke physician)
>
> AF, atrial fibrillation; CTR, cardiothoracic ratio; ESR, erythrocyte sedimentation rate; LV, left ventricular.

Stroke

## Further reading

American Heart Association and American Stroke Association. Guidelines for the early management of patients with ischemic stroke: 2005 guidelines update. *Stroke* website (http://www.strokeaha.org).

Einhaulpl K, et al. European Federation of Neurological Societies guideline on the treatment of cerebral venous and sinus thrombosis. *Eur J Neurol* 2006; 13: 553–9.

Goldstein LB, Simel DL. Is this patient having a stroke? *JAMA* 2005, 293: 2391–402.

Intercollegiate Stroke Working Party. National clinical guidelines for stroke, 2nd edn (2004). Royal College of Physicians website (http://www.rcplondon.ac.uk/pubs/books/stroke/index.htm).

Khaja AM, Grotta JC. Established treatments for acute ischaemic stroke. *Lancet* 2007; 369: 319–30.

Martino R, et al. Dysphagia after stroke: incidence, diagnosis, and pulmonary complications. *Stroke* 2005; 36: 2756–63.

Sacco RL, et al. Experimental treatments for acute ischaemic stroke. *Lancet* 2007; 369: 331–41.

Selim M. Perioperative stroke. *N Engl J Med* 2007; 356: 706–13.

Warlow C, et al. Stroke. *Lancet* 2003; 362: 1211–24.

Stroke

# 48 Transient ischemic attack

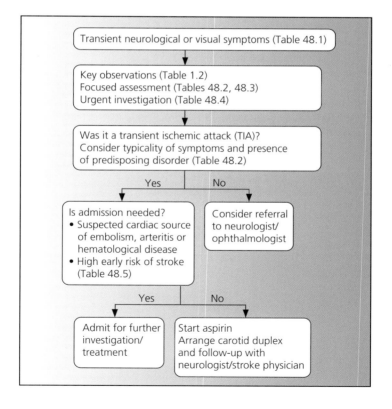

Transient neurological or visual symptoms (Table 48.1)

Key observations (Table 1.2)
Focused assessment (Tables 48.2, 48.3)
Urgent investigation (Table 48.4)

Was it a transient ischemic attack (TIA)?
Consider typicality of symptoms and presence
of predisposing disorder (Table 48.2)

Yes                    No

Is admission needed?
• Suspected cardiac source
  of embolism, arteritis or
  hematological disease
• High early risk of stroke
  (Table 48.5)

Consider referral
to neurologist/
ophthalmologist

Yes                    No

Admit for further
investigation/
treatment

Start aspirin
Arrange carotid duplex
and follow-up with
neurologist/stroke physician

> **TABLE 48.1** Causes of transient neurological or visual symptoms
>
> **Neurological**
> - Arterial disease: atheroembolism or arteritis
> - Embolism from the heart
> - Hematological disease: hyperviscosity syndrome, sickle cell disease
> - Migraine
> - Focal seizure
> - Structural brain lesions causing epilepsy, e.g. subdural hematoma
> - Peripheral nerve lesions
> - Multiple sclerosis
> - Transient global amnesia
> - Labyrinthine disorders
> - Psychological disorders including hyperventilation
> - Metabolic disorders, e.g. hypoglycemia
>
> **Visual**
> - Arterial disease: atheroembolism or arteritis (especially giant cell)
> - Embolism from the heart
> - Hematological disease: hyperviscosity syndrome, sickle cell disease
> - Migraine
> - Glaucoma
> - Raised intracranial pressure
> - Retinal detachment
> - Retinal/vitreous hemorrhage
> - Malignant hypertension
> - Retinal vein thrombosis
> - Orbital tumor
> - Psychological disorders including hyperventilation

**TABLE 48.2** Focused assessment after suspected transient ischemic attack (TIA)

**1 Was this a TIA?**
- The symptoms of TIA are of sudden onset, lack prodromal features such as nausea or palpitation, reach their peak within seconds and usually last for less than 15 min
- TIAs usually cause loss of function. 'Positive' symptoms such as limb movement, paresthesiae or hallucinations are more likely to be due to epilepsy or migraine
- Presyncope or syncope are rarely a result of TIA unless associated with other focal neurological symptoms
- Other causes of transient neurological and visual symptoms are given in Table 48.1

**2 Which arterial territory was affected: carotid or vertebrobasilar?** See Table 48.3

**3 What caused the TIA?** See Table 48.1. Always consider the following:
- Carotid atheroembolism:
  - A carotid bruit is not a sensitive or specific sign of severe carotid disease
  - Carotid duplex scanning is indicated in patients who have had a carotid territory TIA and would be candidates for endarterectomy
- Embolism from the heart, possible in the presence of:
  - Prosthetic heart valve, especially in the mitral position
  - Clinical cardiac abnormality (e.g. pansystolic murmur, mid-diastolic murmur, signs of heart failure)
  - Atrial fibrillation (embolism of left atrial thrombus)
  - Recent anterior myocardial infarction (embolism of LV mural thrombus)
  - Other major ECG abnormality (e.g. Q waves indicative of previous myocardial infarction, LV hypertrophy with strain pattern (?hypertrophic cardiomyopathy), complete left bundle branch block (?dilated cardiomyopathy))
  - Significant cardiac enlargement on chest X-ray

*Continued*

Transient ischemic attack

- Arteritis, suggested by:
  - High ESR or C-reactive protein
  - Headache or systemic symptoms
- Hematological disease:
  - Hyperviscosity syndrome
  - Sickle cell disease

ESR, erythrocyte sedimentation rate; LV, left ventricular.

**TABLE 48.3** Symptoms of carotid and vertebrobasilar transient ischemic attacks (TIAs)

| Symptom | Carotid TIA | Vertebrobasilar TIA |
| --- | --- | --- |
| **Dysphasia** | Yes | No |
| **Loss of vision in one eye** | Yes | No |
| **Loss of vision in both eyes** | No | Yes |
| **Hemianopia** | Yes | Yes |
| **Diplopia** | No | Yes |
| **Dysarthria** | Yes | Yes |
| **Loss of balance** | Yes | Yes |
| **Unilateral motor loss** | Yes | Yes |
| **Unilateral sensory loss** | Yes | Yes |

Transient ischemic attack

**TABLE 48.4** Investigation after transient ischemic attack (TIA)/ monocular visual loss

**All patients**
- Full blood count
- ESR or C-reactive protein (if raised, consider vasculitis, endocarditis, myxoma)
- INR if taking warfarin
- Sickle solubility test if sickle cell disease possible (p. 514)
- Blood glucose
- Sodium, potassium, creatinine and lipids
- Urine stick test
- Blood culture (×2) if febrile or endocarditis is suspected
- ECG (?atrial fibrillation, left ventricular hypertrophy, myocardial infarction)
- Chest X-ray (?lung neoplasm, cardiac enlargement)

**Selected patients**
- CT (or preferably MRI) scan if there is doubt about the diagnosis or symptoms lasted >1 h
- Carotid duplex scanning if transient monocular visual loss or carotid territory TIA (Table 48.3)
- Echocardiography if clinical or ECG evidence of cardiac disease (see Table 47.9)

ESR, erythrocyte sedimentation rate; INR international normalized ratio.

Transient ischemic attack

**Transient ischemic attack**

**TABLE 48.5** Who to admit after a transient ischemic attack (TIA) for urgent investigation/management?

- Patients with suspected cardiac source of embolism, arteritis or hematological disease
- Patients at high early risk of stroke: a score of 4 or more on the scale below

| Characteristics of patient and TIA | Score |
|---|---|
| **Age** >60 years | 1 |
| **Blood pressure** | |
| Systolic BP > 140 mmHg and/or diastolic BP > 90 mmHg | 1 |
| **Clinical features** | |
| Unilateral weakness | 2 |
| Speech disturbance without weakness | 1 |
| **Duration of symptoms** | |
| 60 min or longer | 2 |
| 10–59 min | 1 |
| <10 min | 0 |

From Rothwell, P.M. et al. *Lancet* 2005; **366**: 29–36.

**ALERT**
Patients with carotid territory TIA at high early risk of stroke should have urgent carotid endarterectomy if the duplex scan shows a stenosis of 70–99%.

## Further reading

Flemming KD, et al. Evaluation and management of transient ischemic attack and minor cerebral infarction. *Mayo Clin Proc* 2004; 79: 1071–86.

Johnston SC, et al. Validation and refinement of scores to predict very early stroke risk after transient ischaemic attack. *Lancet* 2007; 369: 283–92.

Rothwell PM, et al. A simple score (ABCD) to identify individuals at high early risk of stroke after transient ischaemic attack. *Lancet* 2005; 366: 29–36.

# 49 Subarachnoid hemorrhage

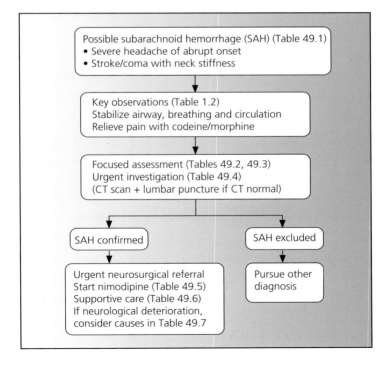

Possible subarachnoid hemorrhage (SAH) (Table 49.1)
• Severe headache of abrupt onset
• Stroke/coma with neck stiffness

Key observations (Table 1.2)
Stabilize airway, breathing and circulation
Relieve pain with codeine/morphine

Focused assessment (Tables 49.2, 49.3)
Urgent investigation (Table 49.4)
(CT scan + lumbar puncture if CT normal)

SAH confirmed

SAH excluded

Urgent neurosurgical referral
Start nimodipine (Table 49.5)
Supportive care (Table 49.6)
If neurological deterioration,
consider causes in Table 49.7

Pursue other
diagnosis

---

**TABLE 49.1** Causes of subarachnoid hemorrhage

**Common**
- Rupture of saccular ('berry') aneurysm of circle of Willis (75% cases)
- Bleeding from arteriovenous malformation
- Primary intracerebral hemorrhage with rupture of the hematoma into the subarachnoid space
- Unknown cause (i.e. cerebral angiography normal and no other cause identified; 20% cases)

**Rare**
- Bleeding tendency
- Bleeding from intracranial tumors, notably metastatic melanoma
- Trauma (most common in the elderly with occipital skull fracture)
- Inflammatory lesions of cerebral arteries (e.g. vasculitis, mycotic aneurysm)
- Sickle cell disease
- Vascular lesions of spinal cord
- Cocaine poisoning

---

**TABLE 49.2** Clinical features of aneurysmal subarachnoid hemorrhage

**History**
- Onset of headache: abrupt, maximal at onset, 'thunderclap' headache
- Severity of headache: usually 'worst of life' or very severe
- Qualitative characteristics: first headache ever of this intensity, unique or different in patients with prior headaches
- Associated symptoms: transient loss of consciousness, diplopia, fit, focal neurological symptoms*

**Background**
- Cigarette smoking
- Hypertension
- Alcohol consumption (especially after recent binge)

*Continued*

- Personal or family history of subarachnoid hemorrhage*
- Risk factors for intracranial aneurysm: polycystic kidney disease*, Ehlers–Danlos syndrome type IV*, pseudoxanthoma elasticum*, fibromuscular dysplasia*, sickle cell disease, alfa1-antitrypsin deficiency

**Examination**
- Retinal or subhyaloid hemorrhages (retinal hemorrhages with curved lower and straight upper borders)*
- Neck stiffness*
- Focal neurological signs
- Low grade fever

* Patients with these features are at very high risk of having an intracranial aneurysm. Ask advice on management from a neurologist, even if CT/lumbar puncture are negative.
From Edlow, J.A. and Caplan, L.R. Avoiding pitfalls in the diagnosis of subarachnoid hemorrhage. *N Engl J Med* 2000; **342**: 29–36.

**TABLE 49.3** Grading scales for patients with subarachnoid hemorrhage

| Grade | World Federation of Neurosurgical Societies Scale | Hunt and Hess Scale |
|---|---|---|
| 1 | GCS 15, no focal deficit | Asymptomatic or mild headache/neck stiffness |
| 2 | GCS 13–14, no focal deficit | Moderate to severe headache, neck stiffness, cranial nerve palsy |
| 3 | GCS 13–14, with focal deficit | Lethargy, confusion or mild focal deficit |
| 4 | GCS 7–12, with or without focal deficit | Stupor, moderate to severe hemiparesis, early decerebrate rigidity |
| 5 | GCS 3–6, with or without focal deficit | Deep coma, decerebrate rigidity, moribund appearance |

GCS, Glasgow Coma Scale (see Table 46.2).

**TABLE 49.4** Urgent investigation in suspected subarachnoid hemorrhage

**CT of the brain**
- Blood in subarachnoid spaces
- May show intracerebral hematoma

**Lumbar puncture if CT is normal**
- Raised opening pressure
- Uniformly blood-stained cerebral spinal fluid (CSF)
- Xanthochromia of the supernatant (always found from 12 h to 2 weeks after the bleed; centrifuge the CSF and examine the supernatant by spectrophotometry if available; if not, compare against a white background with a control tube filled with water)

**Other investigations**
- Full blood count
- Coagulation screen
- Blood glucose
- Sodium, potassium and creatinine
- ECG
- Chest X-ray

**ALERT**
If the CSF findings are equivocal in a patient with suspected subarachnoid hemorrhage, cerebral angiography may be indicated to exclude an intracranial aneurysm: seek advice from a neurologist or neurosurgeon.

---

**TABLE 49.5** Nimodipine after subarachnoid hemorrhage

- To prevent ischemic neurological deficits, give nimodipine 60 mg 4-hourly by mouth or nasogastric tube, for 21 days
- To treat ischemic neurological deficits, give IV via a central line: 1 mg/h initially, increased after 2 h to 2 mg/h if no significant fall in blood pressure. Continue for at least 5 days (max. 14 days)
- Other calcium-channel blockers and beta-blockers should not be given while the patient is receiving nimodipine

---

**TABLE 49.6** Monitoring and supportive care after subarachnoid hemorrhage

- Admit the patient to ITU/HDU
- Monitor conscious level (Glasgow Coma Scale score, see Table 46.2), pupils, respiratory rate, arterial oxygen saturation, heart rate, blood pressure, temperature, fluid balance and blood glucose, initially 2–4-hourly
- Give analgesia as required (e.g. paracetamol 1 g 6-hourly and/or codeine 30–60 mg 4-hourly PO). Add a benzodiazepine if needed for anxiety. Start a stool softener to prevent constipation
- Ensure an adequate fluid intake to prevent hypovolemia: initially 3 L normal saline IV daily. Check electrolytes and creatinine at least every other day
- If conscious level is reduced, place a nasogastric tube for feeding
- Use graduated compression stockings to reduce the risk of DVT
- Antihypertensive therapy is not of proven benefit in preventing rebleeding and may cause cerebral ischemia. If hypertension is sustained and severe (systolic BP >200 mmHg, diastolic BP >110 mmHg), despite adequate analgesia, cautious treatment may be given, e.g. metoprolol initially 25 mg 12-hourly PO: discuss with neurosurgical unit

DVT, deep vein thrombosis; HDU, high-dependency unit; ITU, intensive therapy unit.

**Subarachnoid hemorrhage**

---

**TABLE 49.7** Causes of neurological deterioration after aneurysmal subarachnoid hemorrhage

---

- Recurrent hemorrhage: peak incidence in the first 2 weeks (10% of patients)
- Vasospasm causing cerebral ischemia or infarction: peak incidence between day 4 and day 14 (25% of patients)
- Communicating hydrocephalus: from 1 to 8 weeks after the hemorrhage (15–20% of patients)
- Seizures
- Hyponatremia, due to either inappropriate ADH secretion (p. 442) or cerebral salt wasting

---

## Further reading

Suarez JI, et al. Aneurysmal subarachnoid hemorrhage. *N Engl J Med* 2006; 354: 387–96.

Van Gijn J, et al. Subarachnoid haemorrhage. *Lancet* 2007; 369: 306–18.

# 50 Bacterial meningitis

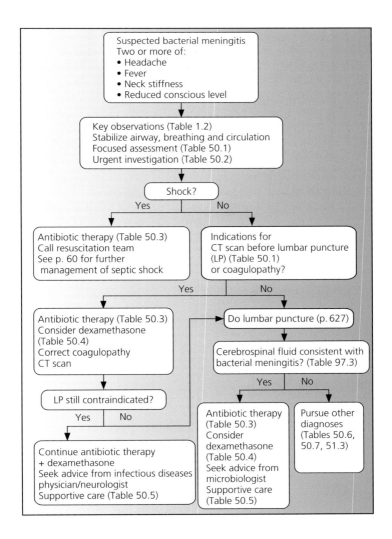

Suspected bacterial meningitis
Two or more of:
- Headache
- Fever
- Neck stiffness
- Reduced conscious level

Key observations (Table 1.2)
Stabilize airway, breathing and circulation
Focused assessment (Table 50.1)
Urgent investigation (Table 50.2)

Shock?

Yes

Antibiotic therapy (Table 50.3)
Call resuscitation team
See p. 60 for further
  management of septic shock

No

Indications for
CT scan before lumbar puncture
(LP) (Table 50.1)
or coagulopathy?

Yes

Antibiotic therapy (Table 50.3)
Consider dexamethasone
(Table 50.4)
Correct coagulopathy
CT scan

No

Do lumbar puncture (p. 627)

Cerebrospinal fluid consistent with
bacterial meningitis? (Table 97.3)

Yes    No

LP still contraindicated?

Yes    No

Antibiotic therapy
(Table 50.3)
Consider
dexamethasone
(Table 50.4)
Seek advice from
microbiologist
Supportive care
(Table 50.5)

Pursue other
diagnoses
(Tables 50.6,
50.7, 51.3)

Continue antibiotic therapy
+ dexamethasone
Seek advice from infectious diseases
physician/neurologist
Supportive care (Table 50.5)

Bacterial meningitis

327

**TABLE 50.1** Focused assessment in suspected bacterial meningitis

**1 Is this meningitis?**
- Consider meningitis in any febrile patient with headache, neck stiffness or a reduced conscious level
- Disorders which can mimic meningitis include subarachnoid hemorrhage (p. 321), viral encephalitis (p. 334), subdural empyema, brain abscess and cerebral malaria (p. 546)

**2 Is immediate antibiotic therapy indicated?**
- If the clinical picture suggests meningitis, and the patient has shock, a reduced conscious level or a petechial/purpuric rash (suggesting meningococcal infection), take blood cultures (×2) and start antibiotic therapy (Table 50.3), plus adjunctive dexamethasone (Table 50.4) if indicated

**3 Should a CT scan be done before lumbar puncture?**
- CT should be done first if there are risk factors for an intracranial mass lesion or signs of raised intracranial pressure:
  - Immunocompromised state (e.g. AIDS, immunosuppressive therapy)
  - History of brain tumor, stroke or focal infection
  - Fits within 1 week of presentation
  - Papilledema
  - Reduced conscious level (Glasgow Coma Scale score <10)
  - Focal neurological signs (not including cranial nerve palsies)
- If CT is needed, take blood cultures (×2) and start antibiotic therapy (Table 50.3), plus adjunctive dexamethasone (Table 50.4) if indicated

---

**TABLE 50.2** Urgent investigation in suspected meningitis

- Blood culture (×2)
- Throat swab
- Lumbar puncture (preceded by CT if indicated, Table 50.1)
- Full blood count
- Coagulation screen if there is petechial/purpuric rash or low platelet count
- C-reactive protein
- Blood glucose
- Sodium, potassium and creatinine
- Arterial blood gases and pH
- Chest X-ray

---

**TABLE 50.3** Initial antibiotic therapy for suspected bacterial meningitis in adults (IV, high dose)

| Setting | No penicillin allergy | Penicillin allergy |
|---------|----------------------|-------------------|
| **Previously healthy adult under 50** | Cefotaxime or ceftriaxone | Minor allergy: cefotaxime or ceftriaxone<br>Severe allergy: chloramphenicol |
| **Age over 50 Immunocompromised (organ transplant, lymphoma, steroid therapy, AIDS) Chronic alcohol abuse** | Cefotaxime or ceftriaxone + ampicillin or amoxycillin | Minor allergy: cefotaxime or ceftriaxone<br>Severe allergy: chloramphenicol |

Bacterial meningitis

---

**ALERT**
Discuss further antibiotic therapy with a microbiologist in the light of the clinical picture and cerebrospinal fluid results.

**TABLE 50.4** Adjunctive dexamethasone in suspected bacterial meningitis

### Indications
- Strong clinical suspicion of bacterial meningitis, especially if CSF is turbid

### Contraindications
- Antibiotic therapy already begun
- Septic shock
- Suspected meningococcal disease (petechial/purpuric rash)
- Immunocompromised (e.g. AIDS, immunosuppressive therapy)

### Regimen
- Give dexamethasone 10 mg IV before or with the first dose of antibiotic therapy (Table 50.3)
- Continue dexamethasone 10 mg 6-hourly IV for 4 days if CSF shows Gram-positive diplococci, or if blood/CSF cultures are positive for *Streptococcus pneumoniae*

CSF, cerebrospinal fluid.

**TABLE 50.5** Supportive treatment of bacterial meningitis

| Element | Comment |
|---|---|
| **Airway, breathing and circulation** | Manage along standard lines (Tables 1.3–1.7) |
| | In patients with septic shock, give low-dose steroid (hydrocortisone 50 mg 6-hourly IV + fludrocortisone 50 µg daily IV) |
| **Raised intracranial pressure** | Manage along standard lines (p. 362) |

*Continued*

| Element | Comment |
|---|---|
| **Fluid balance** | Insensible losses are greater than normal due to fever (allow 500 ml/day/°C) and tachypnea<br>Give IV fluids (2–3 L/day) with daily check of creatinine and electrolytes if abnormal on admission<br>Hyponatremia may occur due to inappropriate ADH secretion (p. 441)<br>Monitor central venous pressure and urine output if patient is oliguric or if plasma creatinine is >200 µmol/L |
| **DVT prophylaxis** | Give DVT prophylaxis with stockings and LWH heparin |
| **Prophylaxis against gastric stress ulceration** | Give proton pump inhibitor |
| **Fits** | Manage along standard lines (p. 349)<br>Prophylactic anticonvulsant therapy not indicated |

ADH, antidiuretic hormone; DVT, deep vein thrombosis; LMW, low molecular weight.

**TABLE 50.6** Tuberculous (TB) meningitis

| Element | Comment |
|---|---|
| **At risk groups** | Immigrants from India, Pakistan and Africa<br>Recent contact with TB<br>Previous pulmonary TB<br>Chronic alcohol abuse<br>IV drug use<br>Immunocompromised (organ transplant, lymphoma, steroid therapy, AIDS) |

*Continued*

Bacterial meningitis

| Element | Comment |
|---|---|
| **Clinical features** | Subacute onset<br>Cranial nerve palsies<br>Retinal tubercles (pathognomonic but rarely seen)<br>Hyponatremia<br>Chest X-ray often normal |
| **CT** | Commonly shows hydrocephalus (~75%)<br>May show cerebral infarction due to arteritis (~15–30%)<br>May show tuberculoma (~5–10%) |
| **Cerebrospinal fluid (CSF)** | High lymphocyte count<br>High protein concentration<br>Acid-fast bacilli may not be seen on Ziehl–Neelsen stain<br>*Mycoplasma tuberculosis* DNA may be detected in CSF by the polymerase chain reaction |
| **Treatment** | Combination chemotherapy with isoniazid (with pyridoxine cover), rifampicin, pyrazinamide and ethambutol or streptomycin<br>Consider adjunctive dexamethasone<br>Seek expert advice |

**TABLE 50.7** Cryptococcal meningitis

| Element | Comment |
|---|---|
| **At risk groups** | Immunocompromised (organ transplant, lymphoma, steroid therapy, AIDS) |
| **Clinical features** | Insidious onset<br>Headache usually major symptom<br>Neck stiffness absent or mild |
| **CT** | Usually normal<br>May show hydrocephalus<br>May show mass lesions (~10%) |

*Continued*

| Element | Comment |
|---|---|
| **Cerebrospinal fluid (CSF)** | Opening pressure usually markedly raised, especially in patients with AIDS<br>Raised lymphocyte count (20–200/mm³)<br>Protein and glucose levels usually only mildly abnormal<br>Cryptococci may be seen on Gram stain<br>India ink preparation positive in 60%<br>CSF culture positive<br>Serological tests for cryptococcal antigen on CSF or blood positive |
| **Treatment** | Amphotericin plus flucytosine<br>Seek expert advice |

## Further reading

British Infection Society. Early management of suspected bacterial meningitis and meninogococcal septicaemia in immunocompetent adults (2005). British Infection Society website (http://www.britishinfectionsociety.org/meningitis.html).

Ginsberg L. Difficult and recurrent meningitis. *J Neurol Neurosurg Psychiatry* 2004; 75 (suppl I): i16–i21.

Van de Beek D, et al. Community-acquired bacterial meningitis in adults. *N Engl J Med* 2006; 354: 44–53.

Bacterial meningitis

# 51 Encephalitis

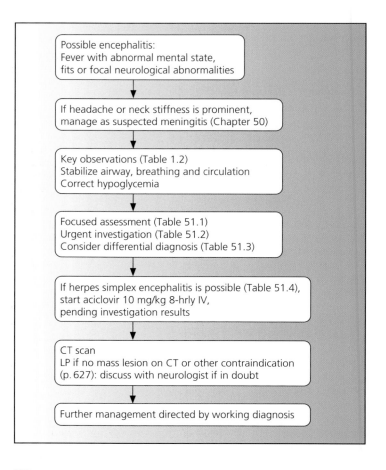

Possible encephalitis:
Fever with abnormal mental state,
fits or focal neurological abnormalities

↓

If headache or neck stiffness is prominent,
manage as suspected meningitis (Chapter 50)

↓

Key observations (Table 1.2)
Stabilize airway, breathing and circulation
Correct hypoglycemia

↓

Focused assessment (Table 51.1)
Urgent investigation (Table 51.2)
Consider differential diagnosis (Table 51.3)

↓

If herpes simplex encephalitis is possible (Table 51.4),
start aciclovir 10 mg/kg 8-hrly IV,
pending investigation results

↓

CT scan
LP if no mass lesion on CT or other contraindication
(p. 627): discuss with neurologist if in doubt

↓

Further management directed by working diagnosis

---

**TABLE 51.1** Focused assessment in suspected encephalitis

- Context: age, sex, comorbidities
- Current major symptoms and their time course (confirm with family or friends)
- Immunocompromised? Consider immunosuppressive therapy, AIDS, cancer, renal failure, liver failure, diabetes, malnutrition, splenectomy, IV drug use
- Recent foreign travel? (See Table 84.1)
- Contact with infectious disease?
- Drug history (if treated with neuroleptic in preceding 2 weeks, consider neuroleptic malignant syndrome (Table 51.5))
- Alcohol history (Chapter 87)
- Poisoning/substance use?
- Sexual history
- Systematic examination (Table 1.9) and neurological examination (Table 46.1)

---

**TABLE 51.2** Urgent investigation in suspected encephalitis

- Blood culture (×2)
- Throat swab
- Full blood count
- Coagulation screen
- C-reactive protein
- Blood glucose
- Sodium, potassium and creatinine
- Liver function tests
- Creatine kinase
- Urinalysis
- Toxicology screen if poisoning is possible (serum (10 ml) + urine (50 ml))
- Arterial blood gases and pH
- Chest X-ray
- Cranial CT
- LP if not contraindicated (send CSF for PCR for HSV-1)
- Serological testing (if indicated) for other causes of encephalitis (Table 51.3)

**TABLE 51.3** Differential diagnosis of viral encephalitis

**Intracranial infection**
- Partially treated bacterial meningitis
- Brain abscess
- Subdural empyema
- Tuberculous meningitis (p. 331)
- Cryptococcal meningitis (p. 332)
- *Toxoplasma* encephalitis

**Systemic infection**
- Infective endocarditis
- *Mycoplasma* and *Legionella* infection
- Syphilis, Lyme disease, leptospirosis
- Fungal infection (coccidiodomycosis, histoplasmosis)
- Cerebral malaria (p. 546)

**Non-infectious**
- Poisoning with amphetamine, cocaine or other psychotropic drug (see Table 11.1)
- Cerebral vasculitis
- Cerebral venous sinus thrombosis
- Acute disseminated encephalomyelitis (in young adults; usually follows infection)
- Malignant meningitis (carcinoma, melanoma, lymphoma, leukemia)
- Non-convulsive status epilepticus
- Brain tumor
- Sarcoidosis
- Drug-induced meningitis
- Neuroleptic malignant syndrome (Table 51.5)
- Behçet's disease
- Acute intermittent porphyria

**TABLE 51.4** Herpes simplex encephalitis

| Element | Comment |
|---|---|
| **Clinical features** | Acute onset (symptoms usually <1 week)<br>Fever<br>Headache<br>Personality change/abnormal behavior<br>Alteration in conscious level<br>Fits<br>Focal neurological abnormalities (cranial nerve palsies, dysphasia, hemiparesis, ataxia) |
| **CT** | May be normal<br>May show generalized brain swelling with loss of cortical sulci and small ventricles<br>May show areas of low attenuation in the temporal and/or frontal lobes |
| **Cerebrospinal fluid (CSF)** | May be normal<br>High lymphocyte count (50–500/mm$^3$), predominance of polymorphs in early phase, red cells often present<br>Protein concentration increased, up to 2.5 g/L<br>Glucose is usually normal but may be low<br>Herpes simplex DNA may be detected in CSF by the polymerase chain reaction |
| **EEG** | Abnormal in two-thirds of cases, with a spike and slow wave pattern localized to the area of brain involved |
| **Treatment** | Aciclovir 10 mg/kg 8-hourly IV<br>Seek expert advice |

**TABLE 51.5** Neuroleptic malignant syndrome

| Element | Comment |
|---|---|
| **Clinical features** | Preceding use of neuroleptic (usually develops within 2 weeks of starting medication) <br> Agitated confusional state progressing to stupor and coma <br> Generalized 'lead-pipe' muscular rigidity, often accompanied by tremor <br> Temperature >38°C (may be >40°C) <br> Autonomic instability: tachycardia, labile or high blood pressure, tachypnea, sweating |
| **CT** | Typically normal |
| **Cerebrospinal fluid** | Typically normal <br> May show raised protein |
| **EEG** | Generalized slow wave activity |
| **Blood tests** | High creatine kinase (typically >1000 units/L, and proportionate to rigidity) <br> High white cell count ($10$–$40 \times 10^9$/L) <br> Electrolyte derangements and raised creatinine common <br> Low serum iron level |
| **Treatment** | Stop neuroleptic <br> Supportive care <br> Use benzodiazepine if needed to control agitation <br> Consider use of dantrolene, bromocriptine or amantadine <br> Seek expert advice |

## Further reading

Adnet P, et al. Neuroleptic malignant syndrome. *Br J Anaesth* 2000; 85: 129–35.

Whitley RJ, Gnann JW. Viral encephalitis: familiar infections and emerging pathogens. *Lancet* 2002; 359: 507–13.

# 52 Spinal cord compression

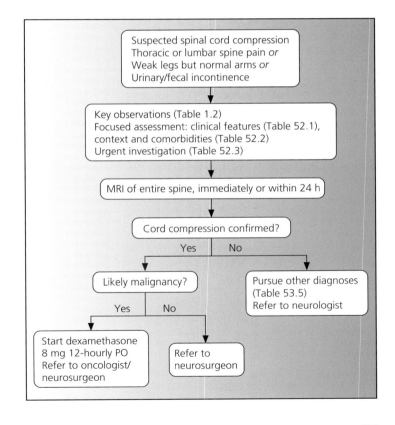

Suspected spinal cord compression
Thoracic or lumbar spine pain *or*
Weak legs but normal arms *or*
Urinary/fecal incontinence

Key observations (Table 1.2)
Focused assessment: clinical features (Table 52.1),
context and comorbidities (Table 52.2)
Urgent investigation (Table 52.3)

MRI of entire spine, immediately or within 24 h

Cord compression confirmed?

Yes     No

Likely malignancy?

Pursue other diagnoses
(Table 53.5)
Refer to neurologist

Yes     No

Start dexamethasone
8 mg 12-hourly PO
Refer to oncologist/
neurosurgeon

Refer to
neurosurgeon

**TABLE 52.1** Typical clinical features of spinal cord and conus/cauda equina compression

| Clinical feature | Site of compression | |
|---|---|---|
| | **Spinal cord** | **Conus and cauda equina** |
| **Site of pain** | Thoracolumbar | Lumbosacral and radicular |
| **Leg weakness** | Symmetrical | Asymmetrical |
| **Knee and ankle reflexes** | Increased | Variable |
| **Plantar responses** | Extensor | Variable |
| **Sensory loss** | Symmetrical with sensory level to pinprick, temperature or vibration | Variable; 'saddle' anesthesia (S3/S4/S5) with conus lesion (Fig. 46.1) |
| **Sphincter involvement** | Late | Early with conus lesion |
| **Progression** | Rapid | Variable |

**ALERT**

Consider spinal cord compression in any patient with spinal pain or weak legs but normal arms. Early diagnosis and treatment are crucial to preserving cord function.

**TABLE 52.2** Causes of non-traumatic extradural spinal cord compression

| Cause | Comment |
|---|---|
| **Malignancy** | Most commonly carcinoma of breast, bronchus or prostate<br>Compression is at thoracic level in 70%, lumbar in 20% and cervical in 10% |

*Continued*

| Spinal extradural abscess | Suspect if there is severe back pain, local spinal tenderness or systemic illness with fever/bacteremia |
|---|---|
| Extradural hematoma | Rare complication of warfarin anticoagulation |
| Prolapse of cervical or thoracic intervertebral disc | Suspect if there is spinal pain accompanied by root pain |
| Atlantoaxial subluxation | Complication of rheumatoid arthritis |

**TABLE 52.3** Urgent investigation in suspected spinal cord compression

- Anteroposterior and lateral X-rays of the spine (look for loss of pedicles, vertebral body destruction, spondylolisthesis, soft-tissue mass; NB normal plain films do not exclude spinal cord compression)
- MRI of the spine (of entire spine, as malignancy often causes multilevel lesions)
- Chest X-ray (look for primary or secondary tumor, or evidence of tuberculosis)
- Full blood count
- Erythrocyte sedimentation rate, C-reactive protein
- Blood culture
- Blood glucose
- Sodium, potassium and creatinine

**TABLE 52.4** Indications for surgery in malignant cord compression

- Single site of spinal cord compression
- Unknown histology with no other lesions for biopsy
- Bone compression or vertebral collapse in a patient with good performance status
- Progression after radiotherapy
- Radioresistant tumor

## Further reading

Darouiche RO. Spinal epidural abscess. *N Engl J Med* 2006; 355: 2012–20.
Gerrard GE, Franks KN. Overview of the diagnosis and management of brain, spine, and meningeal metastases. *J Neurol Neurosurg Psychiatry* 2004; 75 (suppl II): ii37–ii42.

# 53 Guillain–Barré syndrome

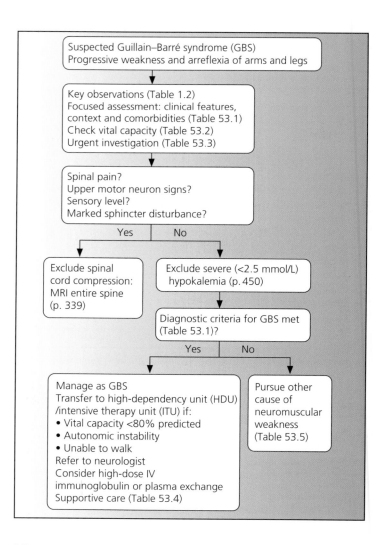

Suspected Guillain–Barré syndrome (GBS)
Progressive weakness and arreflexia of arms and legs

↓

Key observations (Table 1.2)
Focused assessment: clinical features,
context and comorbidities (Table 53.1)
Check vital capacity (Table 53.2)
Urgent investigation (Table 53.3)

↓

Spinal pain?
Upper motor neuron signs?
Sensory level?
Marked sphincter disturbance?

Yes / No

**Yes →**
Exclude spinal
cord compression:
MRI entire spine
(p. 339)

**No →**
Exclude severe (<2.5 mmol/L)
hypokalemia (p. 450)

↓

Diagnostic criteria for GBS met
(Table 53.1)?

Yes / No

**Yes →**
Manage as GBS
Transfer to high-dependency unit (HDU)
/intensive therapy unit (ITU) if:
• Vital capacity <80% predicted
• Autonomic instability
• Unable to walk
Refer to neurologist
Consider high-dose IV
immunoglobulin or plasma exchange
Supportive care (Table 53.4)

**No →**
Pursue other
cause of
neuromuscular
weakness
(Table 53.5)

---

**TABLE 53.1** Making the diagnosis of Guillain–Barré syndrome

**Features required for diagnosis**
- Progressive symmetrical weakness in both arms and both legs (which often begins proximally)
- Arreflexia

**Features strongly supporting diagnosis**
- Progression of symptoms over days to 4 weeks
- Relative symmetry of symptoms
- Mild sensory symptoms or signs
- Cranial nerve involvement, especially bilateral weakness of facial muscles
- Recovery beginning 2–4 weeks after progression ceases
- Autonomic dysfunction
- Absence of fever at onset
- High concentration of protein in cerebrospinal fluid, with fewer than $50/mm^3$ cells
- Typical electrodiagnostic features

**Features excluding diagnosis**
- Diagnosis of botulism, myasthenia, poliomyelitis or toxic neuropathy
- Abnormal porphyrin metabolism
- Recent diphtheria
- Purely sensory syndrome, without weakness

---

**ALERT**
Consider Guillain–Barré syndrome in any patient with paresthesiae in the fingers and toes or weakness of the arms and legs. Respiratory failure and autonomic instability are the major complications.

Guillain–Barré syndrome

**TABLE 53.2** Forced vital capacity (FVC in liters)*

Males†

| Height | | Age (years) | | | | | | | | | | |
|--------|------|-------|------|------|------|------|------|------|------|------|------|------|
| (ft/in) | (cm) | 20–25 | 30 | 35 | 40 | 45 | 50 | 55 | 60 | 65 | 70 |
| 5'3" | 160 | 4.17 | 4.06 | 3.95 | 3.84 | 3.73 | 3.62 | 3.51 | 3.40 | 3.29 | 3.18 |
| 5'6" | 168 | 4.53 | 4.42 | 4.31 | 4.20 | 4.09 | 3.98 | 3.87 | 3.76 | 3.65 | 3.54 |
| 5'9" | 175 | 4.95 | 4.84 | 4.73 | 4.62 | 4.51 | 4.40 | 4.29 | 4.18 | 4.07 | 3.96 |
| 6'0" | 183 | 5.37 | 5.26 | 5.15 | 5.04 | 4.93 | 4.82 | 4.71 | 4.60 | 4.49 | 4.38 |
| 6'3" | 190 | 5.73 | 5.62 | 5.51 | 5.40 | 5.29 | 5.18 | 5.07 | 4.96 | 4.85 | 4.74 |

Continued

Females‡

| Height | | Age (years) | | | | | | | | | |
|---|---|---|---|---|---|---|---|---|---|---|---|
| (ft/in) | (cm) | 20–25 | 30 | 35 | 40 | 45 | 50 | 55 | 60 | 65 | 70 |
| 4'9" | 145 | 3.13 | 2.98 | 2.83 | 2.68 | 2.53 | 2.38 | 2.23 | 2.08 | 1.93 | 1.78 |
| 5'0" | 152 | 3.45 | 3.30 | 3.15 | 3.00 | 2.85 | 2.70 | 2.55 | 2.40 | 2.25 | 2.10 |
| 5'3" | 160 | 3.83 | 3.68 | 3.53 | 3.38 | 3.23 | 3.08 | 2.93 | 2.78 | 2.63 | 2.48 |
| 5'6" | 168 | 4.20 | 4.05 | 3.90 | 3.75 | 3.60 | 3.45 | 3.30 | 3.15 | 3.00 | 2.85 |
| 5'9" | 175 | 4.53 | 4.38 | 4.23 | 4.08 | 3.93 | 3.78 | 3.63 | 3.48 | 3.33 | 3.18 |

\* The values shown are for people of European descent. For races with smaller thoraces (e.g. from the Indian subcontinent or Polynesia), subtract 0.7 L for FVC in males and 0.6 L in females.

† Standard deviation 0.6 L.

‡ Standard deviation 0.4 L.

From Cotes, J.E. *Lung Function*, 4th edn. Oxford: Blackwell Scientific Publications, 1978.

**ALERT**
Arterial blood gases can remain normal despite a severely reduced vital capacity. Pulse oximetry is not a substitute for measuring vital capacity. If no spirometer is available, the breath holding time in full inspiration is a guide to vital capacity (normal >30s), provided there is no coexisting respiratory disease.

---

**TABLE 53.3** Investigation in suspected Guillain–Barré syndrome (GBS)

- Blood glucose
- Biochemical profile
- Creatine kinase
- Full blood count
- Erythrocyte sedimentation rate and C-reactive protein (if high, consider fulminant mononeuritis multiplex, which can mimic GBS)
- ECG
- Chest X-ray
- Measurement of vital capacity with spirometer (Table 53.2)
- Cerebrospinal fluid protein and cell count
- Electrophysiological tests
- Stool culture for *Campylobacter jejuni* (the commonest recognized cause of GBS in the UK) and poliomyelitis
- Acute and convalescent serology for cytomegalovirus, Epstein–Barr virus and *Mycoplasma pneumoniae*

---

**ALERT**
Spinal cord compression is the most important differential diagnosis and must be excluded by MRI if there is spinal pain, a sensory level, marked sphincter disturbance or upper motor neuron signs.

**TABLE 53.4** Monitoring and supportive care in Guillain–Barré syndrome

- Transfer to HDU/ITU if:
  - Vital capacity <80% of predicted
  - Arrhythmia
  - Hypertension/hypotension (indicative of autonomic instability)
  - Unable to walk
- Admit other patients to a general ward for observation and further investigation. Monitor vital capacity, respiratory rate, heart rate and blood pressure 8-hourly
- Give analgesia as required (e.g. paracetamol 1 g 6-hourly and/or dihydrocodeine 30–60 mg 4-hourly PO)
- Start a stool softener to prevent constipation
- Use graduated compression stockings to reduce the risk of DVT

DVT, deep vein thrombosis; HDU, high-dependency unit; ITU, intensive therapy unit.

**TABLE 53.5** Causes of acute neuromuscular weakness

| Site of lesion | Causes |
| --- | --- |
| **Brain** | Stroke |
| | Mass lesion with brainstem compression |
| | Encephalitis |
| | Central pontine myelinolysis |
| | Sedative drugs |
| | Status epilepticus |
| **Spinal cord** | Cord compression |
| | Transverse myelitis |
| | Anterior spinal artery occlusion |
| | Hematomyelia |
| | Poliomyelitis |
| | Rabies |

*Continued*

| Site of lesion | Causes |
|---|---|
| **Peripheral nerve** | Guillain–Barré syndrome |
| | Critical illness neuropathy |
| | Toxins (heavy metals, biological toxins or drug intoxication) |
| | Acute intermittent porphyria |
| | Vasculitis, e.g. polyarteritis nodosa |
| | Lymphomatous neuropathy |
| | Diphtheria |
| **Neuromuscular junction** | Myasthenia gravis |
| | Eaton–Lambert syndrome |
| | Botulism |
| | Biological or industrial toxins |
| **Muscle** | Hypokalemia |
| | Hypophosphatemia |
| | Hypomagnesemia |
| | Inflammatory myopathy |
| | Critical illness myopathy |
| | Acute rhabdomyolysis (see Table 65.4) |
| | Trichinosis |
| | Periodic paralyses |

## Further reading

Hughes RAC, Cornblath DR. Guillain–Barre syndrome. *Lancet* 2005; 366: 1653–66.

# 54 Epilepsy (1): generalized convulsive status epilepticus

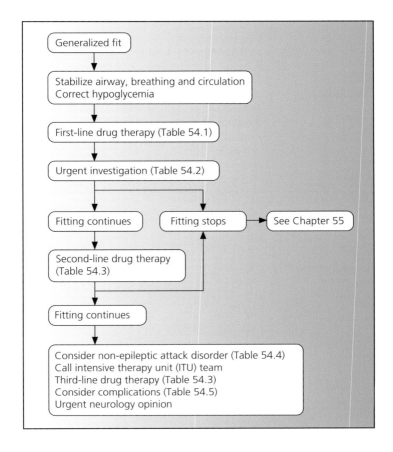

Generalized fit

↓

Stabilize airway, breathing and circulation
Correct hypoglycemia

↓

First-line drug therapy (Table 54.1)

↓

Urgent investigation (Table 54.2)

↓

Fitting continues → Fitting stops → See Chapter 55

↓

Second-line drug therapy
(Table 54.3)

↓

Fitting continues

↓

Consider non-epileptic attack disorder (Table 54.4)
Call intensive therapy unit (ITU) team
Third-line drug therapy (Table 54.3)
Consider complications (Table 54.5)
Urgent neurology opinion

**TABLE 54.1** First-line drug therapy for generalized convulsive status epilepticus

| Drug | Comments |
|------|----------|
| **Lorazepam** | 4 mg IV; dose can be repeated once after 10 min if fitting recurs |
| | Long duration of action and less likely to cause sudden hypotension or respiratory arrest than diazepam |
| | Second-line therapy should be started if control is not achieved within total dose of 8 mg |
| *or* | |
| **Diazepam** | 10–20 mg IV at a rate of <2.5 mg/min |
| | Risk of sudden apnea with faster injection |
| | Dose should not be repeated more than twice, or to a total dose >40 mg, because of the risks of respiratory depression and hypotension |
| | Second-line therapy should be started if control is not achieved within total dose of 40 mg |

**TABLE 54.2** Investigation in convulsive status epilepticus or after generalized fit

**Immediate**
- Blood glucose
- Sodium, potassium, calcium, magnesium and creatinine
- Arterial blood gases and pH

**Urgent**
- Anticonvulsant levels (if on therapy)
- Full blood count
- Coagulation screen
- Serum (10 ml) and urine sample (50 ml) (stored at 4°C) for toxicology screen (e.g. cocaine and amphetamine derivatives) if poisoning suspected or cause of fit is unclear
- Blood culture if febrile
- Liver function tests
- Chest X-ray
- CT scan (see below)
- Lumbar puncture (after CT) if suspected meningitis or encephalitis
- ECG (look for long QT interval, conduction abnormality, Q waves indicative of previous myocardial infarction – if present, consider arrhythmia rather than fit (see Table 19.2))
- EEG

**Indications for urgent CT scan after generalized fit**
- Focal neurological deficit
- Reduced conscious level
- Fever
- Recent head injury
- Persistent headache
- Known malignancy
- Warfarin anticoagulation
- HIV/AIDS

Epilepsy (1): generalized convulsive status epilepticus

**TABLE 54.3** Second- and third-line drug therapy for generalized convulsive status epilepticus

| Drug | Comments |
|---|---|
| **Second-line drug therapy** | |
| **Phenobarbital** | Loading dose: 10 mg/kg to a maximum of 1000 mg, given at 100 mg/min |
| **or** | Maintenance dose: 1–4 mg/kg/day given IV, IM or PO |
| **Phenytoin** (if not already taking phenytoin) | Loading dose: 15 mg/kg IV (for average sized adult, give 1000 mg over 20 min) Infusion rate should not exceed 50 mg/min Administer via IV line used for no other drugs Monitor ECG Maintenance dose: 100 mg 6–8-hourly IV |
| **or** | |
| **Paraldehyde** (if no IV access) | 10–20 ml PR or IM |
| **Third-line drug therapy** | |
| **Propofol** | 2 mg/kg IV bolus, then repeat bolus if necessary Maintenance dose: 5–10 mg/kg/h |
| *or* | |
| **Thiopental** | 100–250 mg IV bolus, then 50 mg bolus every 3 min until burst suppression on EEG Maintenance dose: 2–5 mg/kg/h |

---

**TABLE 54.4** Features of non-epileptic attack disorder (pseudoseizure)

- Asynchronous bilateral movements of the limbs, asymmetrical clonic contractions, pelvic thrusting and side to side movements of the head, often intensified by restraint
- Gaze aversion, resistance to passive limb movement or eye opening, prevention of the hand falling on to the face
- Incontinence, tongue biting and injury rare
- Normal tendon reflexes, plantar responses, blink, corneal and eyelash reflexes
- Absence of metabolic complications
- No postictal confusion (drowsiness may be due to diazepam given to treat suspected fit)

---

**TABLE 54.5** Complications of status epilepticus

**Cerebral**
- Hypoxic/metabolic brain injury
- Cerebral edema and raised intracranial pressure
- Todd paresis

**Systemic**
- Respiratory failure (p. 104)
- Aspiration pneumonia (p. 278)
- Lactic acidosis
- Cardiac arrhythmias
- Neurogenic pulmonary edema
- Hypotension
- Rhabdomyolysis (p. 417)
- Hyperkalemia (p. 446)
- Acute renal failure secondary to rhabdomyolysis (p. 410)
- Acute liver failure
- Disseminated intravascular coagulation

## Further reading

Meierkord H, et al. European Federation of Neurological Societies guideline on the management of status epilepticus (2006). European Federation of Neurological Societies website (http://www.efns.org/content.php?pid=145).

Walker M. Status epilepticus: an evidence based guide. *BMJ* 2005; 33: 673–7.

# 55 Epilepsy (2): management after a generalized fit

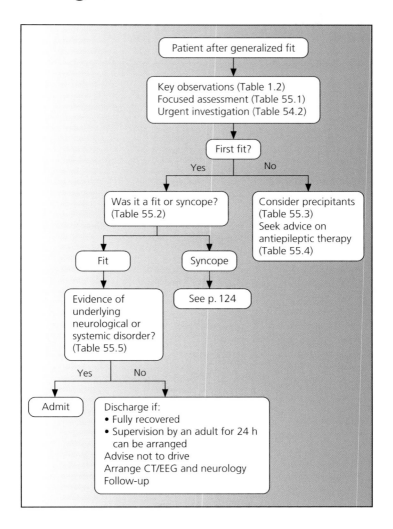

Patient after generalized fit

↓

Key observations (Table 1.2)
Focused assessment (Table 55.1)
Urgent investigation (Table 54.2)

↓

First fit?

Yes → No

**Yes:**
Was it a fit or syncope?
(Table 55.2)

**No:**
Consider precipitants
(Table 55.3)
Seek advice on
antiepileptic therapy
(Table 55.4)

Fit → Syncope

**Fit:**
Evidence of
underlying
neurological or
systemic disorder?
(Table 55.5)

**Syncope:**
See p. 124

Yes → No

**Yes:** Admit

**No:** Discharge if:
• Fully recovered
• Supervision by an adult for 24 h
  can be arranged
Advise not to drive
Arrange CT/EEG and neurology
Follow-up

**TABLE 55.1** Focused assessment after a generalized fit

**History**

**1** *Background*
- Known epilepsy? See Table 55.3 for precipitants of seizures in known epilepsy
- Previous significant head injury (i.e. with skull fracture or loss of consciousness)
- Birth injury, febrile convulsions in childhood, meningitis or encephalitis
- Family history of epilepsy
- Cardiac disease (?previous myocardial infarction, hypertrophic or dilated cardiomyopathy (at risk of ventricular tachycardia))
- Medications
- Alcohol or substance abuse
- Sleep deprivation

**2** *Before the attack*
- Prodromal symptoms: were these cardiovascular (e.g. dizziness, palpitation, chest pain) or focal neurological symptoms (aura)?
- Circumstances, e.g. exercising, standing, sitting or lying, asleep
- Precipitants, e.g. coughing, micturition, head turning

**3** *The attack*
- Were there any focal neurological features at the onset: sustained deviation of the head or eyes or unilateral jerking of the limbs?
- Was there a cry (may occur in tonic phase of fit)?
- Duration of loss of consciousness
- Associated tongue biting, urinary incontinence or injury
- Facial color changes (pallor common in syncope, uncommon with a fit)
- Abnormal pulse (must be assessed in relation to the reliability of the witness)

**4** *After the attack*
- Immediately well or delayed recovery with confusion or headache?

**Examination**
- Key observations (see Table 1.2)
- Conscious level, mental state and speech
- Neck stiffness?
- Focal neurological signs? As a minimum, check visual fields, limb power, tendon reflexes and plantar responses
- Fundi (?papilledema or retinal hemorrhages)
- Heart, lungs and abdomen

**TABLE 55.2** Was it a fit or syncope? Features differentiating a generalized fit from vasovagal and cardiac syncope (Stokes–Adams attack)

| Feature | Generalized fit | Vasovagal syncope | Cardiac syncope |
|---|---|---|---|
| **Occurrence when sitting or lying** | Common | Rare | Common |
| **Occurrence during sleep** | Common | Does not occur | May occur |
| **Prodromal symptoms** | May occur, with focal neurological symptoms, head turning, automatisms | Typical, with dizziness, sweating, nausea, blurring of vision, disturbance of hearing, yawning | Often none. Palpitation may precede syncope in tachyarrhythmias |
| **Focal neurological features at onset** | May occur (and signify focal cerebral lesion) | Never occur | Never occur |
| **Tonic-clonic movements** | Characteristic, occur within 30s of onset | May occur after 30s of syncope (secondary anoxic seizure) | May occur after 30s of syncope (secondary anoxic seizure) |
| **Facial color** | Flush or cyanosis at onset | Pallor at onset and after syncope | Pallor at onset, flush on recovery |
| **Tongue biting** | Common (lateral border) | Rare | Rare |
| **Urinary incontinence** | Common | May occur | May occur |
| **Injury** | May occur | Uncommon | May occur |
| **Postictal confusion** | Common (wakes in ambulance) | Uncommon (wakes on floor) | Uncommon (wakes on floor) |

**Epilepsy (2): management after a generalized fit**

**TABLE 55.3** Precipitants of seizures in known epilepsy

- Poor compliance with therapy, therapy recently reduced or stopped, or altered drug pharmacokinetics (e.g. drug interaction)
- Non-epileptic attack disorder (pseudoseizures) (see Table 54.4)
- Intercurrent infection
- Sleep deprivation
- Severe psychological stress
- Poisoning (Table 55.5)
- Alcohol withdrawal
- Proconvulsive drugs (Table 55.5)
- Progression of underlying structural brain lesion (e.g. glioma)

**TABLE 55.4** Maintenance antiepileptic therapy

| Seizure type | First-line drugs | Second-line drugs | Third-line drugs |
|---|---|---|---|
| **Generalized at onset** | Lamotrigine Valproate* | Levetiracetam Topiramate | Acetazolamide Clonazepam Phenobarbital Clobazam |
| **Focal at onset** | Carbamazepine Lamotrigine Valproate* | Gabapentin Levetiracetam Pregabalin Tiagabine Zonisamide | Acetazolamide Clonazepam Phenobarbital Phenytoin Clobazam |

* Teratogenic, so avoid in young women.

**TABLE 55.5** Causes of generalized seizures

**Neurological disorders**
- Epilepsy
- Stroke
- Meningitis
- Encephalitis
- Cerebral malaria
- Brain tumor
- Brain abscess
- Other cerebral space-occupying lesions
- Acute head injury
- Hypoxic ischemic brain injury (post-cardiopulmonary resuscitation)
- Advanced Alzheimer disease and other dementias
- Hypertensive encephalopathy
- Arteriovenous malformation
- Cerebral vasculitis

**Systemic disorders**
- Poisoning with alcohol, amphetamines, carbon monoxide (HbCO >50%), cocaine, heroin, MDMA ('ecstasy'), phenothiazines, theophylline, tricyclics
- Alcohol withdrawal
- Fulminant hepatic failure
- Advanced renal failure
- Hypoglycemia and hyperglycemia
- Electrolyte disorders: hyponatremia, hypocalcemia, hypomagnesemia
- Proconvulsive drugs: antibiotics in high dose, baclofen, clozapine, cyclosporin, flecainide, lidocaine, maprotiline, theophylline, tramadol

MDMA, methylene dioxymethamfetamine.

*Epilepsy (2): management after a generalized fit*

## Further reading

Brodie MJ, Kwan P. Epilepsy in elderly people. *BMJ* 2005; 331: 1317–22.

Duncan JS, et al. Adult epilepsy. *Lancet* 2006; 367: 1087–100.

Pohlmann-Eden B, et al. The first seizure and its management in adults and children. *BMJ* 2006; 332: 339–42.

# 56 Raised intracranial pressure

**TABLE 56.1** Causes of raised intracranial pressure

| Pathophysiology | Examples |
| --- | --- |
| **Localized mass lesion** | Traumatic hematoma |
| | Neoplasm |
| | Brain abscess |
| | Focal edema secondary to trauma, infarction or neoplasm |
| **Disturbances of CSF circulation** | Obstructive hydrocephalus |
| | Communicating hydrocephalus |
| **Obstruction to major venous sinuses** | Cerebral venous sinus thrombosis |
| | Depressed fracture overlying major venous sinus |
| **Diffuse brain edema** | Meningitis |
| | Encephalitis |
| | Subarachnoid hemorrhage |
| | Fulminant hepatic failure |
| | Hyponatremia |
| | Diabetic ketoacidosis |
| | Hypoxic ischemic brain injury |
| | Drowning |
| **Idiopathic** | Idiopathic intracranial hypertension |

CSF, cerebrospinal fluid.

**TABLE 56.2** Clinical features of raised intracranial pressure

**Clinical**
- Headache (typically throbbing or bursting; worse in the morning; exacerbated by coughing, sneezing, lying down, exertion)
- Nausea and vomiting
- Visual obscurations
- Absence of spontaneous retinal vein pulsation
- Papilledema
- Retinal hemorrhages if abrupt rise in intracranial pressure, e.g. subarachnoid hemorrhage

**Uncal (lateral) syndrome of herniation (typically seen with mass lesion)**
- Unilateral dilated pupil
- Contralateral hemiplegia
- Reduced level of consciousness progressing to coma
- Bilateral up-going plantar responses
- Decerebrate posturing
- Progressive brainstem dysfunction due to distortion/ischemia

**Central syndrome of herniation (typically seen with diffuse brain swelling)**
- Reduced level of consciousness progressing to coma
- Sighs and yawns/Cheyne–Stokes respirations
- Bilateral up-going plantar responses
- Decorticate posturing
- Progressive brainstem dysfunction due to distortion/ischemia

**TABLE 56.3** Factors which may exacerbate raised intracranial pressure

- Upper airway obstruction
- Obstruction of neck veins
- Hypoxia/hypercapnia
- Fits
- Fever
- Hypovolemia
- Hyponatremia

Raised intracranial pressure

---

**TABLE 56.4** Management of raised intracranial pressure

- Identify and treat the cause, and seek urgent advice on management from a neurologist or neurosurgeon
- Secure the airway and maintain a normal $PaO_2$ and $PaCO_2$. Ask for urgent help from an anesthetist with management of the airway and ventilation
- Maintain normal blood pressure
- Maintain normal blood glucose and electrolytes
- Control fits
- Nurse head-up 30° to optimize cerebral venous drainage
- Treat fever
- Ensure adequate analgesia and sedation
- Give dexamethasone 8 mg 12-hourly IV/PO for tumor-related cerebral edema
- Consider mannitol to reduce raised intracranial pressure due to diffuse cerebral edema. Give mannitol 20% 100–200 ml (0.5 g/kg) IV over 10 min, provided urine output is >30 ml/h. Check plasma osmolality: further mannitol may be given until plasma osmolality is 320 mosmol/kg

---

## Further reading

Dunn LT. Raised intracranial pressure. *J Neurol Neurosurg Psychiatry* 2002; 73 (suppl I): i23–i27.

# Gastrointestinal/liver/renal

# 57 Acute upper gastrointestinal hemorrhage

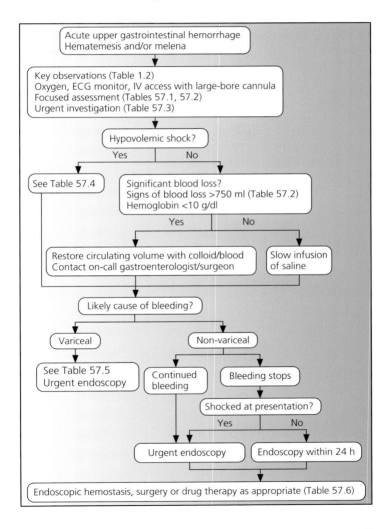

Acute upper gastrointestinal hemorrhage
Hematemesis and/or melena

Key observations (Table 1.2)
Oxygen, ECG monitor, IV access with large-bore cannula
Focused assessment (Tables 57.1, 57.2)
Urgent investigation (Table 57.3)

Hypovolemic shock?

Yes — See Table 57.4

No

Significant blood loss?
Signs of blood loss >750 ml (Table 57.2)
Hemoglobin <10 g/dl

Yes — Restore circulating volume with colloid/blood
Contact on-call gastroenterologist/surgeon

No — Slow infusion of saline

Likely cause of bleeding?

Variceal — See Table 57.5
Urgent endoscopy

Non-variceal

Continued bleeding

Bleeding stops

Shocked at presentation?

Yes — Urgent endoscopy

No — Endoscopy within 24 h

Endoscopic hemostasis, surgery or drug therapy as appropriate (Table 57.6)

**TABLE 57.1** Focused assessment in upper gastrointestinal (GI) hemorrhage

- Volume of blood lost (Table 57.2)?
- Variceal bleeding possible (known varices, known chronic liver disease, signs of chronic liver disease, signs of portal hypertension (splenomegaly, ascites))?
- Previous upper GI bleeding and endoscopy findings?
- Current and recent drug therapy (ask specifically about non-steroidal anti-inflammatory drugs (NSAIDs), aspirin and other antiplatelet agents, and warfarin)
- Usual and recent alcohol intake
- Did vomiting preceded the first hematemesis (suggesting Mallory–Weiss tear)?
- Other medical problems (especially cardiovascular and renal disease)?

**ALERT**

A good outcome in upper GI hemorrhage requires vigorous fluid resuscitation, and close collaboration between the admitting team, interventional endoscopist and GI surgeon.

**TABLE 57.2** Upper gastrointestinal hemorrhage: estimating the size of bleed*

**Major bleed (>1500 ml, >30% of blood volume)**
- Pulse >120/min
- Systolic BP <120 mmHg
- Cool or cold extremities with slow or absent capillary refill
- Tachypnea (respiratory rate >20/min)
- Abnormal mental state: agitation, confusion, reduced conscious level

**Minor bleed (<750 ml, <15% of blood volume)**
- Pulse <100/min
- Systolic BP >120 mmHg, with postural fall <20 mmHg from lying to sitting
- Normal perfusion of extremities
- Normal respiratory rate
- Normal mental state

* Bear in mind that the cardiovascular responses to blood loss are affected by rate of bleeding, age, associated cardiovascular disease and therapy (e.g. beta-blockers).

**TABLE 57.3** Urgent investigation in upper gastrointestinal hemorrhage

- Full blood count
- Group and save serum: cross-match 6 units of whole blood if there is shock or signs of major bleed
- Prothrombin time
- Sodium, potassium, creatinine and urea
- Liver function tests
- ECG if age >50 or known cardiac disease
- Chest X-ray
- Arterial blood gases and pH if there is shock

Acute upper gastrointestinal hemorrhage

**TABLE 57.4** Management of acute massive gastrointestinal hemorrhage with hypovolemic shock

| Goal | Procedures | Comments |
|------|-----------|----------|
| **Obtain help** | Call for help from:<br>• Senior colleague in medicine<br>• Duty gastroenterologist/surgeon<br>• Duty hematologist | Nominated coordinator should take responsibility for communication and documentation |
| **Secure airway and breathing** | Give oxygen 60–100%<br>Call anesthetist to assess airway if conscious level is impaired | Endotracheal intubation may be needed to protect airway and prevent pulmonary aspiration |
| **Restore circulating volume** | Put in a large-bore peripheral IV cannula (e.g. gray Venflon)<br>Rapidly infuse colloid until systolic BP is >90mmHg<br>If systolic BP is <90mmHg despite 1 L of colloid, use uncrossmatched O Rh− blood (no more than 2 units)<br>Use blood warmer | Monitor ECG<br>Put in bladder catheter and central venous cannula when patient is stable, to monitor urine output and central venous pressure<br>Aim for systolic BP >90mmHg and urine output >30ml/h<br>Keep patient warm (may require Bair-Hugger) |
| **Investigation** | See Table 57.3<br>Recheck FBC, PT, APTT and fibrinogen every 4 h or after one-third blood volume (>3 units) replacement or after blood component infusion | Clotting screen may be affected by colloid infusion<br>Misidentification is commonest transfusion risk |

Continued

| Goal | Procedures | Comments |
|------|-----------|----------|
| **Red cell replacement** | Give uncrossmatched O Rh– blood in extreme emergency (no more than 2 units)<br><br>Give uncrossmatched ABO-specific blood when blood group known<br><br>Use fully cross-matched blood if irregular antibodies are present<br><br>Use blood warmer if infusing at >50ml/kg/h | Rh+ is acceptable if male or postmenopausal female patient<br><br>Lab will complete cross-match after issue<br><br>Further cross-match not required until after replacement of one blood volume (8–10 units)<br><br>Packed red cells do not contain coagulation factors or platelets |
| **Request platelets if platelet count <50 × $10^9$/L** | Allow for delivery time (which may be 1–2 h if obtained from another center)<br><br>Anticipate platelet count <50 × $10^9$/L after two times blood volume replacements (>16 units) | Target platelet count >50 × $10^9$/L |
| **Request fresh frozen plasma (10–15ml/kg, ~1L or 4 units) if PT >20s and/orAPTT >48s** | Allow for delivery time plus 30min thawing time<br><br>Reverse warfarin anticoagulation with vitamin K 10mg IV; consider prothrombin complex concentrate (discuss with hematologist) | Aim for PT and APTT <1.5 × control |
| **Request cryoprecipitate (1–1.5 pack/10kg) if fibrinogen <1g/L** | Allow for delivery time plus 30min thawing time | Aim for fibrinogen >1g/L |
| **Arrest bleeding** | Plan interventional endoscopy or surgery | See Tables 57.5, 57.6 |

APTT, activated partial thromboplastin time; FBC, full blood count; PT, prothrombin time.

**Acute upper gastrointestinal hemorrhage**

---

**TABLE 57.5** Management of variceal bleeding

---

- Ask for help from a gastroenterologist
- Correct hypovolemia and clotting abnormalities. Give blood as soon as it is available, to minimize the sodium load from colloid or saline infusions
- Give terlipressin (to reduce portal pressure by splanchnic vasoconstriction) (causes less myocardial ischemia than vasopressin, and is more effective than octreotide): 2 mg IV followed by 1–2 mg every 4–6 h until bleeding is controlled, for up to 72 h
- If bleeding continues, put in a Sengstaken–Blakemore tube (p. 638)
- Arrange for urgent endoscopy with a view to injection sclerotherapy or banding of varices. To prevent inhalation, this is best done with a cuffed endotracheal tube
- Give a proton pump inhibitor orally or via the gastric channel of a Sengstaken–Blakemore tube or IV to prevent stress ulceration, and lactulose initially at 30 ml 3-hourly to prevent encephalopathy (p. 394)
- Infection is common in patients with variceal bleeding, and the incidence is reduced by prophylactic antibiotic therapy, begun before endoscopy. Give ciprofloxacin or equivalent IV, followed by oral therapy for a total of 7–10 days

---

**ALERT**

The mortality of variceal bleeding is around 50%. Urgent endoscopy is required to define the source of bleeding. Therapeutic endoscopy (injection sclerotherapy or banding) is the best treatment of bleeding varices.

**TABLE 57.6** Management of non-variceal upper gastrointestinal (GI) hemorrhage

**Peptic ulcer**
- Bleeding from a peptic ulcer usually stops spontaneously
- The mortality is highest in patients over 60 years who continue to bleed or rebleed; bleeding may be reduced by endoscopic hemostasis or surgery
- Drug treatment to heal the ulcer (e.g. proton pump inhibitor or $H_2$-receptor antagonist) should be given. In elderly patients, long-term treatment with a gastric antisecretory drug may be advisable to prevent recurrent bleeding
- Treatment to eradicate *Helicobacter pylori* should be given; nearly all duodenal ulcers, and most gastric ulcers not due to NSAIDs, are associated with *H. pylori* infection
- Patients with gastric ulcers (some of which are malignant) should have endoscopy repeated at 6–8 weeks

**Erosive gastritis**
There are two groups of patients:
- Previously well patients in whom erosive gastritis is related to aspirin, NSAIDs or alcohol. Bleeding usually stops quickly and no specific treatment is needed
- Critically ill patients with stress ulceration, in whom the mortality is high. Give a proton pump inhibitor IV and correct clotting abnormalities. As a last resort, if bleeding is catastrophic, surgery with partial gastric resection can be done but carries a high mortality

**Mallory–Weiss tear**
- Bleeding usually stops spontaneously and rebleeding is rare
- If bleeding continues, the options are endoscopic hemostasis, interventional radiology or surgery

**Esophagitis and esophageal ulcer**
- Give a proton pump inhibitor for 4 weeks, followed by a further 4–8 weeks treatment if not fully healed

*Continued*

**Upper GI hemorrhage with 'negative' endoscopy**

- In a significant proportion of patients, a first endoscopy does not reveal a source of bleeding
- Discuss repeating the endoscopy, especially if blood or food obscured the views obtained, or the patient has chronic liver disease (as varices which have recently bled may not be visible)
- Patients who presented with melena only should be investigated for a small bowel or proximal colonic source of bleeding if no upper GI source is found. A normal blood urea suggests a colonic cause of melena, except in patients with chronic liver disease
- Visceral angiography can be useful after two negative endoscopies, but only if done when the patient is actively bleeding

NSAIDs, non-steroidal anti-inflammatory drugs.

## Further reading

Barkun A, et al. Consensus recommendations for managing patients with nonvariceal upper gastrointestinal bleeding. *Ann Intern Med* 2003; 139: 843–57.

Bosch J, Garcia-Pagan JC. Prevention of variceal rebleeding. *Lancet* 2003; 361: 952–4.

Jalan R, Hayes PC. UK guidelines on the management of variceal haemorrhage in cirrhotic patients. *Gut* 2000; 6 (suppl III): iii1–iii15.

Sharara AI, Rockey DC. Gastroesophageal variceal hemorrhage. *N Engl J Med* 2001; 345: 669–81.

Stainsby D, et al. Management of massive blood loss: a template guideline. *Br J Anaesth* 2000; 85: 487–91.

# 58 Esophageal rupture

---

**TABLE 58.1** Causes of esophageal perforation/rupture

- Spontaneous esophageal rupture, typically associated with vomiting (Boerhaave syndrome) (usually occurs in the left posterolateral wall of the lower third of the esophagus, with leak into the left pleural cavity)
- Blunt trauma to the chest
- Instrumentation of the esophagus (risk with diagnostic endoscopy very low; risk increased with procedures such as dilatation of stricture or sclerotherapy of varices)
- Surgery to esophagus or adjacent structures
- Left atrial radiofrequency ablation for atrial fibrillation (causing atrioesophageal fistula)

---

**TABLE 58.2** Features of spontaneous esophageal rupture (Boerhaave syndrome)

**History**
- Typical presentation is vomiting followed by severe lower retrosternal chest pain in a middle-aged male, often with a background of heavy alcohol intake
- Esophageal rupture may occur without vomiting, and may follow straining (e.g. in labor or with weight-lifting), coughing or hiccoughing

**Examination**
- Pneumomediastinum may result in subcutaneous emphysema (found in ~25% patients) and crackling sounds on auscultation of the heart
- There may be signs of pleural effusion/pneumothorax
- Signs of septic shock (from mediastinitis) may dominate the clinical picture and are seen in ~25% of patients at presentation

**Differential diagnosis**
- Includes myocardial infarction, aortic dissection, pulmonary embolism, pericarditis, pneumonia, spontaneous pneumothorax, perforated peptic ulcer, acute pancreatitis
- Misdiagnosis of spontaneous esophageal rupture is common

**Esophageal rupture**

**TABLE 58.3** Urgent investigation in suspected Boerhaave syndrome

| Test | Comment |
| --- | --- |
| **Chest X-ray** | Almost always abnormal in Boerhaave syndrome although changes may be subtle at presentation<br>Abnormalities seen include pneumomediastinum, mediastinal widening, subcutaneous emphysema, pleural effusion (usually on left), pneumothorax, free peritoneal gas |
| **CT thorax** | Indicated if chest X-ray is non-diagnostic and other diagnoses such as aortic dissection or pulmonary embolism are more likely<br>In Boerhaave syndrome, CT may show extraesophageal gas, periesophageal fluid, mediastinal widening, and gas and fluid in pleural spaces, retroperitoneum and lesser sac |
| **Water-soluble (Gastrografin) contrast swallow** | Definitive test. Reveals location and extent of extravasation of contrast medium<br>If negative despite high clinical index of suspicion, barium swallow should be done |
| **Aspiration of pleural effusion** | Exudative pleural effusion with low pH, high amylase level, purulent; may contain undigested food |
| **Tests to exclude other diagnoses and needed in management** | ECG, arterial blood gases and pH, full blood count, group and save, biochemistry, blood culture |

---

**TABLE 58.4** Management of Boerhaave syndrome

- Urgent surgical opinion
- Admit to high-dependency unit (HDU)/intensive therapy unit (ITU)
- Nil by mouth
- Nasogastric drainage
- Opioid analgesia + antiemetic
- IV fluids
- Antibiotic therapy to cover anaerobic and Gram-positive/Gram-negative aerobic bacteria: e.g. piperacillin/tazobactam + metronidazole + gentamicin
- Management of septic shock if present (p. 60)

---

## Further reading

Henderson JAM, Peloquin AJM. Boerhaave revisited: spontaneous esophageal perforation as a diagnostic masquerade. *Am J Med* 1989; 86: 559–67.

Khan AZ, Strauss D, Mason RC. Boerhaare's syndrome: diagnosis and surgical management. *Surgeon* 2007; 5: 39–44.

Younes Z, Johnson D. The spectrum of spontaneous and iatrogenic esophageal injury: perforations, Mallory–Weiss tears, and hematomas. *J Clin Gastroenterol* 1999; 29: 306–17.

Esophageal rupture

# 59  Acute diarrhea

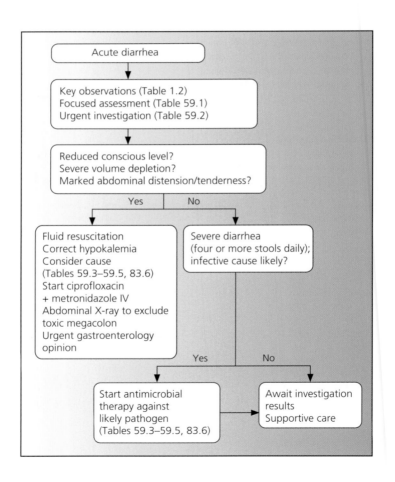

Acute diarrhea

↓

Key observations (Table 1.2)
Focused assessment (Table 59.1)
Urgent investigation (Table 59.2)

↓

Reduced conscious level?
Severe volume depletion?
Marked abdominal distension/tenderness?

Yes — No

**Yes:**
Fluid resuscitation
Correct hypokalemia
Consider cause
(Tables 59.3–59.5, 83.6)
Start ciprofloxacin
+ metronidazole IV
Abdominal X-ray to exclude
toxic megacolon
Urgent gastroenterology
opinion

**No:**
Severe diarrhea
(four or more stools daily);
infective cause likely?

Yes — No

**Yes:**
Start antimicrobial
therapy against
likely pathogen
(Tables 59.3–59.5, 83.6)

**No:**
Await investigation
results
Supportive care

---

**TABLE 59.1** Focused assessment in acute diarrhea

**History**
- Mode of onset (abrupt, subacute or gradual) and duration
- Frequency and nature of the stools (watery or containing blood and mucus). Severe diarrhea is defined as four or more stools daily; bloody stools are a common feature of shigellosis, salmonellosis, severe *Campylobacter* enteritis and ulcerative colitis, and are rare (5%) in *Clostridium difficile* infection
- Have others in the same household or who have shared the same food also developed diarrhea?
- Other symptoms (malaise, fever, vomiting, abdominal pain)?
- Current or recent hospital inpatient (at risk of *C. difficile* infection)?
- Travel abroad in the past 6 months?
- Previous significant gastrointestinal symptoms or known gastrointestinal diagnosis?
- Medications (in particular antibiotics) taken in the 6 weeks before the onset of diarrhea?
- Any other medical problems? (Causes of acute diarrhea in HIV/AIDS are given in Table 83.6)

**Examination**
- Severity of illness and degree of volume depletion (mental state, temperature, heart rate, blood pressure lying and sitting)
- Signs of toxic megacolon (marked abdominal distension and tenderness)? (May complicate many forms of infective colitis (including *C. difficile*) as well as colitis due to inflammatory bowel disease)
- Extra-abdominal features (e.g. rash and arthropathy)?

**Acute diarrhea**

**ALERT**
Diarrhea in the HIV-positive patient: see Table 83.6, p. 541.

---

**TABLE 59.2** Urgent investigation in acute severe diarrhea

- Stool microscopy and culture
- Test for *Clostridium difficile* toxin in stool
- Full blood count
- Erythrocyte sedimentation rate and C-reactive protein
- Blood glucose
- Sodium, potassium and creatinine
- Albumin and liver function tests
- Blood culture if febrile
- Sigmoidoscopy if bloody diarrhea
- Abdominal X-ray if marked distension or tenderness (?toxic megacolon)

---

**TABLE 59.3** Community-acquired diarrhea

| Cause | Clinical features | Diagnosis/treatment (if indicated) |
|---|---|---|
| **Campylobacter enteritis (C. jejuni)** | Incubation period 2–6 days<br>Associated fever and abdominal pain<br>Diarrhea initially watery, later may contain blood and mucus<br>Usually self-limiting, lasting 2–5 days<br>May be followed after 1–3 weeks by Guillain–Barré syndrome (p. 342) | Culture of *C. jejuni* from stool<br>Ciprofloxacin 500 mg 12-hourly PO for 5 days *or* Erythromycin 500 mg 12-hourly PO for 5 days |
| **Non-typhoid salmonellosis** | Incubation period 1–2 days | Culture of *Salmonella* species from stool. |

*Continued*

| Cause | Clinical features | Diagnosis/treatment (if indicated) |
|-------|-------------------|-----------------------------------|
| *(Salmonella* **species)** | Associated fever, vomiting and abdominal pain<br>Diarrhea may become bloody if colon is involved<br>Usually self-limiting<br>More severe in immunosuppressed | Ciprofloxacin 500 mg 12-hourly PO for 5 days *or*<br>Trimethoprim 200 mg 12-hourly PO for 5 days |
| *Escherichia coli* **O157:H7 (enterohemorrhagic** *E. coli***)** | Incubation period 1–3 days<br>Associated vomiting and abdominal pain<br>May have low grade fever<br>Watery diarrhea, which may become bloody<br>May be complicated by hemolytic uremic syndrome from 2–14 (mean 7) days after onset of illness | Culture of *E. coli* O157 from stool (using sorbitol MacConkey agar; missed by standard culture)<br>Serological tests<br>Supportive treatment: antibiotic therapy is unhelpful |
| *Clostridium difficile* **colitis** | Typically causes diarrhea in hospital, but may occur in community (see Table 59.4) | |
| **Ulcerative colitis** | May present with acute diarrhea, usually bloody<br>Vomiting does not occur, and abdominal pain is not a prominent feature | Exclusion of infective causes of diarrhea and typical histological appearances on rectal biopsy<br>IV and rectal steroid |
| **Fecal impaction with overflow diarrhea** | At risk of fecal impaction<br>No vomiting or systemic illness | Rectal examination discloses hard impacted feces<br>Laxatives/enemas |

Acute diarrhea

**Acute diarrhea**

TABLE 59.4 Hospital-acquired diarrhea

| Cause | Clinical features | Diagnosis/treatment |
|---|---|---|
| **Clostridium difficile colitis** | Diarrhea usually begins within 4–10 days of antibiotic treatment, but may not appear for 4–6 weeks<br><br>Presentations range from mild self-limiting watery diarrhea to (rarely) acute fulminating toxic megacolon<br><br>Low grade fever and abdominal tenderness are common<br><br>Although the rectum and sigmoid colon are usually involved, in 10% of cases colitis is confined to the more proximal colon | Diagnosis is based on detection of C. difficile toxins A and B in the stool. In severe colitis, sigmoidoscopy may show adherent yellow plaques (2–10 mm in diameter)<br><br>Supportive treatment and isolation of the patient to reduce the risk of spread<br><br>Stop antibiotic therapy if possible. If diarrhea is mild (1–2 stools daily), symptoms may resolve within 1–2 weeks without further treatment<br><br>If antibiotic therapy needs to be continued, or if moderate/severe diarrhea (three or more stools daily), give metronidazole 400 mg 8-hourly PO for 7–10 days<br><br>Around 20% of patients will have a relapse after completing a course of metronidazole, due to germination of residual spores within the colon, reinfection with C. difficile, or further antibiotic treatment: give either a further course of metronidazole or vancomycin 125 mg 6-hourly PO for 7–10 days<br><br>If the patient is severely ill and unable to take oral medication, give metronidazole 500 mg 8-hourly IV (IV vancomycin should not be used as significant excretion into the gut does not occur). |
| **Drugs** | Many drugs may cause diarrhea, including chemotherapeutic agents, proton pump inhibitors and laxatives in excess | Diarrhea resolves after treatment is completed or with withdrawal of the causative drug |

**TABLE 59.5** Acute diarrhea following recent travel abroad

| Cause | Clinical features | Diagnosis/treatment |
|---|---|---|
| **Giardiasis (*Giardia lamblia*)** | Widespread distribution Explosive onset of watery diarrhoea 1–3 weeks after exposure | Identification of cysts or trophozoites in stool or jejunal biopsy Metronidazole 400 mg 8-hourly for 5 days |
| **Amoebic dysentery (*Entamoeba histolytica*)** | Mexico, South America, South Asia, West and South-East Africa Diarrhea may be severe with blood and mucus | Identification of cysts in stools Metronidazole 800 mg 8-hourly for 5 days |
| **Schistosomiasis (*Schistosoma mansoni* and *S. japonicum*)** | *S. mansoni*: South America and Middle East *S. japonicum*: China and the Philippines Diarrhea onset 2–6 weeks or longer after exposure | Identification of ova in stool Praziquantel (seek expert advice) |
| **Shigellosis (*Shigella* species)** | Incubation period 1–2 days Associated fever and abdominal pain Diarrhea may be watery or bloody | Culture of *Shigella* species from stool Ciprofloxacin 500 mg 12-hourly PO for 5 days *or* Trimethoprim 200 mg 12-hourly PO for 5 days |
| **Non-typhoid salmonellosis** | See Table 59.3 | |

Acute diarrhea

## Further reading

Musher DM, Musher BL. Contagious acute gastrointestinal infections. *N Engl J Med* 2004; 351: 2417–27.

Starr J. *Clostridium difficile* associated diarrhoea: diagnosis and treatment. *BMJ* 2005; 331: 498–501.

# 60 Acute jaundice

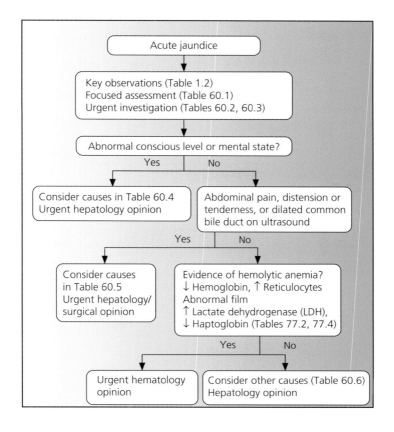

Acute jaundice

Key observations (Table 1.2)
Focused assessment (Table 60.1)
Urgent investigation (Tables 60.2, 60.3)

Abnormal conscious level or mental state?

Yes     No

Consider causes in Table 60.4
Urgent hepatology opinion

Abdominal pain, distension or tenderness, or dilated common bile duct on ultrasound

Yes     No

Consider causes in Table 60.5
Urgent hepatology/ surgical opinion

Evidence of hemolytic anemia?
↓ Hemoglobin, ↑ Reticulocytes
Abnormal film
↑ Lactate dehydrogenase (LDH),
↓ Haptoglobin (Tables 77.2, 77.4)

Yes     No

Urgent hematology opinion

Consider other causes (Table 60.6)
Hepatology opinion

**TABLE 60.1** Focused assessment of the jaundiced patient

**History**
- Duration and time course of jaundice and other symptoms (e.g. fever, abdominal pain)
- Known liver or biliary tract disease?
- Full drug history, to include all prescription and non-prescription drugs, herbal remedies and dietary supplements taken over the past year
- Risk factors for viral hepatitis (foreign travel, IV drug use, men who have sex with men, multiple sexual partners, body piercing and tattoos, blood transfusion and blood products, needle-stick injury in health-care worker)?
- Sexual history
- Pregnancy?
- Usual and recent alcohol intake (see Table 87.1)?
- Foreign travel in past 6 months?
- Other medical problems (e.g. cardiovascular disease, transplant recipient, cancer, HIV/AIDS, hematological disease)?
- Family history of jaundice/liver disease?

**Examination**
- Key observations (see Table 1.2) and systematic examination (see Table 1.9)
- Conscious level and mental state; grade of encephalopathy if present:

**Grading of hepatic encephalopathy**

| | |
|---|---|
| **Subclinical** | Impaired work, personality change, sleep disturbance. Impaired psychomotor testing |
| **Grade 1** | Mild confusion, agitation, apathy. Fine tremor, asterixis |
| **Grade 2** | Drowsiness, lethargy, disorientation. Asterixis, dysarthria |
| **Grade 3** | Sleepy but rousable. Marked confusion. Hyperreflexia, hyperventilation |
| **Grade 4** | Unrousable: 4a, responsive to painful stimuli; 4b, unresponsive. Decerebrate posturing, oculocephalic reflexes intact |

- Depth of jaundice?
- Signs of chronic liver disease?
- Right upper quadrant tenderness?
- Liver enlargement (seen in early viral hepatitis, alcoholic hepatitis, malignant infiltration, congestive heart failure, acute Budd–Chiari syndrome)?
- Splenomegaly?
- Ascites?

**TABLE 60.2** Urgent investigation in acute jaundice

- Prothrombin time
- Full blood count
- Reticulocyte count and blood film if suspected hemolysis
- Blood glucose
- Sodium, potassium, creatinine and urea
- Liver function tests: bilirubin (total and unconjugated), aspartate transaminase, alanine transaminase, gamma-glutamyl transferase, alkaline phosphatase, albumin (see Table 60.3)
- Serum LDH and haptoglobin if suspected hemolysis
- Blood culture
- Urine stick test, microscopy and culture
- Markers of viral hepatitis (anti-HAV IgM, HBsAg, anti-HBc IgM, anti-HCV, anti-HEV)
- Microscopy and culture of ascites if present (aspirate 10 ml for cell count (use EDTA tube) and culture (inoculate blood culture bottles) (see p. 389)
- Ultrasound of liver, biliary tract and hepatic/portal veins
- Pregnancy test in women of child-bearing age
- Consider copper studies in young adults (Wilson disease, see Table 62.1)

EDTA, ethylene diaminetetra-acetic acid; HAV, hepatitis A virus; HBc, hepatitis B core; HBsAG, hepatitis B surface antigen; HCV, hepatitis C virus; HEV, hepatitis E virus; IgM, immunoglobulin M; LDH, lactate dehydrogenase.

**ALERT**
Acute Jaundice is due to biliary obstruction by stones or cancer in ~50% of cases.

Acute jaundice

**TABLE 60.3** Causes of plasma aspartate and alanine transaminase levels of more than 1000 units/L

**Common**
- Acute viral hepatitis
- Ischemic hepatitis
- Acute drug- or toxin-related liver injury

**Rare**
- Acute exacerbation of autoimmune chronic active hepatitis
- Reactivation of chronic hepatitis B
- Acute Budd–Chiari syndrome (see Table 62.1)
- Veno-occlusive disease
- HELLP syndrome (hemolysis, elevated liver enzymes, low platelet count; p. 553)
- Acute fatty liver of pregnancy
- Hepatic infarction (may complicate HELLP syndrome)
- Hepatitis delta in a chronic carrier of hepatitis B
- Acute Wilson disease (see Table 62.1)
- Massive lymphomatous infiltration of the liver

**TABLE 60.4** Jaundice with abnormal conscious level/mental state

- Fulminant hepatic failure (see Table 62.1)
- Decompensated chronic liver disease (see Table 62.2)
- Postcardiac arrest: ischemic hepatitis plus hypoxic ischemic brain injury
- Sepsis with multiple organ failure
- Severe acute cholangitis (see Table 64.1)
- Alcoholic hepatitis (see Table 63.1)
- Falciparum malaria (see Table 84.4)

---

**TABLE 60.5** Jaundice with abdominal pain, distension or tenderness

- Acute cholangitis (see Table 64.1)
- Intra-abdominal sepsis
- Paracetamol poisoning (p. 75)
- Congestive heart failure
- Liver abscess
- Viral hepatitis
- Alcoholic hepatitis (see Table 63.1)
- Acute pancreatitis (see Table 64.2)
- HELLP syndrome of pregnancy (hemolysis, elevated liver enzymes, low platelet count) (p. 553)
- Budd–Chiari syndrome (see Table 62.1)

---

**TABLE 60.6** Causes of intrahepatic cholestasis

- Viral hepatitis (some cases)
- Alcoholic hepatitis
- Drugs and toxins
- Sepsis
- Primary biliary cirrhosis
- Primary sclerosing cholangitis
- Liver infiltration (e.g. sarcoidosis, tuberculosis, lymphoma)
- Intrahepatic cholestasis of pregnancy
- Syphilitic hepatitis
- End-stage liver disease

**Acute jaundice**

## Further reading

Beckingham IJ, Ryder SD. Investigation of liver and biliary disease. *BMJ* 2001; 322: 33–6.

# 61 Ascites

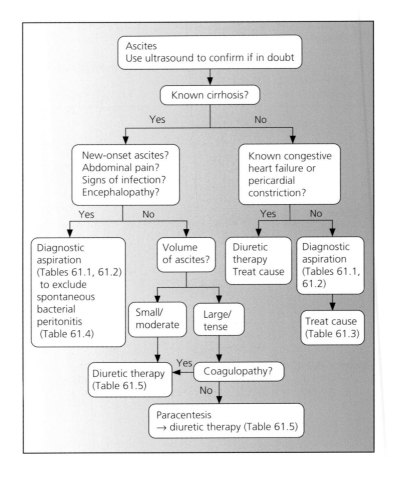

Ascites
Use ultrasound to confirm if in doubt

Known cirrhosis?

Yes — New-onset ascites?
Abdominal pain?
Signs of infection?
Encephalopathy?

No — Known congestive
heart failure or
pericardial
constriction?

Yes — Diagnostic
aspiration
(Tables 61.1, 61.2)
to exclude
spontaneous
bacterial
peritonitis
(Table 61.4)

No — Volume
of ascites?

Yes — Diuretic
therapy
Treat cause

No — Diagnostic
aspiration
(Tables 61.1,
61.2)

Small/
moderate

Large/
tense

Treat cause
(Table 61.3)

Diuretic therapy
(Table 61.5)

Yes — Coagulopathy?

No — Paracentesis
→ diuretic therapy (Table 61.5)

---

**TABLE 61.1** Diagnostic aspiration of ascites

---

**1** Confirm the indications for aspiration of ascites. Explain the procedure to the patient and obtain consent
- Deranged clotting (common in patients with cirrhosis and ascites) is not a contraindication, but ask advice from a hematologist if the patient has disseminated intravascular coagulation (see Table 78.4)
- Complications of the procedure (hematoma, hemoperitoneum, infection) are rare. Inadvertent puncture of the intestine may occur but rarely leads to secondary infection
**2** The patient should lie relaxed in a supine position, having emptied the bladder
- Select a site for puncture in the right or left lower quadrant, away from scars and the inferior epigastric artery (whose surface marking is a line drawn from the femoral pulse to the umbilicus)
**3** Put on gloves. Prepare the skin with chlorhexidine or povidone-iodine. Anesthetize the skin with 2 ml of lidocaine 1% using a 25 G (orange) needle. Then infiltrate a further 5 ml of lidocaine along the planned needle path through the abdominal wall and down to the peritoneum
**4** Give the local anesthetic time to work. Mount a 21 G (green) needle on a 50 ml syringe and then advance along the anesthetized path. Aspirate as you advance. Having entered the peritoneal cavity, aspirate 30–50 ml of ascites. Remove the needle and place a small dressing over the puncture site
**5** Send samples for:
- Albumin concentration (plain tube)
- Total and differential white cell count (EDTA tube)
- Bacterial culture (inoculate aerobic and anaerobic blood culture bottles with 10 ml each)
- Other tests if indicated (Table 61.2)
**6** Clear up and dispose of sharps safely. Write a note of the procedure in the patient's record: approach/appearance of ascites/volume aspirated/samples sent. Ensure the samples are sent promptly for analysis

---

EDTA, ethylene diaminetetra-acetic acid.

Ascites

**TABLE 61.2** Ascites: tests

| Test | Comment |
|------|---------|
| **Visual inspection** | Ascites due to cirrhosis is usually clear yellow, but may be cloudy when complicated by spontaneous bacterial peritonitis |
| **Albumin concentration** | Measure the albumin concentration in ascites and serum and calculate the serum–ascites albumin gradient (SAAG) (serum minus ascitic albumin concentration) |
| | A SAAG of 11 g/L or greater indicates portal hypertension with 97% accuracy, while a SAAG of <11 g/L indicates the absence of portal hypertension |
| | Causes of ascites according to the SAAG are given in Table 61.3 |
| **Total and differential white cell count** | Send a sample in an EDTA tube to the hematology lab for total and differential white cell count |
| | In uncomplicated cirrhosis, the total white cell count is <500/mm$^3$ and neutrophil count <250/mm$^3$ |
| | Spontaneous bacterial peritonitis is associated with a neutrophil count of >250/mm$^3$ |
| | In peritoneal tuberculosis, the white cell count is usually 150–4000/mm$^3$, predominantly lymphocytes |
| **Bacterial culture** | Send ascites for culture in patients with new-onset ascites or if you suspect infection (fever, abdominal pain, confusion, renal failure or acidosis) |
| | Inoculate aerobic and anaerobic blood culture bottles with 10 ml per bottle of ascites |
| **Cytology** | Send a sample for cytology if you suspect malignancy or if the SAAG is <11 g/L |
| | Cytology is usually positive in the presence of |

*Continued*

| Test | Comment |
|------|---------|
| | peritoneal metastases, but these are found in only about two-thirds of patients with ascites related to malignancy |
| **Other tests** | Total protein, glucose, LDH |
| | Gram stain |
| | Ziehl–Neelsen stain and testing for *Mycobacterium tuberculosis* DNA if suspected tuberculosis |
| | Amylase if suspected pancreatitis |

EDTA, ethylene diaminetetra-acetic acid; LDH, lactate dehydrogenase.

---

**TABLE 61.3** Causes of ascites according to the serum–ascites albumin gradient (SAAG)

**High SAAG (11 g/L or greater)** (associated with portal hypertension)
- Cirrhosis
- Alcoholic hepatitis
- Hepatic outflow obstruction:
  - Budd–Chiari syndrome (thrombosis of one or more of the large hepatic veins, the inferior vena cava, or both)
  - Hepatic veno-occlusive disease
- Cardiac ascites:
  - Tricuspid regurgitation
  - Constrictive pericarditis
  - Right-sided heart failure

**Low SAAG (<11 g/L)** (associated with peritoneal neoplasms, infection and inflammation)
- Peritoneal carcinomatosis
- Peritoneal tuberculosis
- Pancreatitis
- Serositis
- Nephrotic syndrome
- Myxedema
- Meig syndrome

**TABLE 61.4** Spontaneous bacterial peritonitis

- Defined as spontaneous infection of ascitic fluid in the absence of an intra-abdominal source of infection
- It is a common complication of ascites due to cirrhosis
- Prevalence among patients with ascites is between 10% and 30%
- Causes fever (70%), abdominal pain (60%), abdominal tenderness (50%) and change in mental state (50%)
- Diagnosis based on finding of >250 neutrophils/mm$^3$ of ascitic fluid
- Aerobic Gram-negative bacteria, especially *Escherichia coli*, are the commonest organisms
- May be complicated by hepatorenal syndrome (in up to 30% of patients, see Table 62.5): IV albumin solution 1.5 g/kg at diagnosis and 1 g/kg 48 h later may reduce the likelihood of hepatorenal syndrome developing, and improve prognosis
- Treat with third-generation cephalosporin, e.g. cefotaxime 2 g 8-hourly IV daily for 5 days, followed by quinolone PO for 5 days
- Recurrence is common (estimated 70% probablility of recurrence at 1 year). Consider prophylaxis with quinolone or co-trimoxazole.

**TABLE 61.5** Management of ascites due to cirrhosis

- Restrict dietary sodium intake to ~50 mmol/day
- Start diuretic therapy with spironolactone 100 mg daily + furosemide 40 mg daily PO, as single morning doses
- Monitor daily weight. Target weight loss is 0.5 kg daily in patients without peripheral edema and 1 kg daily in those with peripheral edema
- Increase the doses of spironolactone (by 100 mg steps) and furosemide (by 40 mg steps) every 3–5 days if target weight loss is not achieved, to maximum doses of spironolactone 400 mg daily and furosemide 160 mg daily (as single or divided doses)
- Reduce the spironolactone dose if there is hyperkalemia
- Amiloride (10–40 mg daily) can be substituted for spironolactone if there is symptomatic gynecomastia
- If there is tense ascites, consider a single paracentesis (to remove 5 L), followed by dietary sodium restriction and diuretic therapy. Albumin solution (8 g albumin per liter of ascites removed) should be given IV during paracentesis. Seek advice from a hepatologist/ gastroenterologist

**ALERT**

Patients who develop ascites as a complication of cirrhosis have a poor prognosis (2-year survival ~50%), and should be referred to a hepatologist for consideration of liver transplantation.

## Further reading

Gines P, et al. Management of cirrhosis and ascites. *N Engl J Med* 2004; 350: 1646–54.

Menon KVN, et al. The Budd–Chiari syndrome. *N Engl J Med* 2004; 350: 578–85.

Soares-Weiser K, et al. Antibiotic treatment for spontaneous bacterial peritonitis. *BMJ* 2002; 324: 100–2.

Thomsen TW. Paracentesis. *N Engl J Med* 2006; 355: e21.

# 62 Acute liver failure

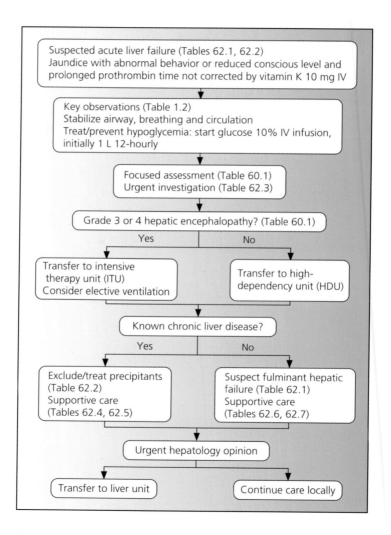

Suspected acute liver failure (Tables 62.1, 62.2)
Jaundice with abnormal behavior or reduced conscious level and prolonged prothrombin time not corrected by vitamin K 10 mg IV

↓

Key observations (Table 1.2)
Stabilize airway, breathing and circulation
Treat/prevent hypoglycemia: start glucose 10% IV infusion, initially 1 L 12-hourly

↓

Focused assessment (Table 60.1)
Urgent investigation (Table 62.3)

↓

Grade 3 or 4 hepatic encephalopathy? (Table 60.1)

Yes → Transfer to intensive therapy unit (ITU)
Consider elective ventilation

No → Transfer to high-dependency unit (HDU)

↓

Known chronic liver disease?

Yes → Exclude/treat precipitants (Table 62.2)
Supportive care (Tables 62.4, 62.5)

No → Suspect fulminant hepatic failure (Table 62.1)
Supportive care (Tables 62.6, 62.7)

↓

Urgent hepatology opinion

Transfer to liver unit          Continue care locally

| **TABLE 62.1** Causes of fulminant hepatic failure (FHF) | |
|---|---|
| **Cause** | **Comment** |
| **Drug-related** | Paracetamol poisoning (p. 75): the commonest cause of FHF in the UK; AST/ALT typically >3500 units/L<br>Idiosyncratic reaction (usually occurs within 6 months of starting drug; many drugs implicated, e.g. co-amoxiclav) |
| **Viral hepatitis** | Hepatitis A, B, C, D or E virus<br>Herpes simplex virus (a rare cause; usually seen in patients taking immunosuppressive therapy or in third trimester of pregnancy) |
| **Ischemic hepatitis** | 'Shock liver'<br>May occur after cardiac arrest or prolonged hypotension, or in severe congestive heart failure, and therefore often associated with acute renal failure<br>Markedly raised AST/ALT |
| **Budd–Chiari syndrome** | Due to acute hepatic vein thrombosis<br>Typically occurs in women age 20–40 years<br>Presents with right upper quadrant pain, hepatomegaly and ascites<br>Underlying hematological disorder (e.g. polycythemia rubra vera, paroxysmal nocturnal hemoglobinuria) or other cause of thrombophilia (p. 227)<br>Diagnose by duplex ultrasound of hepatic veins and IVC |
| **Acute fatty liver of pregnancy** | Occurs in last trimester of pregnancy<br>Often associated with pre-eclampsia (p. 552) |

*Continued*

**Acute liver failure**

| Cause | Comment |
|---|---|
| **Autoimmune hepatitis** | Consider if there are other autoimmune disorders (e.g. hemolytic anemia, idiopathic thrombocytopenic purpura, type 1 diabetes, thyroiditis, celiac disease) Autoantibodies (antinuclear antibodies, antismooth muscle antibodies) and hypergammaglobulinemia usually present |
| ***Amanita phalloides* poisoning** | Suspect if the patient has eaten wild mushrooms Usually associated with severe gastrointestinal symptoms (nausea, vomiting, diarrhea, abdominal pain), which develop within hours to one day of ingestion |
| **Wilson disease** | Suspect in a patient age <30 with liver failure and hemolytic anemia (giving markedly elevated bilirubin) Kayser–Fleischer rings are present in ~50% Serum ceruloplasmin is typically low (but may be normal in ~15% and is often reduced in other forms of ALF) and serum/urinary copper levels high Alkaline phosphatase and urate are low |
| **Malignant infiltration** | May occur in breast cancer, small cell lung cancer, lymphoma and melanoma Associated with hepatomegaly Diagnosis made by imaging and biopsy |
| **Cause unclear** | Retake the drug history Consider transjugular liver biopsy |

ALF, acute liver failure; ALT, alanine aminotransferase; AST, aspartate aminotransferase; IVC, inferior vena cava.

**ALERT**

Contact your regional liver unit urgently if you suspect fulminant hepatic failure, to discuss management and transfer.

---

**TABLE 62.2** Causes of decompensation of chronic liver disease

- Infection, especially spontaneous bacterial peritonitis (p. 392)
- Alcoholic hepatitis (p. 404)
- Acute gastrointestinal hemorrhage (p. 365)
- Acute viral hepatitis
- Major surgery and anesthesia
- Drugs: diuretics, hypnotics, sedatives and narcotic analgesics
- Hypokalemia and hypoglycemia
- Constipation

**TABLE 62.3** Urgent investigation in acute liver failure

**Needed urgently**
- Prothrombin time and coagulation screen
- Full blood count and reticulocyte count
- Blood glucose
- Sodium, potassium, creatinine and urea*
- Liver function tests: bilirubin, aspartate transaminase, alanine transaminase, gamma-glutamyl transferase, alkaline phosphatase, albumin
- Amylase and lipase
- Paracetamol level if unexplained acute liver failure or paracetamol poisoning is suspected
- Arterial blood gases, pH and lactate
- Blood culture
- Urine stick test, microscopy and culture
- Microscopy and culture of ascites if present (aspirate 10 ml for cell count (use EDTA tube) and culture (inoculate blood culture bottles) (see p. 389)
- Chest X-ray
- Ultrasound of liver, biliary tract and hepatic/portal veins
- Pregnancy test in women of child-bearing age

**For later analysis (if suspected fulminant hepatic failure)**
- Markers of viral hepatitis (anti-HAV IgM, HBsAg, anti-HBc IgM, anti-HCV, anti-HEV)
- HIV test
- Autoimmune profile (antinuclear antibodies, antismooth muscle antibodies, immunoglobulins)
- Plasma ceruloplasmin in patients aged <50 (to exclude Wilson disease)
- Serum (10 ml) and urine (50 ml) for toxicological analysis if needed
- Blood group

EDTA, ethylene diaminetetra-acetic acid; HAV, hepatitis A virus; HBc, hepatitis B core; HBsAG, hepatitis B surface antigen; HCV, hepatitis C virus; HEV, hepatitis E virus; IgM, immunoglobulin M.
* Urea may be low because of reduced hepatic synthesis; if markedly elevated with a normal creatinine, suspect upper gastrointestinal hemorrhage.

**TABLE 62.4** Management of decompensated chronic liver disease

## Look for and treat precipitants (Table 62.2)
- If there is ascites, aspirate 10 ml for cell count (use an EDTA tube) and culture (inoculate blood culture bottles) (p. 389)
- Assume spontaneous bacterial peritonitis (see Table 61.4) is present if ascitic fluid shows >250 neutrophils/mm³, and treat with cefotaxime 2 g 8-hourly IV
- Start empirical antibiotic therapy with cefotaxime 2 g 8-hourly IV if there is fever, even in the absence of focal signs of infection, after taking blood cultures

## Maintain blood glucose >3.5 mmol/L
- Give glucose 10% by IV infusion initially 1 L 12-hourly
- Check blood glucose 1–4-hourly and immediately if conscious level deteriorates

## Maintain fluid and electrolyte balance
- Low sodium diet (~50 mmol/day)
- Potassium supplements to maintain plasma level >3.5 mmol/L
- If IV fluid is needed, use albumin solution or dextrose 5% or 10%. Avoid saline
- Treat ascites with spironolactone (plus a loop diuretic if necessary) aiming for weight loss of 0.5 kg/day (see Table 61.5). If ascites is refractory to diuretic therapy, use paracentesis with IV infusion of salt-poor albumin (p. 392)
- Check sodium, potassium and creatinine daily. A rising creatinine may reflect hypovolemia, sepsis, nephrotoxic drugs or hepatorenal syndrome (Table 62.5)

## Nutrition
- Early feeding by mouth or fine-bore nasogastric tube, with protein intake 60 g/day

*Continued*

**Drugs**

- Start lactulose 30 ml 3-hourly PO until diarrhea begins, then reduce to 30 ml 12-hourly
- Give a proton pump inhibitor, ranitidine or sucralfate to reduce the risk of gastric stress ulceration
- Give vitamin supplements IV or PO (thiamine and other B group vitamins, vitamin C, vitamin K, folate)
- Avoid sedatives and opioids. Other drugs that are contraindicated are listed in the *British National Formulary*

EDTA, ethylene diaminetetra-acetic acid.

---

**TABLE 62.5** Hepatorenal syndrome

**Criteria for diagnosis**

- Chronic or acute liver disease with liver failure and portal hypertension
- Plasma creatinine concentration >133 µmol/L, with progressive increase over days to weeks, and oliguria
- Exclusion of other causes of renal failure (p. 414)
- Urine sodium concentration <10 mmol/L (if not taking diuretic), urine osmolality greater than plasma osmolality, urinary protein excretion <0.5 g/day, urine red cell count <50 mm$^3$

**Management**

- Treat underlying liver disease
- Exclude/treat spontaneous bacterial peritonitis (p. 392)
- General management of acute renal failure (p. 410)
- Consider treatment with terlipressin (0.5–2.0 mg IV every 4–12 h) for 5–15 days plus albumin solution (1 g/kg IV on day 1, followed by 20–40 g daily) for 5–15 days: discuss with hepatologist/gastroenterologist

**TABLE 62.6** Supportive care in fulminant hepatic failure before transfer to regional liver unit

**Ask for help**
- Ask for help from your local gastroenterologist/hepatologist or discuss management with the regional liver unit

**Monitoring and general care**
- Nurse the patient with 30° head-up tilt in a quiet area of an intensive therapy unit or high-dependency unit
- Monitor the conscious level 1–4-hourly, pulse and blood pressure 1–4-hourly and temperature 8-hourly
- Check blood glucose 1–4-hourly and immediately if conscious level deteriorates
- Monitor blood oxygen saturation by pulse oximeter and give oxygen by mask to maintain $SaO_2$ >92%
- Give platelet concentrate before placing central venous and arterial lines if the platelet count is <50 × $10^9$/L. Avoid giving fresh frozen plasma unless there is active bleeding, as this affects coagulation tests – the best prognostic marker – for several days
- If encephalopathy is grade 2 or more, or if systolic BP is <90 mmHg, put in central venous and radial arterial lines and urinary catheter
- Give blood if hemoglobin is <10 g/dl. Fluid therapy should be with albumin solution or glucose 5% or 10%. Saline should not be used
- If encephalopathy progresses to grade 3 or 4, arrange elective endotracheal intubation and ventilation
- Put in a nasogastric tube for gastric drainage if the patient is vomiting or is ventilated.

**Management of complications**
- See Table 62.7

**TABLE 62.7** Management of complications of acute liver failure

| Complication | Management |
|---|---|
| **Cerebral edema** | Cerebral edema occurs in 75–80% of patients with grade 4 encephalopathy and is often fatal<br><br>It may result in paroxysmal hypertension, dilated pupils, sustained ankle clonus and sometimes decerebrate posturing (papilledema is usually absent). If these occur:<br>• Give mannitol 20% 100–200 ml (0.5 g/kg) IV over 10 min, provided urine output is >30 ml/h and pulmonary artery wedge pressure is <15 mmHg. Check plasma osmolality: further mannitol may be given until plasma osmolality is 320 mosmol/kg<br>• Hyperventilate to an arterial $PCO_2$ of 4.0 kPa (30 mmHg)<br>• If there is no response to these measures, give thiopental 125–250 mg IV over 15 min, followed by an infusion of 50–250 mg/h for up to 4 h |
| **Hypotension** | Correct hypovolemia with blood or 4.5% human albumin solution<br>Use epinephrine, norepinephrine or dopamine infusion (p. 58) to maintain mean arterial pressure >60 mmHg |
| **Oliguria/renal failure** | Correct hypovolemia<br>Avoid high-dose furosemide<br>Start renal replacement therapy if anuric or oliguric with plasma creatinine >400 μmol/L |
| **Hypoglycemia** | Give glucose 10% IV 1 L 12-hourly<br>Check blood glucose 1–4 hourly and give stat doses of glucose 25 g IV if <3.5 mmol/L |

*Continued*

| Complication | Management |
|---|---|
| **Coagulopathy** | Give vitamin K 10 mg IV daily<br>Give platelet transfusion if count $<50 \times 10^9$/L<br>Give fresh frozen plasma only if there is active bleeding |
| **Gastric stress ulceration** | Prophylaxis with proton pump inhibitor, ranitidine or sucralfate |
| **Hypoxemia** | Many possible causes: inhalation, infection, pulmonary edema, atelectasis, intrapulmonary hemorrhage<br>Increase inspired oxygen<br>Ventilate with positive end-expiratory pressure if $SaO_2$ remains <92% |
| **Infection** | Daily culture of blood, sputum and urine<br>Early treatment of presumed infection with broad-spectrum antibiotic therapy: discuss with microbiologist<br>Consider antifungal therapy if fever with negative blood cultures |

Acute liver failure

## Further reading

Bailey B, et al. Fulminant hepatic failure secondary to acetaminophen poisoning: a systematic review and meta-analysis of prognostic criteria determining the need for liver transplantation. *Crit Care Med* 2003; 31: 299–305.

Polson J, Lee WM. American Association for the Study of Liver Diseases position paper: the management of acute liver failure. *Hepatology* 2005; 41: 1179–97.

# 63 Alcoholic hepatitis

**TABLE 63.1** Alcoholic hepatitis: diagnosis and management

**Clinical features and blood results**
- Malaise
- Jaundice
- Nausea and vomiting
- Stigmata of chronic liver disease may be present
- Fever (low grade)
- Tender hepatomegaly
- Ascites
- Raised white cell count (may be >20 × 10$^9$/L) and C-reactive protein
- Prothrombin time prolonged >5 s over control
- Mildy raised AST and ALT (typically <200 units/L, AST > ALT: increases of >10 times suggests viral hepatitis or drug toxicity)
- Raised gamma-glutamyl transferase and serum IgA
- Raised bilirubin (may be >750 μmol/L)
- Raised ferritin (often >1000 μg/L)
- Low sodium, low potassium, low urea, variable creatinine, low hemoglobin, high MCV, low platelet count

**Identification of clinically severe alcoholic hepatitis**
- An index of severity ('discriminant function', DF) can be calculated: DF = ([patient's prothrombin time − control] × 4.6) + (bilirubin (μmol/L) ÷ 17.1)
- A DF of >32 identifies patients with severe alcoholic hepatitis (mortality ~50%) who will need intensive care and who may benefit from corticosteroid

*Continued*

**Management of alcoholic hepatitis**

- Seek advice from a gastroenterologist/hepatologist
- Avoid diuretics and ensure adequate volume replacement (use 4.5% human albumin solution and/or salt-poor albumin; avoid normal saline)
- Supportive management of alcohol withdrawal (p. 563)
- Start nasogastric feeding early
- Give oral/IV thiamine
- Start broad-spectrum antibiotic (e.g. cefotaxime 1 g 8-hourly IV) after taking cultures of blood, urine and ascites
- Check renal function and prothrombin time daily until there is a consistent improvement
- Consider corticosteroid therapy in patients with DF >32

ALT, alanine aminotransferase; AST, aspartate aminotransferase; IgA, immunoglobulin A; MCV, mean corpuscular volume.

**ALERT**
Suspect alcoholic hepatitis in the jaundiced patient known to abuse alcohol.

## Further reading

Mathurin P. Corticosteroids for alcoholic hepatitis: what's next? *J Hepatol* 2005; 43: 526–33.

Stewart SF, Day CP. The management of alcoholic liver disease. *J Hepatol* 2003; 38 (suppl I): S2–S13.

# 64 Biliary tract disorders and acute pancreatitis

**TABLE 64.1** Biliary tract disorders: clinical features and management

| Disorder | Clinical features and blood results | Management |
|---|---|---|
| **Biliary colic** | Severe pain, typically in right upper quadrant or epigastrium, but may be retrosternal, lasts 20 min to 6 h<br>Nausea and vomiting | Analgesia (e.g. pethidine)<br>Elective ultrasound of biliary tract |
| **Acute cholecystitis due to gallstones** | Severe pain, typically in right upper quadrant, lasts >12 h<br>Often previous biliary colic<br>Nausea and vomiting<br>Often afebrile at presentation or only low grade fever<br>Right upper quadrant tenderness<br>Raised white cell count (usually $12-15 \times 10^9$/L) in ~60%<br>Liver function tests and amylase normal or only mildly raised; ALT rises before alkaline phosphatase | Analgesia (e.g. pethidine)<br>Nil by mouth<br>Nasogastric drainage if there is vomiting<br>Fluid replacement<br>Antibiotic therapy (e.g. third-generation cephalosporin or quinolone; in severe case, add metronidazole)<br>Surgical opinion<br>Urgent ultrasound of biliary tract<br>*Continued* |

| Disorder | Clinical features and blood results | Management |
|---|---|---|
| **Acute cholangitis** | Pain, typically in right upper quadrant, may be mild<br>May follow ERCP<br>Jaundice (in ~60%)<br>Fever with rigors<br>Raised white cell count<br>Abnormal liver function tests and raised amylase<br>Postive blood culture (in ~30%) | Analgesia (e.g. pethidine)<br>Nil by mouth<br>Nasogastric drainage if there is vomiting<br>Fluid replacement<br>Antibiotic therapy (e.g. third-generation cephalosporin or quinolone + metronidazole; if recent ERCP, give piperacillin/tazobactam (or ciprofloxacin if penicillin allergy) + metronidazole + gentamicin)<br>Surgical opinion<br>Urgent ultrasound of biliary tract<br>Biliary drainage by ERCP |

ALT, alanine aminotransferase; ERCP, endoscopic retrograde cholangiopancreatography.

Biliary tract disorders and acute pancreatitis

**TABLE 64.2** Acute pancreatitis: clinical features and management

| Element | Comment |
|---|---|
| **Common causes** | Gallstones<br>Alcohol |
| **Less common causes** | Complication of ERCP<br>Hyperlipidemia<br>Drugs<br>Hypercalcemia<br>Pancreas divisum<br>Abdominal trauma<br>HIV infection |
| **Clinical features and blood results** | Epigastric pain, typically sudden in onset when due to gallstones, may increase in severity over a few hours in other causes, may last for several days<br>Nausea and vomiting<br>Abdominal tenderness/guarding<br>Fever at presentation may reflect cytokine-mediated systemic inflammation or acute cholangitis<br>Shock, respiratory failure, renal failure and multiorgan failure may occur<br>Raised amylase and lipase<br>Raised white cell count and C-reactive protein<br>Abnormal liver function tests (elevated ALT more than three times the upper limit of normal is highly predictive of gallstone pancreatitis if alcohol is excluded)<br>Hypoglycemia, hypocalcemia, hypomagnesemia and disseminated intravascular coagulation may occur |
| **Identification of severe acute pancreatitis** | APACHE II score of 8 or more<br>Organ failure (shock, respiratory failure, renal failure) |

*Continued*

| Element | Comment |
|---|---|
| | Pleural effusion on admission chest X-ray |
| | C-reactive protein >150 mg/L |
| | Substantial pancreatic necrosis (at least 30% glandular necrosis on contrast-enhanced CT) |
| **Management of acute pancreatitis** | Fluid resuscitation |
| | Cardiovascular/respiratory support |
| | Analgesia with opioid and antiemetic |
| | Antibiotic therapy with meropenem for radiographically documented pancreatic necrosis |
| | Surgery for infected pancreatic necrosis |
| | Value of prophylactic antibiotic therapy uncertain |
| | ERCP/sphincterotomy for patients with gallstone pancreatitis in whom biliary obstruction is suspected on the basis of raised bilirubin and clinical cholangitis |
| | Nutritional support (enteral feeding by nasoenteric tube beyond the ligament of Treitz, in the absence of substantial ileus) |

ALT, alanine aminotransferase; APACHE II, severity of illness scoring system based on acute physiology and chronic health evaluation; ERCP, endoscopic retrograde cholangiopancreatography.

Biliary tract disorders and acute pancreatitis

## Further reading

Indar AA, Beckingham IJ. Acute cholecystitis. *BMJ* 2002; 325: 639–43.

Miura F. Flow charts for the diagnosis and treatment of acute cholangitis and cholecystitis: Tokyo guidelines. *J Hepatobiliary Pancreatic Surg* 2007; 14: 27–34.

UK Working Party on Acute Pancreatitis. UK guidelines for the management of acute pancreatitis. *Gut* 2005; 54 (suppl III): iii1–iii9.

Wada K, et al. Diagnostic criteria and severity assessment of acute cholangitis: Tokyo guidelines. *J Hepatobiliary Pancreatic Surg* 2007; 14: 52–8.

Whitcomb DC. Acute pancreatitis. *N Engl J Med* 2006; 354: 2142–50.

# 65 Acute renal failure

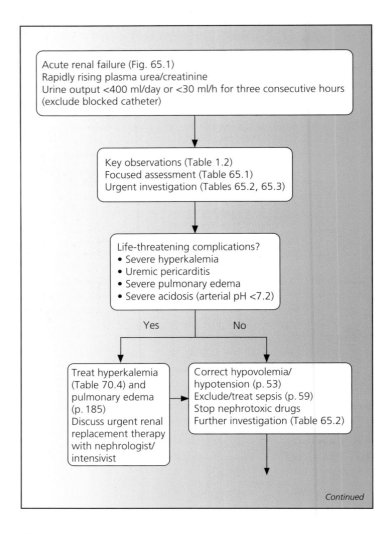

Acute renal failure (Fig. 65.1)
Rapidly rising plasma urea/creatinine
Urine output <400 ml/day or <30 ml/h for three consecutive hours
(exclude blocked catheter)

Key observations (Table 1.2)
Focused assessment (Table 65.1)
Urgent investigation (Tables 65.2, 65.3)

Life-threatening complications?
• Severe hyperkalemia
• Uremic pericarditis
• Severe pulmonary edema
• Severe acidosis (arterial pH <7.2)

Yes        No

Treat hyperkalemia
(Table 70.4) and
pulmonary edema
(p. 185)
Discuss urgent renal
replacement therapy
with nephrologist/
intensivist

Correct hypovolemia/
hypotension (p. 53)
Exclude/treat sepsis (p. 59)
Stop nephrotoxic drugs
Further investigation (Table 65.2)

*Continued*

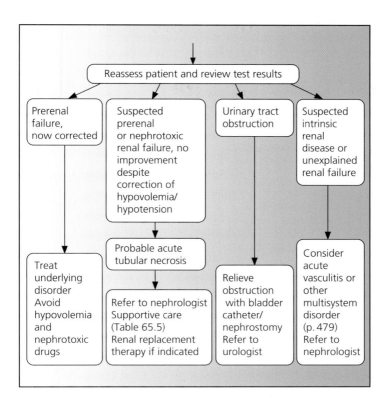

**TABLE 65.1** Focused assessment in acute renal failure

### History

- Review the notes, and drug, observation and fluid balance charts
- Has there been anuria, oliguria or polyuria? Anuria is seen in severe hypotension or complete urinary tract obstruction. More rarely it may be due to bilateral renal artery occlusion (e.g. with aortic dissection), renal cortical necrosis or necrotizing glomerular disease
- Has the blood pressure been normal, high or low, and if low, for how long?
- Is hypovolemia likely? Has there been hemorrhage, vomiting, diarrhea, recent surgery or the use of diuretics?
- Is sepsis possible? What are the results of recent blood, urine and other cultures?
- Is there a past history of renal or urinary tract disease? Are there previous biochemistry results to establish when renal function was last normal? Over how long has renal function been deteriorating?
- Is there known cardiac disease with heart failure, hypertension or peripheral arterial disease (commonly associated with atherosclerotic renal artery stenosis, p. 223)?
- Is there liver disease (associated with the hepatorenal syndrome, p. 400)?
- Is there diabetes, or other multisystem disorder which might involve the kidneys? Do not forget endocarditis (p. 203) and myeloma as causes of renal failure
- Has renal failure followed cardiac catheterization via the femoral artery (raising the possibility of renal atheroembolism)?
- Has the patient been exposed to any nephrotoxic drugs (including contrast media) or poisons? Consider occupational exposure to toxins.

### Examination

- Key observations (see Table 1.2) and systematic examination (see Table 1.9)
- Are there signs of fluid depletion (tachycardia, low JVP with flat neck veins, hypotension or postural hypotension) or fluid overload (high JVP, triple cardiac rhythm, hypertension, lung crackles, pleural effusions, ascites, peripheral edema)?

*Continued*

- Is there purpura? If so, consider:
  - Sepsis with disseminated intravascular coagulation (see Table 78.4)
  - Meningococcal sepsis
  - Thrombotic thrombocytopenic purpura (see Table 78.3)
  - Henoch–Schönlein purpura
  - Other vasculitides (Table 76.3)
- Is the patient jaundiced? If so, consider:
  - Hepatorenal syndrome (see Table 62.5)
  - Paracetamol poisoning (p. 75)
  - Severe congestive heart failure
  - Sepsis with disseminated intravascular coagulation (see Table 78.4)
  - Leptospirosis
- Check for palpable kidneys or bladder. A rectal examination should be done to assess the prostate and to check for a pelvic mass. Check the major pulses: is there evidence of peripheral arterial disease?

JVP, jugular venous pressure.

**ALERT**
Acute renal failure developing in hospital is usually due to hypotension, sepsis or nephrotoxic drugs (including contrast media).

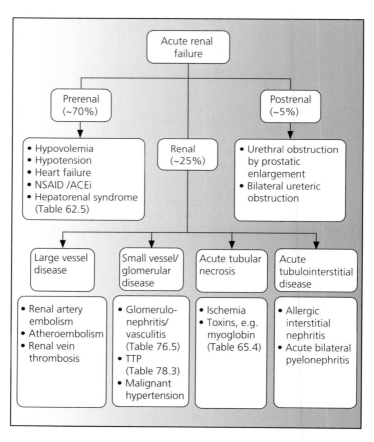

**FIGURE 65.1** Causes of acute renal failure. ACEi, angiotensin-converting-enzyme inhibitor; NSAID, non-steroidal anti-inflammatory drug; TTP, thrombotic thrombocytopenic purpura.

---

**TABLE 65.2** Investigation in acute renal failure

---

### Needed urgently in all patients
- Creatinine, urea, sodium, potassium and calcium
- Blood glucose
- Arterial blood gases and pH
- Full blood count
- Coagulation screen if the patient has purpura or jaundice, or the blood film shows hemolysis or a low platelet count
- Blood culture if sepsis possible or cannot be excluded
- Urine stick test for glucose, blood and protein
- Urine microscopy and culture
- ECG
- Chest X-ray
- Ultrasound of the kidneys and urinary tract if the diagnosis is not clear from clinical assessment and examination of the urine

### For later analysis
- Full biochemical profile, including urate
- Creatine kinase if suspected rhabdomyolysis (urine stick test positive for blood, but no red blood cells on microscopy)
- Erythrocyte sedimentation rate and C-reactive protein
- Serum and urine protein electrophoresis
- Serum complement and other immunological tests (antinuclear antibodies, antineutrophil cytoplasmic antibodies, antiglomerular basement membrane antibodies) if suspected acute glomerulonephritis
- Ultrasound of kidneys and urinary tract if not already done
- Echocardiography if clinical cardiac abnormality, major ECG abnormality, or suspected endocarditis (p. 203)
- Serology for HIV and hepatitis B and C if clinically indicated or dialysis is needed

**Acute renal failure**

**TABLE 65.3** Urinalysis and urine microscopy in acute renal failure*

**Red cells, red cell casts, proteinuria (2+ or more)**
- Acute glomerulonephritis
- Acute vasculitis

**Stick test positive for blood, but no red cells on microscopy**
- Rhabdomyolysis

**Tubular cell casts, granular casts, tubular casts**
- Acute tubular necrosis

**White cells**
- Urinary tract infection
- Interstitial nephritis

**Normal or near normal**
- Prerenal causes
- Urinary tract obstruction
- Some cases of acute tubular necrosis (more commonly in nephrotoxic or non-oliguric acute tubular necrosis)
- Hypercalcemia
- Tubular obstruction (myeloma, acute uric acid nephropathy, aciclovir, methotrexate, ethylene glycol poisoning)
- Renal atheroembolism (consider in the elderly patient with renal failure and skin lesions (especially livedo reticularis), or after cardiac catheterization)

* In patients with a bladder catheter, red and white cells in the urine may be due to the catheter itself.

## Further reading

Chadban SJ, Atkins RC. Glomerulonephritis. *Lancet* 2005; 365: 1797–86.

Esson ML, Schrier RW. Diagnosis and treatment of acute tubular necrosis. *Ann Intern Med* 2002; 137: 744–52.

Hilton R. Acute renal failure. *BMJ* 2006; 333: 786–90.

Lameire N, et al. Acute renal failure. *Lancet* 2005; 365: 417–30.

Maeder M, et al. Contrast nephropathy: review focusing on prevention. *J Am Coll Cardiol* 2004; 44: 1763–71.

Schrier RW, Wang W. Acute renal failure and sepsis. *N Engl J Med* 2004; 351: 159–69.

| TABLE 65.4 Rhabdomyolysis | |
|---|---|
| **Element** | **Comment** |
| **Definition** | Syndrome resulting from skeletal muscle injury with release of myocyte contents into plasma |
| **Traumatic causes** | Trauma<br>Crush injury<br>Electrical injury (p. 574) |
| **Non-traumatic causes** | |
| Infection | Bacterial pyomyositis<br>*Legionella* infection<br>Viral infections<br>Falciparum malaria |
| Electrolyte abnormalities | Hypokalemia<br>Hypocalcemia<br>Hypophosphatemia<br>Hyponatremia |
| Immune-mediated | Dermatomyositis<br>Pyomyositis |
| Drugs | Alcohol<br>Statins<br>Cocaine |
| Metabolic disorders | Myophosphorylase deficiency<br>Phosphofructase deficiency<br>Carnitine palmitoyltransferase deficiency |
| Others | Status epilepticus<br>Coma of any cause with muscle compression<br>Hypothermia (p. 566)<br>Diabetic ketoacidosis (p. 429) and hyperosmolar non-ketotic hyperglycemia (p. 436)<br>Neuroleptic malignant syndrome<br>Malignant hyperthermia<br>Drowning (p. 571)<br>Prolonged strenuous exercise |

*Continued*

**Acute renal failure**

**Acute renal failure**

| Element | Comment |
|---|---|
| **Biochemical markers** | Raised plasma creatine kinase: levels >5000 units/L are associated with an incidence of acute renal failure of >50%<br>Myoglobinuria: myoglobin gives positive result on stick test of urine for blood |
| **Complications** | Hypovolemia due to extravasation of fluid into muscle<br>Acute renal failure from hypovolemia and renal tubular obstruction, tubular damage and renal vasoconstriction<br>Metabolic effects of muscle injury: hyperkalemia, hypocalcemia, hyperphosphatemia, hyperuricemia |
| **Management of severe rhabdomyolysis** | Diagnose and treat underlying cause<br>Vigorous fluid resuscitation with normal saline<br>Transfer the patient to high-dependency unit.<br>Put in a bladder catheter to monitor urine output and, in patients over 60 or with cardiac disease, a central venous catheter so that central venous pressure can be monitored to guide fluid replacement<br>Manage acute renal failure along standard lines (Table 65.5) |

**ALERT**
Contact your renal unit early about patients with acute renal failure, before the plasma creatinine is >400 μmol/L.

**TABLE 65.5** Supportive care in acute renal failure (ARF) due to acute tubular necrosis before renal replacement therapy is started

**Fluid balance**
- Restrict the daily fluid intake to 500 ml plus the previous day's measured losses (urine, nasogastric drainage, etc.), allowing more if the patient is febrile (500 ml for each °C of fever)
- The patient's fluid status should be assessed twice daily (by weighing and fluid balance chart) and the next 12 h of fluids adjusted appropriately

**Diet**
- Aim for an energy content >2000 kcal/day (>8400 kJ/day)
- Restrict protein content to 20–40 g/day
- Restrict dietary phosphate to <800 mg/day
- Consider enteral feeding (by nasoenteric tube) or parenteral nutrition if renal failure is prolonged or the patient is hypercatabolic

**Potassium**
- Stop potassium supplements and potassium-retaining drugs
- Restrict dietary potassium intake to <40 mmol/day
- If plasma potassium rises above 5 mmol/L despite dietary restriction, start calcium resonium which may be given orally (15 g 8-hourly PO) or by retention enema (30 g)

**Infection**
- Patients with ARF are vulnerable to infection, especially pneumonia and urinary tract infection
- Urinary catheters and vascular lines should be removed wherever possible
- If the patient develops fever or unexplained hypotension, search for a focus of infection, send blood and urine for culture and start antibiotic therapy to cover both Gram-positive and -negative organisms; discuss choice of antibiotics with a microbiologist

**Gastrointestinal bleeding**
- Gastrointestinal bleeding occurs in 10–30% of patients with ARF
- Start prophylactic therapy with a proton pump inhibitor

**Drugs**
- Avoid potentially nephrotoxic drugs, such as non-steroidal anti-inflammatory drugs, ACE inhibitors and nephrotoxic antibiotics
- Make sure all drug dosages are adjusted appropriately: consult the section on drug therapy in renal impairment in the *British National Formulary* (www.bnf.org)

# Endocrine/metabolic

# 66 Hypoglycemia and hyperglycemic states

**TABLE 66.1** Causes of hypoglycemia

**In patients with diabetes**
- Excess insulin
- Excess sulfonylurea
- Development of renal failure (with reduced clearance of insulin and sulfonylurea)
- Development of other endocrine disorder (adrenal insufficiency, hypothyroidism, hypopituitarism)
- Gastroparesis and malabsorption

**In patients with or without diabetes**
- Alcoholic binge (inhibits hepatic gluconeogenesis)
- Starvation
- Severe liver disease (p. 394)
- Sepsis (p. 59)
- Salicylate poisoning (p. 75)
- Adrenal insufficiency (p. 457)
- Hypopituitarism
- Falciparum malaria (p. 546)
- Quinine/quinidine for malaria
- Pentamidine for *Pneumocystis* pneumonia
- Salicylate poisoning
- Insulinoma
- Prescribing/dispensing error with substitution of sulfonylurea

---

**TABLE 66.2** Management of hypoglycemia

---

**1** If the patient is drowsy or fitting (this may sometimes occur with mild hypoglycemia, especially in young diabetic patients):
- Give 50 ml of 50% glucose IV via a large vein (if not available give 250 ml of 10% glucose over 15–30 min) or glucagon 1 mg IV/IM/SC
- Recheck blood glucose after 5 min and again after 30 min
- In patients with chronic alcohol abuse, there is a remote risk of precipitating Wernicke encephalopathy by a glucose load; prevent this by giving thiamine 100 mg IV before or shortly after glucose administration

**2** Identify and treat the cause (Table 66.1)

**3** If hypoglycemia recurs or is likely to recur (e.g. liver disease, sepsis, excess sulfonylurea):
- Start an IV infusion of glucose 10% at 1 L 12-hourly via a central or large peripheral vein
- Adjust the rate to keep the blood glucose level at 5–10 mmol/L
- After excess sulfonylurea therapy, maintain the glucose infusion for 24 h

**4** If hypoglycemia is only partially responsive to glucose 10% infusion:
- Give glucose 20% IV via a central vein
- If the cause is intentional insulin overdose, consider local excision of the injection site

**TABLE 66.3** Causes of blood glucose levels above 11 mmol/L

| Diagnosis | Blood glucose (mmol/L) | Venous bicarbonate (mmol/L) | Arterial pH | Urinary ketones | Dehydration | Drowsiness | Management |
|---|---|---|---|---|---|---|---|
| DKA | >11 | <15 | <7.25 | +++ | ++ | – to +++ | See p. 429 |
| HONK | >30 | >15* | >7.30* | + | ++++ | +++ | See p. 436 |
| Poorly controlled diabetes | >11 | >15 | >7.30 | – to ++ | –/+ | – | Treat with insulin infusion if significant intercurrent illness (see Table 66.5) |
| Newly diagnosed diabetes | >11 | >15 | >7.30 | – to ++ | –/+ | – | See Table 66.4 |

DKA, diabetic ketoacidosis; HONK, hyperosmolar non-ketotic hyperglycemia.
* May be lower if intercurrent illness has caused lactic acidosis.

**TABLE 66.4** Management of newly diagnosed diabetes

| Clinical state | Blood glucose | Urinary ketones | Management |
|---|---|---|---|
| **Well** | >11 | ++ | Insulin* |
| | 11–20 | –/+ | Diet |
| | >20 | –/+ | Oral hypoglycemic |
| **Unwell or vomiting** | >11 | ++ | Insulin infusion (see Table 66.5) |
| **Acute coronary syndrome** | >11 | – to ++ | See Table 66.6 |
| **Other significant intercurrent illness** | 11–15 | + | Check laboratory glucose in 2 h; start insulin infusion if >15 mmol/L (see Table 66.5) |
| | >15 | +/++ | Insulin infusion (see Table 66.5) |

\* The patient has insulin-dependent diabetes with mild ketoacidosis caught early before major fluid loss has occurred. Insulin can be given as an IV infusion (Table 66.5) or as a four-times daily SC regimen (see Table 66.7): ask advice from a diabetologist.

---

**TABLE 66.5** Continuous insulin infusion using a syringe pump

**1** Make 50 units of soluble insulin up to 50 ml with normal saline (i.e. 1 unit/ml). Flush 10 ml of the solution through the line before connecting to the patient (as some insulin will be adsorbed onto the plastic)

**2** Check blood glucose and start the infusion at the appropriate rate (see below)

**3** Glucose 5% should be infused concurrently at an appropriate rate (e.g. 1 L 12-hourly IV (500 ml 12-hourly after myocardial infarction))

**4** Check blood glucose after 1 h and then at least 2-hourly. Adjust the insulin infusion rate as needed, aiming to keep blood glucose between 5 and 10 mmol/L

| **Blood glucose (mmol/L)** | **Insulin infusion rate (units/h) and action** |
|---|---|
| **<5***  | Stop insulin |
|  | Check blood glucose every 15 min and restart infusion at 1 unit/h when blood glucose is >7 mmol/L |
|  | Call doctor to review scale |
| **5–7** | 1 |
| **7–10** | 2 |
| **10–15** | 3 |
| **15–20**[+] | 4 |
| **>20** | 6 |
|  | Call doctor to review scale |

* If blood glucose is repeatedly <5 mmol/L, reduce the insulin infusion rates by 0.5–1 units/h.

[+] If blood glucose is repeatedly >15 mmol/L, increase the insulin infusion rates by 2–4 units/h.

---

**TABLE 66.6** Management of diabetes/hyperglycemia after acute coronary syndrome

---

**Known diabetes or blood glucose >11 mmol/L**

- Confirm initial stick test result with laboratory measurement of blood glucose, and check HbA1c.
- If blood glucose is >11 mmol/L, start an insulin infusion (Table 66.5) and continue insulin by infusion for 24 h or until there is stability of the blood glucose and cardiovascular system, whichever is the longer. While the patient is receiving insulin by infusion, also give dextrose 5% 500 ml 12-hourly IV
- If blood glucose is <11 mmol/L in a patient with known diabetes, continue usual treatment and monitor blood glucose preprandially and at 2200 h. If blood glucose rises above 11 mmol/L, start an insulin infusion (Table 66.5)
- After insulin has been given by infusion for 24 h, change to SC insulin

**Management after insulin infusion has been discontinued**

- Estimate the daily insulin requirement from the total dose given by infusion over the previous 24 h. Give one-third as intermediate-acting (isophane) insulin SC at 2200 h. Divide the remaining two-thirds into three and give as short-acting (soluble) insulin SC before meals
- Monitor blood glucose preprandially and at 2200 h, and adjust doses of insulin as needed
- Ask advice from a diabetologist on long-term management. In general:
  - Insulin treated, with good control (HbA1c <7.5%): return to usual regimen
  - Insulin treated, with poor control (HbA1c >7.5%): review regimen
  - Oral therapy with good control (HbA1c <7.5%): return to usual therapy
  - Oral therapy with poor control (HbA1c >7.5%): transfer to insulin
  - Previously undiagnosed: individualized management

---

## Further reading

Cavanagh PR. Treatment for diabetic foot ulcers. *Lancet* 2005; 366: 1725–35.
Inzucchi SE. Management of hyperglycemia in the hospital setting. *N Engl J Med* 2006; 355: 1903–11.
Service FJ. Hypoglycemic disorders. *N Engl J Med* 1995; 332: 1144–52.

# 67 Diabetic ketoacidosis

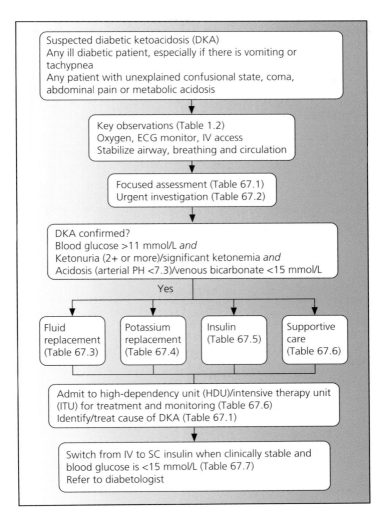

Suspected diabetic ketoacidosis (DKA)
Any ill diabetic patient, especially if there is vomiting or tachypnea
Any patient with unexplained confusional state, coma, abdominal pain or metabolic acidosis

↓

Key observations (Table 1.2)
Oxygen, ECG monitor, IV access
Stabilize airway, breathing and circulation

Focused assessment (Table 67.1)
Urgent investigation (Table 67.2)

↓

DKA confirmed?
Blood glucose >11 mmol/L *and*
Ketonuria (2+ or more)/significant ketonemia *and*
Acidosis (arterial PH <7.3)/venous bicarbonate <15 mmol/L

Yes

| Fluid replacement (Table 67.3) | Potassium replacement (Table 67.4) | Insulin (Table 67.5) | Supportive care (Table 67.6) |

Admit to high-dependency unit (HDU)/intensive therapy unit (ITU) for treatment and monitoring (Table 67.6)
Identify/treat cause of DKA (Table 67.1)

↓

Switch from IV to SC insulin when clinically stable and blood glucose is <15 mmol/L (Table 67.7)
Refer to diabetologist

Diabetic ketoacidosis

**TABLE 67.1** Focused assessment in suspected diabetic ketoacidosis (DKA)

**1 Is this DKA?**
Confirmation of the diagnosis of DKA depends on the biochemistry (see flow diagram above), but you should suspect DKA in any diabetic patient with:
- Nausea, vomiting and abdominal pain
- Tachypnea/hyperventilation
- Acetone on the breath
- Thirst and polyuria (reflecting poorly controlled diabetes)

**2 What has caused DKA?**
- Sepsis is a common precipitant (~30% cases) and complication of DKA and may not cause fever. Check carefully for a focus of sepsis, including examination of the feet and perineum
- Other causes are inappropriate reduction in or non-compliance with insulin therapy (~20% cases), surgery, myocardial infarction, alcohol/substance abuse and emotional stress.
- DKA may also be the first presentation of type 1 insulin-dependent diabetes (~25% cases)

**ALERT**
DKA typically occurs in patients with type 1 diabetes but may also be seen in patients with type 2 diabetes (ketosis-prone type 2 diabetes).

**ALERT**

Rhinocerebral mucormycosis is a fungal infection of the paranasal sinuses particularly associated with DKA, and should be suspected in patients with headache, ocular or facial pain. Seek an urgent ears, nose and throat (ENT) opinion.

---

**TABLE 67.2** Urgent investigation in suspected diabetic ketoacidosis

- Blood glucose (laboratory measurement)
- Plasma or urinary ketones (stick test of plasma or urine with Ketostix)
- Venous plasma bicarbonate
- Sodium, potassium and creatinine
- Arterial blood gases and pH
- Full blood count (high white count may be due to acidosis, rather than infection)
- C-reactive protein
- Blood culture
- Urine stick test, microscopy and culture
- Chest X-ray
- ECG

**Diabetic ketoacidosis**

---

**TABLE 67.3** Fluid replacement in diabetic ketoacidosis

This must take account of:
- The likely fluid deficit (typically 100 ml/kg body weight)
- The blood pressure, central venous pressure and urine output
- Coexisting renal or cardiac disease

**1** Give normal saline 1 L IV over 30–60 min (give the faster rate if systolic BP is <90 mmHg), followed by 1 L over 1 h, without added potassium
- Put in a central line (after initial fluid replacement) to monitor central venous pressure (CVP) if plasma creatinine is >200 μmol/L or the patient has cardiac disease
- Reduce the infusion rate if the CVP rises >+10 cm $H_2O$

**2** Give further normal saline (with potassium added according to the plasma level, see Table 67.4):
- 1 L over 2 h
- Then individualized to the patient, e.g. 1 L 4–8-hourly until the fluid deficit has been corrected, as shown by warm extremities with a normal pulse and blood pressure and normal creatinine. Aim to correct the fluid deficit over 36 h, half in the first 12 h and the rest over the next 24 h

**3** When blood glucose is <15 mmol/L, change to glucose (with potassium added according to the plasma level, see Table 67.4):
- Use glucose 10% 1 L 8-hourly if significant metabolic correction is still needed (persisting acidosis)
- Otherwise use glucose 5% 1 L 8-hourly
- Give concurrent normal saline (without potassium added) if still hypovolemic

**4** Bicarbonate should only be given if arterial pH is <7.0 and systolic BP is <90 mmHg despite fluid replacement. Give 50 ml of 8.4% sodium bicarbonate over 30 min and recheck arterial pH, giving further doses if needed to increase arterial pH >7.0

**TABLE 67.4** Potassium replacement in diabetic ketoacidosis*

| Plasma potassium (mmol/L) | Potassium added (mmol/L) |
|---|---|
| <4 | 40 |
| 4–5.4 | 20 |
| >5.5 | None |

* Check plasma potassium on admission, after 2 h, and then 4-hourly until the rate of fluid infusion is 8-hourly or slower.

**TABLE 67.5** Insulin infusion in diabetic ketoacidosis using a syringe pump

**1** Give 10 units soluble insulin IV stat while the infusion is being prepared
**2** Make 50 units of soluble insulin up to 50 ml with normal saline (i.e. 1 unit/ml). Flush 10 ml of the solution through the line before connecting to the patient (as some insulin will be adsorbed onto the plastic)
**3** Start the infusion at 6 units/h. Check blood glucose by hourly stick test, and 2-hourly laboratory measurement, and adjust the infusion rate as below. Blood glucose will usually fall by around 5 mmol/L/h
**4** If there is no fall in blood glucose after 2 h, confirm that the pump is working and the IV line is connected properly and double the infusion rate. Recheck blood glucose after a further 2 h and double the insulin infusion rate again if necessary

| Blood glucose (mmol/L) | Insulin infusion rate (units/h) | IV fluid* |
|---|---|---|
| <5[†] | Stop insulin<br>Check blood glucose every 15 min and restart infusion at 1 unit/h when blood glucose is >7 mmol/L<br>Call doctor to review scale | Glucose |

*Continued*

| | | |
|---|---|---|
| **5–7** | 1 | Glucose |
| **7–10** | 2 | Glucose |
| **10–15** | 3 | Glucose |
| **15–20** | 4 | Saline |
| **>20** | 6 Call doctor to review scale | Saline |

\* Use glucose 10% 1 L 8-hourly if significant metabolic correction is still needed (persisting acidosis), otherwise use glucose 5% 1 L 8-hourly. Give concurrent normal saline (without potassium added) if still hypovolemic.
† If blood glucose is repeatedly <5 mmol/L, reduce the insulin infusion rates by 0.5–1 units/h. If blood glucose is repeatedly >15 mmol/L, increase the insulin infusion rates by 2–4 units/h.

**TABLE 67.6** Supportive care and monitoring in diabetic ketoacidosis (DKA)

**Supportive care**
- Admit to intensive therapy unit or high-dependency unit
- Give oxygen (35% or more, as needed) if arterial oxygen saturation is <92%, or $PaO_2$ is <10 kPa
- Place a nasogastric tube if the patient is too drowsy to answer questions or there is a gastric succussion splash. Aspirate the stomach and leave on continuous drainage. Inhalation of vomit is a potentially fatal complication of DKA
- Put in a bladder catheter if no urine has been passed after 4 h, or if the patient is incontinent, but not otherwise
- Use graduated compression stockings and prophylactic low molecular weight heparin to reduce the risk of deep vein thrombosis

**Monitoring**
- Continous display:
  - ECG
  - Arterial oxygen saturation

*Continued*

- Check hourly:
  - Conscious level (e.g. Glasgow Coma Scale, p. 297) until fully conscious
  - Respiratory rate until stable and then 4-hourly
  - Blood pressure until stable and then 4-hourly
  - Central venous pressure until the infusion rate is 1 L 8-hourly or less
  - Blood glucose by stick test
  - Fluid balance
- Check 2-hourly:
  - Blood glucose by laboratory measurement until <20 mmol/L then check 4-hourly
- Check 4-hourly:
  - Plasma potassium until the infusion rate is 1 L 8-hourly or less
  - Venous bicarbonate until >15 mmol/L and then monitor ketogenesis from the urine ketone level

**TABLE 67.7** Switching from IV to SC insulin after treatment of diabetic ketoacidosis

**1** Estimate the daily insulin requirement from double the total dose given by infusion over the last 12 h
**2** Give one-third of the total daily dose as intermediate-acting (isophane) insulin SC at 2200 h. Divide the remaining two-thirds into three, and give as short-acting (soluble) insulin SC before meals
**3** Check blood glucose before meals and at 2200 h, and adjust doses of insulin as needed, aiming for levels 4–7 mmol/L
**4** Ask advice from a diabetologist on a suitable long-term regimen

## Further reading

Chiasson J-L, et al. Diagnosis and treatment of diabetic ketoacidosis and the hyperglycaemic hyperosmolar state. *J Can Med Assoc* 2003; 168: 859–66.
Savage MW, Kilvert A. ABCD guidelines for the management of hyperglycaemic emergencies in adults. *Pract Diabetes Int* 2006; 23: 227–31.

**Diabetic ketoacidosis**

# 68 Hyperosmolar non-ketotic hyperglycemia

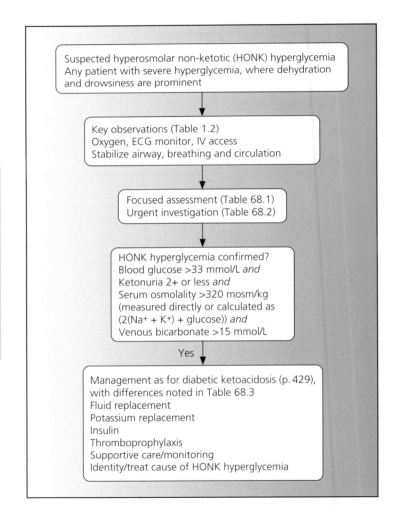

Suspected hyperosmolar non-ketotic (HONK) hyperglycemia
Any patient with severe hyperglycemia, where dehydration and drowsiness are prominent

↓

Key observations (Table 1.2)
Oxygen, ECG monitor, IV access
Stabilize airway, breathing and circulation

↓

Focused assessment (Table 68.1)
Urgent investigation (Table 68.2)

↓

HONK hyperglycemia confirmed?
Blood glucose >33 mmol/L *and*
Ketonuria 2+ or less *and*
Serum osmolality >320 mosm/kg
(measured directly or calculated as
($2(Na^+ + K^+)$ + glucose)) *and*
Venous bicarbonate >15 mmol/L

Yes ↓

Management as for diabetic ketoacidosis (p. 429), with differences noted in Table 68.3
Fluid replacement
Potassium replacement
Insulin
Thromboprophylaxis
Supportive care/monitoring
Identity/treat cause of HONK hyperglycemia

**TABLE 68.1** Focused assessment in suspected hyperosmolar non-ketotic (HONK) hyperglycemia

**1 Is this HONK hyperglycemia?**
Confirmation of the diagnosis of HONK hyperglycemia depends on the biochemistry (see flow diagram above), but you should suspect it in any patient with type 2 diabetes who has:
- Marked thirst and polyuria
- Drowsiness (progressing to coma), which develops as plasma osmolality rises >320 mosmol/kg

**2 What has caused HONK hyperglycemia?**
- Sepsis is the commonest precipitant, usually pneumonia or urinary tract infection. Check carefully for a focus of sepsis
- Myocardial infarction, stroke, and corticosteroid therapy may also precipitate HONK hyperglycemia

**TABLE 68.2** Urgent investigation in suspected hyperosmolar non-ketotic hyperglycemia

- Blood glucose (laboratory measurement)
- Plasma or urinary ketones (stick test with Ketostix)
- Venous plasma bicarbonate
- Sodium, potassium and creatinine
- Plasma osmolality (measured directly or calculated from the formula: plasma osmolality = [2(Na + K) + urea + glucose]; normal range is 285–295 mosmol/kg)
- Arterial blood gases and pH
- Full blood count
- C-reactive protein
- Blood culture
- Urine stick test, microscopy and culture
- Chest X-ray
- ECG

Hyperosmolar non-ketotic hyperglycemia

**TABLE 68.3** Management of hyperosmolar non-ketotic (HONK) hyperglycemia

This is broadly the same as for diabetic ketoacidosis (DKA, see Chapter 67), with the differences noted below:

- The fluid deficit in HONK hyperglycemia is typically 100–200 ml/kg body weight (greater than in DKA, where it is typically 100 ml/kg). Aim to correct the fluid deficit over 36 h, half in the first 12 h (with initial rapid fluid replacement if needed to restore circulating blood volume/blood pressure) and the rest over the next 24 h
- If plasma sodium concentration is >155 mmol/L, use 0.45% saline in place of normal saline
- Insulin sensitivity is greater in the absence of severe acidosis: halve the infusion rate
- The risk of thromboembolism is high. Use graduated compression stockings and, unless contraindicated (e.g. recent stroke), give full dose low molecular weight heparin until mobile
- Total body potassium is lower and the plasma level more variable as treatment begins. Check the level 30 min after starting insulin and then 2-hourly
- Most patients can subsequently be maintained on oral hypoglycemic therapy, although recovery of endogenous insulin production may be delayed. Continue insulin (SC regimen, see Table 67.7) unless the total daily requirement falls below 20 units, when an oral hypoglycemic can be tried
- Arrange early follow-up with a diabetologist to review therapy

## Further reading

Chiasson J-L, et al. Diagnosis and treatment of diabetic ketoacidosis and the hyperglycaemic hyperosmolar state. *J Can Med Assoc* 2003; 168: 859–66.

Savage MW, Kilvert A. ABCD guidelines for the management of hyperglycaemic emergencies in adults. *Pract Diabetes Int* 2006; 23: 227–31.

# 69 Sodium disorders

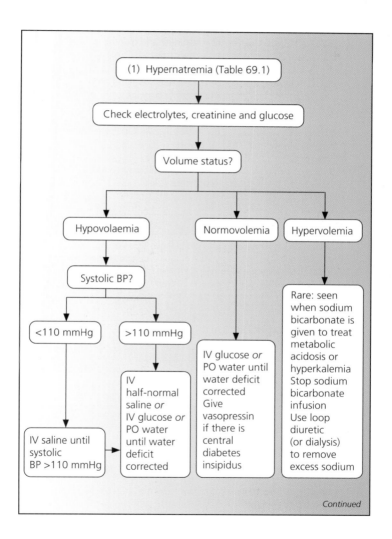

(1) Hypernatremia (Table 69.1)

↓

Check electrolytes, creatinine and glucose

↓

Volume status?

- **Hypovolaemia**
  - Systolic BP?
    - <110 mmHg
      - IV saline until systolic BP >110 mmHg
    - >110 mmHg
      - IV half-normal saline *or* IV glucose *or* PO water until water deficit corrected

- **Normovolemia**
  - IV glucose *or* PO water until water deficit corrected Give vasopressin if there is central diabetes insipidus

- **Hypervolemia**
  - Rare: seen when sodium bicarbonate is given to treat metabolic acidosis or hyperkalemia Stop sodium bicarbonate infusion Use loop diuretic (or dialysis) to remove excess sodium

*Continued*

**Sodium disorders**

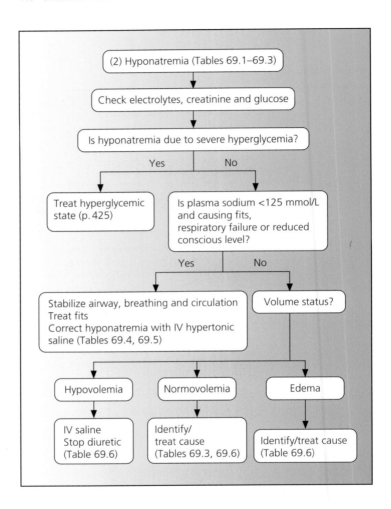

**ALERT**
IV hypertonic saline to correct hyponatremia may be hazardous:
seek expert advice first.

| TABLE 69.1 Plasma sodium concentration | | |
|---|---|---|
| **Plasma sodium concentration (mmol/L)** | **Classification** | **Clinical features** |
| >**155** | Severe hypernatremia | Confusional state, coma |
| **150–155** | Moderate hypernatremia | Muscle weakness, confusional state |
| **143–149** | Mild hypernatremia | Typically asymptomatic |
| **138–142** | Normal range | |
| **130–137** | Mild hyponatremia | Typically asymptomatic |
| **124–129** | Moderate hyponatremia | Headache, nausea, vomiting, muscle weakness, confusional state |
| <**125** | Severe hyponatremia | Coma, respiratory failure and seizures (reflecting cerebral edema) especially when hyponatremia has developed rapidly |

**Sodium disorders**

---

TABLE 69.2 Causes of hyponatremia

**With normal or elevated plasma osmolality**
- Severe hyperglycemia

**With increased plasma ADH**
- Effective depletion of circulating volume
  - True volume depletion
  - Congestive heart failure
  - Cirrhosis
  - Thiazides

*Continued*

- Syndrome of inappropriate ADH secretion (Table 69.3)
- Endocrine disorders
  - Adrenal insufficiency
  - Hypothyroidism
  - Pregnancy

**With reduced plasma ADH**
- Advanced renal failure (acute or chronic)
- Primary polydipsia

ADH, antidiuretic hormone.

**TABLE 69.3** Syndrome of inappropriate ADH secretion (SIADH)

**Criteria**
- Plasma sodium concentration <130 mmol/L and plasma osmolality <275 mosmol/kg
- Urine sodium concentration >40 mmol/L and urine osmolality >100 mosmol/kg
- No edema and no signs of hypovolemia
- Normal renal, thyroid and adrenal function (checked by Synacthen test, p. 461)
- Not taking diuretics or purgatives

**Causes**
- Malignant disease: small cell carcinoma of bronchus, thymoma, lymphoma, sarcoma, mesothelioma, carcinoma of pancreas and duodenum
- Intrathoracic disorders: pneumonia, tuberculosis, empyema, asthma, pneumothorax, positive-pressure ventilation
- Neurological disorders: meningitis, encephalitis, head injury, brain tumor, cerebral abscess, subarachnoid hemorrhage, Guillain–Barré syndrome, acute intermittent porphyria
- Drugs: antidepressants, carbamazepine, cytotoxics, MDMA ('ecstasy'), opioids, oxytocin, phenothiazines, thiazides
- Other causes: postoperative state, adrenal insufficiency, idiopathic, HIV infection

ADH, antidiuretic hormone; MDMA, methylene dioxymethamfetamine.

**TABLE 69.4** Hyponatremia with severe neurological symptoms: targets and treatment

| Rate of development of hyponatremia and volume status | Target/treatment |
|---|---|
| **Acute hyponatraemia** (developing in <48h): usually due to administration of hypotonic fluids after surgery | Target: increase plasma sodium by 2 mmol/L/h until symptoms resolve or it has reached 130 mmol/L<br>Treatment: hypertonic saline IV (Table 69.5) plus loop diuretic IV |
| **Chronic hyponatremia** | Target: increase plasma sodium by no more than 1 mmol/L/h, and no more than 10–15 mmol/L in 24h, until symptoms resolve or it has reached 130 mmol/L |
| Volume depleted | Treatment: isotonic saline IV guided by measurement of central venous pressure |
| Normovolemic with normal cardiac function | Treatment: hypertonic saline IV (Table 69.5) |
| Volume overloaded (edematous) or with impaired cardiac function | Treatment: hypertonic saline IV (Table 69.5) plus loop diuretic IV or hemofiltration/dialysis |

Sodium disorders

## Further reading

Adrogue H, Madias NE. Hypernatraemia. *N Engl J Med* 2000; 342: 1493–9.
Adrogue H, Madias NE. Hyponatraemia. *N Engl J Med* 2000; 342: 1581–9.
Ellison DH, Berl T. The syndrome of inappropriate antidiuresis. *N Engl J Med* 2007; 356: 2064–72.
Reynolds RM, et al. Disorders of sodium balance. *BMJ* 2006; 332: 702–5.

**TABLE 69.5** Hyponatremia with severe neurological symptoms: hypertonic saline regimen (NB seek expert advice first.)

**1** Estimate the patient's total body water volume (liters) (roughly 50% of body weight)

**2** Subtract the patient's plasma sodium from 130: this number is the required correction of plasma sodium in mmol/L, and the number of hours over which plasma sodium should be corrected in patients with chronic hyponatremia

**3** Multiply the total body water volume (liters) by the required correction of plasma sodium (mmol/L). This gives the number of millimoles of sodium needed to correct the patient's plasma sodium to 130 mmol/L

**4** Divide the number of millimoles of sodium needed for correction by 514 (the number of mmol of sodium in 1 L of 514 mM sodium chloride). Multiply by 1000 to give the number of milliliters of 514 mM sodium chloride needed to correct plasma sodium to 130 mmol/L

**5** Divide the number of milliliters of 514 mM sodium chloride to be given by the number of hours needed for correction of the plasma sodium. This gives the infusion rate in ml/h. Hypertonic saline should be given by a volumetric pump

**6** Give a loop diuretic IV (or consider hemofiltration/dialysis in severe renal failure) if the patient is edematous or has impaired cardiac function

**7** Monitor central venous pressure, blood pressure, conscious level and urine output hourly. Check plasma sodium 2-hourly, and modify the infusion rate as appropriate:
  - Acute hyponatremia (due to administration of hypotonic fluids after surgery): aim for an increase in plasma sodium of 2 mmol/L/h until symptoms resolve or plasma sodium reaches 130 mmol/L
  - Chronic hyponatremia: aim for an increase in plasma sodium of no more than 1 mmol/L/h, and no more than 10–15 mmol/L in 24 h, until symptoms resolve or plasma sodium reaches 130 mmol/L

| TABLE 69.6 Hyponatremia without severe neurological symptoms | |
| --- | --- |
| **Type of hyponatremia** | **Management** |
| **Hypovolemic hyponatremia** | Give normal saline IV (with potassium supplements if required) until the volume deficit has been corrected |
| | In asymptomatic patients in whom hyponatremia is due to diuretic therapy, withdrawal of the diuretic and a normal diet is usually sufficient to correct plasma sodium to normal |
| **Normovolemic hyponatremia** | Causes include adrenal insufficiency, treatment with thiazide diuretics and the syndrome of inappropriate ADH secretion (SIADH) (Table 69.3) |
| | Management depends on the cause. In patients with SIADH, plasma sodium can be increased by fluid restriction (to 800 ml/day), treatment with demeclocycline (which inhibits the renal response to ADH) or a loop diuretic (e.g. furosemide 40 mg daily PO) combined with a high sodium diet (2–3 g NaCl daily) |
| **Edematous hyponatremia** | The combination of hyponatremia and edema can occur in congestive heart failure, liver failure and advanced renal failure (acute or chronic) |
| | Correction of the hyponatremia (if indicated) requires treatment of the underlying disease. Management is often difficult and expert advice should be sought |

ADH, antidiuretic hormone.

**ALERT**
If the patient has no symptoms attributable to hyponatremia or is only mildly symptomatic (e.g. headache, nausea, lethargy), hypertonic saline should not be given.

Sodium disorders

# 70 Potassium disorders

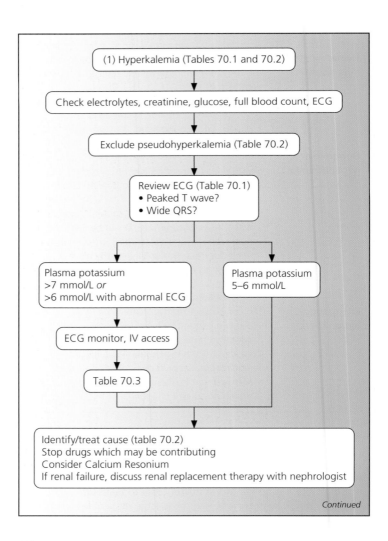

(1) Hyperkalemia (Tables 70.1 and 70.2)

Check electrolytes, creatinine, glucose, full blood count, ECG

Exclude pseudohyperkalemia (Table 70.2)

Review ECG (Table 70.1)
• Peaked T wave?
• Wide QRS?

Plasma potassium
>7 mmol/L *or*
>6 mmol/L with abnormal ECG

Plasma potassium
5–6 mmol/L

ECG monitor, IV access

Table 70.3

Identify/treat cause (table 70.2)
Stop drugs which may be contributing
Consider Calcium Resonium
If renal failure, discuss renal replacement therapy with nephrologist

*Continued*

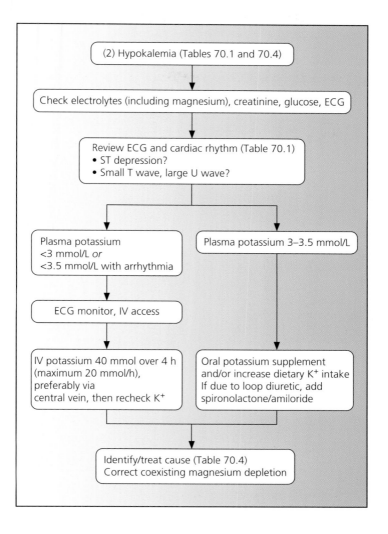

**Potassium disorders**

TABLE 70.1 Plasma potassium concentration

| Plasma potassium concentration (mmol/L) | Classification | Clinical features | ECG features |
|---|---|---|---|
| >6.0 | Severe hyperkalemia | Often asymptomatic Muscle weakness may occur | Tall peaked T wave with shortened QT interval → Progressive lengthening of the PR interval and QRS duration → Sine wave QRS pattern → Ventricular standstill or fibrillation |
| 5.6–6.0 | Moderate hyperkalemia | Usually asymptomatic | |
| 5.1–5.5 | Mild hyperkalemia | Usually asymptomatic | |
| 3.5–5.0 | Normal range | | |
| 3.0–3.4 | Mild hypokalemia | Usually asymptomatic | Extrasystoles, atrial fibrillation, atrioventricular block, ST depression, reduced T wave amplitude, increased U wave amplitude |
| 2.5–2.9 | Moderate hypokalemia | Arrhythmias may occur, especially in patients with underlying cardiac disorders or taking antiarrhythmic drugs | |
| <2.5 | Severe hypokalemia | Arrhythmias commonly occur Muscle necrosis may occur Below 2 mmol/L there may be ascending paralysis, resembling Guillain–Barré syndrome | |

---

**TABLE 70.2** Causes of true hyperkalemia and pseudohyperkalemia

**True hyperkalemia**
*Increased intake (rarely the cause unless there is reduced urinary potassium excretion)*
- Dietary (e.g. fruit juices)
- Prescribed potassium supplement

*Increased potassium release from cells*
- Metabolic acidosis
- Insulin deficiency, hyperglycemia and hyperosmolality
- Rhabdomyolysis
- Trauma and burns
- Hyperkalemic periodic paralysis

*Reduced urinary potassium excretion*
- Renal failure
- Drugs: ACE inhibitors, angiotensin-receptor blockers, potassium-retaining diuretics, non-steroidal anti-inflammatory drugs
- Adrenal insufficiency

**Pseudohyperkalemia**
- Delayed processing of specimen
- Hemolysis
- Leucocytosis >$100 \times 10^9$/L
- Thrombocytosis >$1000 \times 10^9$/L

ACE, angiotensin-converting enzyme.

---

Potassium disorders

## Further reading

Alazami M. Unusual causes of hypokalaemia and paralysis. *Q J Med* 2005; 99: 181–92.

Gennari FJ. Hypokalemia. *N Engl J Med* 1998; 339: 451–8.

Palmer BF. Managing hyperkalemia caused by inhibitors of the rennin–angiotensin–aldosterone system. *N Engl J Med* 2004; 31: 585–92.

**TABLE 70.3** Management of severe hyperkalemia with ECG abnormalities

**1** Give 10 ml of calcium chloride 10% IV over 5 min. This can be repeated every 5 min up to a total dose of 40 ml. Calcium chloride is more toxic to veins than calcium gluconate, but provides more calcium per ampoule (272 mg of calcium in 10 ml of calcium chloride 10%; 94 mg of calcium in 10 ml of calcium gluconate 10%)

**2** Give 25 g of glucose (50 ml of glucose 50%) with 10 units of soluble insulin IV over 30 min. This will usually reduce plasma potassium for several hours. Check blood glucose after glucose/insulin has been given to exclude rebound hypoglycemia

**3** If hyperkalemia is associated with a severe metabolic acidosis (arterial pH <7.2), give sodium bicarbonate 50 mmol (50 ml of 8.4% solution) IV over 30 min preferably via a central line. Bicarbonate should not be given if alveolar ventilation is impaired (as shown by a raised $PaCO_2$)

**4** Stop potassium supplements or any drugs (e.g. ACE inhibitors, potassium-retaining diuretics) which may be contributing to hyperkalemia. Start Calcium Resonium (15 g 8-hourly PO or 30 g by retention enema)

**5** Recheck plasma potassium after 2 h. If hyperkalemia is due to acute renal failure, renal replacement therapy may need to be started to prevent a recurrence: discuss this with a nephrologist

**TABLE 70.4** Causes of hypokalemia

**Decreased potassium intake**
- Intake of <25 mmol/day

**Increased potassium entry into cells**
- Beta-adrenergic agonists
- Theophylline

**Increased gastrointestinal loss of potassium**
- Vomiting, nasogastric drainage
- Diarrhea

**Increased urinary loss of potassium**
- Diuretics, mineralocorticoids, high-dose glucocorticoids
- High-dose penicillins
- Metabolic alkalosis (p. 116)
- Type 1 distal renal tubular acidosis
- Magnesium depletion

# 71 Calcium disorders

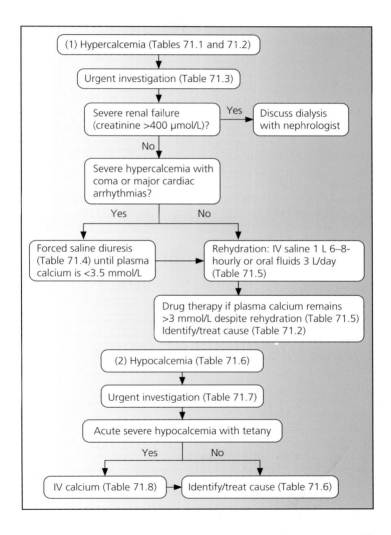

(1) Hypercalcemia (Tables 71.1 and 71.2)

↓

Urgent investigation (Table 71.3)

↓

Severe renal failure (creatinine >400 μmol/L)? — Yes → Discuss dialysis with nephrologist

No ↓

Severe hypercalcemia with coma or major cardiac arrhythmias?

Yes / No

Yes → Forced saline diuresis (Table 71.4) until plasma calcium is <3.5 mmol/L

No → Rehydration: IV saline 1 L 6–8-hourly or oral fluids 3 L/day (Table 71.5)

↓

Drug therapy if plasma calcium remains >3 mmol/L despite rehydration (Table 71.5) Identify/treat cause (Table 71.2)

(2) Hypocalcemia (Table 71.6)

↓

Urgent investigation (Table 71.7)

↓

Acute severe hypocalcemia with tetany

Yes / No

Yes → IV calcium (Table 71.8) → Identify/treat cause (Table 71.6)

**TABLE 71.1** Classification of plasma calcium concentration*

| Plasma total calcium concentration (mmol/L) | Classification | Clinical features |
|---|---|---|
| >3.5 | Severe hypercalcemia | Confusional state and coma |
| 3.0–3.5 | Moderate hypercalcemia | Polyuria (from hypercalciuria-induced nephrogenic diabetes insipidus), vomiting, constipation, abdominal pain |
| 2.65–3.0 | Mild hypercalcemia | Usually asymptomatic |
| 2.20–2.64 | Normal range | |
| 1.9–2.2 | Mild hypocalcemia | Usually asymptomatic |
| 1.5–1.9 | Moderate hypocalcemia | Paresthesiae, muscle cramps, positive Chvostek and Trousseau signs |
| <1.5 | Severe hypocalcemia | Tetany, seizures, QT prolongation which may progress to ventricular fibrillation or heart block |

* Derangements of plasma calcium concentration result from disordered handling of calcium by the gut, kidneys or bone. Calcium exists in the extracellular fluid in three forms: the physiologically important ionized fraction (50%), the protein-bound fraction (40%) and a small fraction (10%) complexed to anions. Most laboratories measure total calcium, which should be corrected for the plasma albumin concentration (a major determinant of the ionized calcium fraction): add/subtract 0.2 mmol/L from the total calcium for each 10 g by which plasma albumin is below/above 40 g/L.

Calcium disorders

---

**TABLE 71.2** Causes of hypercalcemia

**Common**
- Malignancy involving bone (carcinoma of breast or bronchus, myeloma and lymphoma)
- Primary hyperparathyroidism
- Chronic renal failure with hyperparathyroidism or treatment with calcium and vitamin D metabolites

**Rare**
- Sarcoidosis
- Thyrotoxicosis
- Other malignancies
- Vitamin D therapy
- Familial hypocalciuric hypercalcemia
- Thiazides

---

**TABLE 71.3** Urgent investigation in hypercalcemia

- Full blood count
- Creatinine, sodium and potassium
- Blood glucose
- Uncuffed sample for calcium, phosphate, total protein, albumin, alkaline phosphatase
- Chest X-ray
- ECG

*If the cause of hypercalcemia is not known*:
- Serum and urine protein electrophoresis
- Parathyroid hormone (measure after overnight fast)
- Erythrocyte sedimentation rate and C-reactive protein
- Thyroid function tests

**TABLE 71.4** Management of severe hypercalcemia with coma or major cardiac arrhythmias

- Admit to intensive therapy unit (ITU) or high-dependency unit (HDU)
- Put in a central venous line to monitor central venous pressure (CVP) and a urinary catheter to monitor urine output
- Give normal saline 1 L 2-hourly IV until the patient is rehydrated (CVP +5 to 10 cmH$_2$O)
- Then give furosemide 20–40 mg IV
- If the CVP rises above +10 cmH$_2$O, slow the infusion rate or give additional diuretic
- Check plasma potassium and calcium 2-hourly. Give IV potassium as required
- When plasma calcium is <3.5 mmol/L, stop the forced saline diuresis and give normal saline without diuretic 1 L 6–8-hourly IV
- Further management is given in Table 71.5

**TABLE 71.5** Management of hypercalcemia

1 The first-line treatment is rehydration
   - In patients with mild symptoms, oral rehydration (a fluid intake of at least 2–3 L/day) may be sufficient
   - Patients with more severe symptoms should receive normal saline IV 1 L 6–8-hourly IV
2 If plasma calcium remains >3 mmol/L despite rehydration, drug therapy to inhibit osteoclast-mediated bone resorption is indicated. The most commonly used agents are given below:

| Class of drug | Indication |
|---|---|
| **Biphosphonate** | First choice in hypercalcemia due to non-hematological malignancy or primary hyperparathyroidism |
| **Calcitonin** | Failure to respond to biphosphonate |
| **Glucocorticoid** | Hypercalcemia due to lymphoma, myeloma, vitamin D toxicity and sarcoidosis |

3 Specific treatment will be needed to prevent a recurrence of hypercalcemia (e.g. chemotherapy for cancer, surgery for primary hyperparathyroidism)

**TABLE 71.6** Causes of hypocalcemia (not due to hypoalbuminemia)

### Loss of calcium from the circulation
- Acute pancreatitis
- Malignancy (either involving bone, with increased osteoblastic activity, or in response to chemotherapy, with phosphate released from tumor cells forming complexes with plasma calcium)
- Multiple citrated blood transfusions
- Rhabdomyolysis (p. 417)
- Septic shock

### Hypoparathyroidism
- After parathyroid, thyroid or radical neck surgery
- Idiopathic (may be associated with chronic mucocutaneous candidiasis and primary adrenal insufficiency)

### Vitamin D deficiency

### Disorders of magnesium

---

**TABLE 71.7** Urgent investigation in hypocalcemia

- Full blood count
- Creatinine, sodium and potassium
- Blood glucose
- Uncuffed sample for calcium, phosphate, magnesium, total protein, albumin, alkaline phosphatase, gamma-glutamyl transferase
- ECG

*If the cause of hypocalcemia is not known:*
- Parathyroid hormone (measure after overnight fast)
- Serum 25-hydroxyvitamin D level

Calcium disorders

| **TABLE 71.8** Management of acute severe hypocalcemia |
| --- |
| **1** Give 10 ml of calcium gluconate 10% IV over 5 min, followed by a continuous infusion of calcium gluconate<br>**2** Add the contents of ten 10 ml ampoules of calcium gluconate to 900 ml of dextrose 5% (withdraw 100 ml from a 1 L bag), giving a concentration of roughly 1 mg elemental calcium per milliliter, and infuse at 50 ml/h until symptoms are relieved or corrected plasma calcium is >1.9 mmol/L<br>**3** Seek expert advice on further management |

## Further reading

Stewart AF. Hypercalcemia associated with cancer. *N Engl J Med* 2005; 352: 373–9.

# 72 Acute adrenal insufficiency

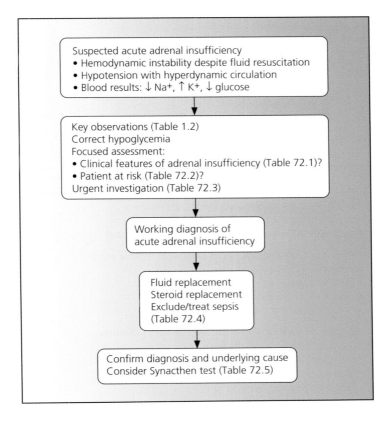

Suspected acute adrenal insufficiency
- Hemodynamic instability despite fluid resuscitation
- Hypotension with hyperdynamic circulation
- Blood results: ↓ Na+, ↑ K+, ↓ glucose

Key observations (Table 1.2)
Correct hypoglycemia
Focused assessment:
- Clinical features of adrenal insufficiency (Table 72.1)?
- Patient at risk (Table 72.2)?
Urgent investigation (Table 72.3)

Working diagnosis of
acute adrenal insufficiency

Fluid replacement
Steroid replacement
Exclude/treat sepsis
(Table 72.4)

Confirm diagnosis and underlying cause
Consider Synacthen test (Table 72.5)

---

**TABLE 72.1** Clinical features of adrenal insufficiency

**Primary (Addison disease) and secondary adrenal insufficiency**
- Tiredness, weakness, anorexia, weight loss
- Hypotension/postural hypotension
- Nausea, vomiting, diarrhea
- Hyponatremia, hypoglycemia, mild normocytic anemia, lymphocytosis, eosinophilia

**Primary adrenal insufficiency and associated disorders only**
- Hyperpigmentation
- Hyperkalemia
- Vitiligo
- Autoimmune thyroid disease

**Secondary adrenal insufficiency and associated disorders only**
- Pale skin without marked anemia
- Amenorrhea, decreased libido and potency
- Scanty axillary and pubic hair
- Small testicles
- Secondary hypothyroidism
- Headache, visual symptoms
- Diabetes insipidus

---

**TABLE 72.2** Causes of acute adrenal insufficiency

**Rapid withdrawal of chronic corticosteroid therapy**

**Sepsis or surgical stress in patients with chronic adrenal dysfunction from**
- Chronic corticosteroid therapy
- Autoimmune adrenalitis
- Other causes, e.g. tuberculosis, AIDS-related infections

**Bilateral adrenal hemorrhage, necrosis or thrombosis**
- Fulminant meningococcal sepsis (Waterhouse–Friderichsen syndrome)
- Coagulation disorders (e.g. antiphospholipid antibody syndrome)
- Heparin or warfarin therapy (including heparin-induced thrombocytopenia, see p. 505)

*Continued*

**Pituitary/hypothalamic disorders:**
- Postpartum pituitary necrosis (Sheehan syndrome)
- Necrosis or bleeding into a pituitary macroadenoma
- Head trauma (often associated with diabetes insipidus)
- Sepsis or surgical stress in patients with hypopituitarism

**TABLE 72.3** Urgent investigation in suspected acute adrenal insufficiency

- Blood glucose
- Sodium, potassium and creatinine
- Plasma cortisol and corticotropin (10 ml blood in a heparinized tube, for later analysis)*
- Full blood count
- Coagulation screen
- Erythrocyte sedimentation rate and C-reactive protein
- Blood culture
- Urine stick test, microscopy and culture
- Chest X-ray
- ECG

*Typical biochemical findings in acute adrenal insufficiency:*
- Raised creatinine
- Low sodium (120–130 mmol/L)
- Raised potassium (5–7 mmol/L)
- Low glucose
- Eosinophilia, lymphocytosis

* A plasma cortisol level of >700 nmol/L in a critically ill patient effectively excludes adrenal insufficiency. Corticotropin is high in primary and low in secondary adrenal insufficiency.

**TABLE 72.4** Management of suspected acute adrenal insufficiency

| Action | Comment |
|---|---|
| **Investigation** | Take blood for measurement of cortisol and corticotropin levels (for later analysis), and other investigations (Table 72.3) |
| **Exclude/treat hypoglycemia** | Check blood glucose: if <3.5 mmol/L, give 50 ml of 50% glucose IV via a large vein |
| **Fluid replacement** | 1 L of normal saline over 30 min *then*<br>1 L of normal saline over 60 min<br>If systolic BP remains <90 mmHg after 2 L saline, put in a central line and infuse saline to keep the central venous pressure 5–10 cmH$_2$O<br>If systolic BP is >90 mmHg, give normal saline 1 L every 6–8 h IV until the fluid deficit has been corrected, as judged by clinical improvement and the absence of postural hypotension<br>Hyperkalemia is common in acute adrenal insufficiency and potassium should not be added if plasma potassium is >5 mmol/L |
| **Steroid replacement** | Give hydrocortisone 100 mg IV, followed by a continuous infusion of 10 mg/h over the first 24 h<br>Continue hydrocortisone 100 mg IV daily until vomiting has stopped<br>Maintenance therapy is with hydrocortisone 30 mg PO daily which is given in divided doses (20 mg in the morning and 10 mg in the evening) and fludrocortisone 50–300 µg PO daily |
| **Exclude/treat sepsis** | Start antibiotic therapy for suspected sepsis (p. 59) if a source of sepsis is evident; or if the white cell count is <3 or >20 × 10$^9$/L; or if the temperature is <36 or >38°C |
| **Confirm the diagnosis and underlying cause** | To confirm the diagnosis in equivocal cases (where the initial plasma cortisol level is borderline), use the short tetracosactrin (Synacthen) test (Table 72.5) |

---

**TABLE 72.5** Short tetracosactrin (Synacthen) test

- The test should be done when the patient has recovered from acute illness, as hydrocortisone (but not fludrocortisone) must be stopped for 24h before the test. The patient should be resting quietly but need not fast prior to the test
- Give 250 µg of tetracosactrin IV or IM before 10 a.m. Measure plasma cortisol immediately before, and 30 and 60 min after the injection
- With normal adrenal function, the baseline plasma cortisol is over 140 nmol/L, and the 30 or 60 min level is over 500 nmol/L and at least 200 nmol/L above the baseline level
- In patients with primary hypoadrenalism, tetracosactrin does not stimulate cortisol secretion, because the adrenal cortex is already maximally stimulated by endogenous corticotropin. In severe secondary hypoadrenalism, plasma cortisol does not increase because of adrenocortical atrophy. However, in secondary hypoadrenalism which is mild or of recent onset, the test may be normal

---

## Further reading

Arlt W, Allolio B. Adrenal insufficiency. *Lancet* 2003; 361: 1881–93.

Cooper MS, Stewart PM. Corticosteroid insufficiency in acutely ill patients. *N Engl J Med* 2003; 348: 727–34.

Dorin RI, et al. Diagnosis of adrenal insufficiency. *Ann Intern Med* 2003; 139: 194–204.

Vella A, et al. Adrenal hemorrhage: a 25-year experience at the Mayo Clinic. *Mayo Clin Proc* 2001; 76: 161–8.

# 73 Thyroid emergencies

---

**TABLE 73.1** Thyrotoxic crisis: recognition

**Clinical features**
- Fever, abnormal mental state, sinus tachycardia or atrial fibrillation
- Signs of thyrotoxicosis, which may not be prominent in the elderly, or may be masked by other illness: check for goitre, thyroid bruit and ophthalmopathy

**Precipitants**
- Sepsis
- Surgical stress
- Trauma
- Iodine: amiodarone; radiographic contrast media; radioiodine
- Pulmonary embolism, myocardial infarction

**Urgent investigation**
- Thyroid hormones (free T3 and free T4*) and TSH (for later analysis)
- Blood glucose
- Creatinine, sodium and potassium, liver function tests
- Full blood count
- C-reactive protein
- Blood culture
- Urine stick test, microscopy and culture
- Chest X-ray
- ECG
- Arterial blood gases and pH

---

T3, tri-iodothyronine; T4, thyroxine; TSH, thyroid-stimulating hormone.
* If severely ill, increased production of reverse T3 may lead to near normal thyroxine levels.

**ALERT**

The mortality of untreated thyrotoxic crisis is high. If the diagnosis is suspected, antithyroid treatment must be started before biochemical confirmation.

---

**TABLE 73.2** Thyrotoxic crisis: management

**Start antithyroid treatment**
- Start either propylthiouracil 15–30 mg 6-hourly by mouth or nasogastric tube, reducing to 10–20 mg 8-hourly or after 24 h, or carbimazole (which acts principally by inhibiting thyroxine synthesis) 150–300 mg 6-hourly by mouth or nasogastric tube, reducing to 100–200 mg 8-hourly plus after 24 h
- After 4 h, start iodine (which inhibits secretion of thyroxine). If iodine is started before antithyroid drugs, excess thyroxine may be produced leading to an exacerbation of the crisis. Give 0.1–0.3 ml of aqueous iodine oral solution (Lugol solution) 8-hourly by mouth or nasogastric tube. Stop after 2 days if propylthiouracil is used or after 1 week with carbimazole
- Give dexamethasone 2 mg 6-hourly PO to inhibit hormone release from the thyroid and reduce the peripheral conversion of thyroxine to tri-iodothyronine
- Exchange transfusion or hemodialysis may be considered in a patient who fails to improve within 24–48 h. Seek advice from an endocrinologist

**Treat heart failure**
- This is usually associated with fast atrial fibrillation. Cardioversion of atrial fibrillation is very unlikely to be successful until the patient is euthyroid: give digoxin to control the ventricular rate
- There is relative digoxin resistance (increased renal excretion and reduced action on AV conduction) so high doses are needed. Loading dose: 0.5 mg IV over 30 min followed by 0.25 mg IV over 30 min every 2 h until the heart rate is <100/min or up to a total dose of 1.5 mg. Maintenance dose: 0.25–0.5 mg daily PO
- Give loop diuretic IV as required

*Continued*

**Start beta-blockade**
- If there is no pulmonary edema, give propranolol 40–160 mg 6-hourly PO, aiming to reduce the heart rate to <100/min
- Diltiazem 60–120 mg 6-hourly PO can be used if beta-blockade is contraindicated because of asthma

**Start anticoagulation**
- Give heparin by IV infusion or LMW heparin SC to patients with atrial fibrillation or if pulmonary embolism is suspected (p. 231)
- Other patients should receive LMW heparin SC as prophylaxis against venous thromboembolism.

**Other supportive care**
- Treat severe agitation with chlorpromazine (50 mg 8-hourly PO; or 25 mg 8-hourly IM; or by rectal suppository 100 mg 6–8 hourly)
- Exclude/treat sepsis.
- Reduce fever by fanning, tepid sponging or paracetamol (avoid aspirin as it displaces thyroxine from thyroid-binding globulin)
- Give fluid replacement guided by measurement of central venous pressure

AV, atrioventricular; LMW, low molecular weight.

---

**TABLE 73.3** Myxedema coma: recognition and management

| Element | Comments |
| --- | --- |
| **Clinical features** | Features suggesting myxedema in the patient with hypothermia:<br>• Preceding symptoms of hypothyroidism: weight gain with reduced appetite, dry skin and hair loss<br>• Previous radio-iodine treatment for thyroxicosis<br>• Thyroidectomy scar<br>• Hyponatremia (plasma sodium <130 mmol/L)<br>• Macrocytosis<br>• Failure of core temperature to rise >0.5°C per hour with external rewarming<br>(Slowly relaxing tendon reflexes are a non-specific feature of hypothermia) |

*Continued*

| **Investigation** | Thyroid hormones (free T3 and free T4) and TSH (for later analysis)<br>Cortisol (for later analysis)<br>Blood glucose<br>Creatinine, sodium and potassium, liver function tests<br>Full blood count<br>C-reactive protein<br>Blood culture<br>Urine stick test, microscopy and culture<br>Chest X-ray<br>ECG<br>Arterial blood gases and pH |
|---|---|
| **Thyroid and corticosteroid hormone replacement** | Start thyroid hormone replacement with T3 or T4<br>Give hydrocortisone 100 mg 12-hourly IV in case there is panhypopituitarism<br>T3 has a shorter half-life than T4 which is an advantage if hemodynamic problems develop and the dose has to be reduced<br>• Day 1–3: T3 10 μg 8-hourly IV<br>• Day 4–6: T3 20 μg 12-hourly IV<br>• Day 7–14: T3 20 μg 8-hourly IV<br>An alternative regimen is T4 400–500 μg as a bolus IV or via a nasogastric tube. No further replacement therapy should be given for 1 week |
| **Supportive care** | See management of hypothermia, p. 566 |

T3, tri-iodothyronine; T4, thyroxine; TSH, thyroid-stimulating hormone.

## Further reading

Cooper DS. Hyperthyroidism. *Lancet* 2003; 362: 459–68.
Roberts CGP, Ladenson PW. Hypothyroidism. *Lancet* 2004; 363: 793–803.
Young R, Worthley LIG. Diagnosis and management of thyroid disease and the critically ill patient. *Crit Care Resusc* 2004; 6: 295–305.

# Dermatology/rheumatology

# 74 Cellulitis

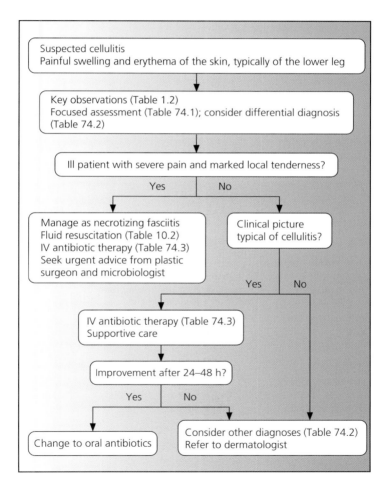

Cellulitis

Suspected cellulitis
Painful swelling and erythema of the skin, typically of the lower leg

Key observations (Table 1.2)
Focused assessment (Table 74.1); consider differential diagnosis (Table 74.2)

Ill patient with severe pain and marked local tenderness?

Yes | No

Manage as necrotizing fasciitis
Fluid resuscitation (Table 10.2)
IV antibiotic therapy (Table 74.3)
Seek urgent advice from plastic surgeon and microbiologist

Clinical picture typical of cellulitis?

Yes | No

IV antibiotic therapy (Table 74.3)
Supportive care

Improvement after 24–48 h?

Yes | No

Change to oral antibiotics

Consider other diagnoses (Table 74.2)
Refer to dermatologist

**TABLE 74.1** Urgent investigation in suspected cellulitis

- Full blood count
- C-reactive protein
- Creatinine and electrolytes
- Blood culture
- Microscopy and culture of blister fluid if present
- Duplex scan if deep venous thrombosis is possible (p. 224)

**TABLE 74.2** Disorders which may be mistaken for cellulitis

| Disorder | Distinguishing features |
|---|---|
| **Necrotizing fasciitis** | Ill patient<br>Severe pain, disproportionate to physical signs<br>Skin may be very tender, with blue-black discoloration and blistering<br>Rapid clinical progression |
| **Leg eczema (venous eczema or contact dermatitis)** (NB cellulitis may complicate eczema) | Longer history<br>May be bilateral (bilateral cellulitis is rare)<br>No fever or systemic symptoms<br>Itching rather than tenderness of the skin<br>History of varicose veins or DVT<br>Crusting or scaling (in cellulitis the skin is typically smooth and shiny) |
| **Deep vein thrombosis (DVT)** (NB cellulitis may complicate DVT) | Proximal margin of erythema usually not well demarcated<br>If clinical setting suggests DVT (p. 224), duplex scan of leg veins needed to exclude this |
| **Allergic reaction to insect sting or bite** | No ascending lymphangitis<br>Itching |

*Continued*

| Disorder | Distinguishing features |
|---|---|
| **Chronic edema/ lymphedema** (NB cellulitis may complicate chronic edema or lymphedema) | Usually bilateral<br>Erythema may be feature<br>No fever |
| **Gouty arthritis** | Arthritis prominent<br>Typically involves first metatarsophalangeal joint (p. 477) |

**TABLE 74.3** Initial antibiotic therapy in cellulitis

| Setting | Organisms to be covered in addition to *Streptococcus pyogenes* and *Staphylococcus aureus* | Antibiotic therapy IV | |
|---|---|---|---|
| | | Not allergic to penicillin | Penicillin allergy |
| **Otherwise well** | Strep. pyogenes is commonest causative organism, but Staph. aureus should also be covered if cellulitis is severe | Benzylpenicillin + flucloxacillin | Clarithromycin |
| **Diabetes with foot ulcer** | Gram-negative and anaerobic bacteria | Co-amoxiclav | Ciprofloxacin + clindamycin |

*Continued*

Cellulitis

| Setting | Organisms to be covered in addition to *Streptococcus pyogenes* and *Staphylococcus aureus* | Antibiotic therapy IV | |
|---|---|---|---|
| | | Not allergic to penicillin | Penicillin allergy |
| **Possible necrotizing fasciitis** | Streptococci spp. Gram-negative and anaerobic bacteria | Benzylpenicillin + gentamicin + metronidazole | Vancomycin or teicoplanin + gentamicin + metronidazole |
| **Hospital- or nursing-home acquired** | Meticillin-resistant *Staph. aureus* (MRSA) | Vancomycin or teicoplanin | Vancomycin or teicoplanin |
| **Human bite** | Mixed oral flora including anaerobes | Co-amoxiclav | Clarithromycin + metronidazole |

**ALERT**
Necrotizing fasciitis is a life-threatening disorder which may be confused with cellulitis in its early stages. Severe pain is the diagnostic clue. If suspected, seek urgent advice from a plastic surgeon and microbiologist.

## Further reading

Falgas ME, Vergidis PI. Narrative review: diseases that masquerade as infectious cellulitis. *Ann Intern Med* 2005; 142: 47–55.

Hasham S, et al. Necrotising fasciitis. *BMJ* 2005; 330: 830–3.

Swartz MN. Cellulitis. *N Engl J Med* 2004; 350: 904–12.

# 75 Acute arthritis

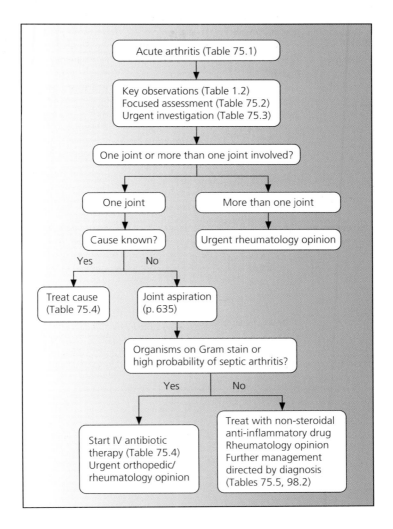

Acute arthritis (Table 75.1)

↓

Key observations (Table 1.2)
Focused assessment (Table 75.2)
Urgent investigation (Table 75.3)

↓

One joint or more than one joint involved?

- One joint
- More than one joint

**More than one joint** → Urgent rheumatology opinion

**One joint** → Cause known?

Yes → Treat cause (Table 75.4)

No → Joint aspiration (p. 635)

↓

Organisms on Gram stain or high probability of septic arthritis?

Yes → Start IV antibiotic therapy (Table 75.4) Urgent orthopedic/rheumatology opinion

No → Treat with non-steroidal anti-inflammatory drug Rheumatology opinion Further management directed by diagnosis (Tables 75.5, 98.2)

Acute arthritis

| Cause | Monoarthritis | Usually oligoarthritis (2–4 joints) | Usually polyarthritis (5 or more joints) |
|---|---|---|---|
| **TABLE 75.1** Causes of acute arthritis | | | |
| **Common** | Gout<br>Pseudogout<br>Septic arthritis<br>Trauma*<br>Hemarthrosis<br>  secondary to<br>  warfarin<br>  anticoagulation<br>Flare of<br>  osteoarthritis<br>  (overuse or<br>  minor trauma) | Ankylosing<br>  spondylitis<br>Inflammatory<br>  bowel disease<br>Reactive arthritis<br>  following gut<br>  or genitourinary<br>  infection<br>Psoriatic arthritis<br>Endocarditis<br>  (acute synovitis<br>  or tenosynovitis) | Rheumatoid arthritis<br>Systemic lupus<br>  erythematosus<br>Viral diseases (e.g.<br>  rubella, hepatitis<br>  B and C,<br>  infectious<br>  mononucleosis) |
| **Uncommon or rare** | Osteonecrosis<br>Pigmented<br>  villonodular<br>  synovitis<br>Tuberculosis<br>Hemophilia<br>Palindromic<br>  rheumatism | Sarcoidosis<br>Whipple disease | Poststreptococcal<br>  infection<br>Leukemia<br>Vasculitis<br>Syphilis<br>Adult Still disease<br>Familial<br>  Mediterranean<br>  fever |

\* Causing internal derangement, hemarthrosis or fracture, or acute synovitis from penetrating injury.

**TABLE 75.2** Focused assessment of acute arthritis

**History**
- Duration and time course of arthritis and other symptoms (e.g. fever, rash, diarrhea, urethritis, uveitis)
- Known arthritis or prosthetic joint?
- Previous similar attacks of arthritis?
- History of trauma?
- Possible septic arthritis? Septic arthritis usually follows a bacteremia (e.g. from IV drug use) in a patient at risk because of rheumatoid arthritis, the presence of a prosthetic joint or immunocompromise
- Risk of gonococcal arthritis?
- Other illness?
- Current medication

**Examination**
- Key observations (see Table 1.2) plus systematic examination (see Table 1.9)
- Pattern of joint involvement: monoarthritis, oligoarthritis (two to four joints) or polyarthritis (five joints or more) (see Table 75.1)
- Arthritis or periarticular inflammation (bursitis, tendinitis or cellulitis)? Painful limitation of movement of the joint suggests arthritis
- Extra-articular signs (e.g. fever, rash, mouth ulcers, anterior uveitis, urethritis)

**TABLE 75.3** Urgent investigation in acute arthritis

- Joint aspiration (p. 635)
- X-ray joint for baseline and to exclude osteomyelitis (rare)
- Blood glucose
- Sodium, potassium and creatinine
- Liver function tests
- Full blood count
- Erythrocyte sedimentation rate and C-reactive protein
- Viral serology if indicated
- Blood culture (×2)
- Urine stick test, microscopy and culture
- Swab of urethra, cervix and anorectum if gonococcal infection is possible

Acute arthritis

**TABLE 75.4** Initial antibiotic therapy for suspected septic arthritis

| Organisms on Gram stain | Antibiotic therapy (IV, high dose) | |
| --- | --- | --- |
| | Not allergic to penicillin | Penicillin allergy |
| **Gram-positive cocci Gram-negative cocci (gonococci)** | Flucloxacillin Ceftriaxone | Clindamycin Minor allergy: ceftriaxone Major allergy: meropenem |
| **Gram-negative rods** | Ciprofloxacin + gentamicin | Ciprofloxacin + gentamicin |
| **None seen: gonococcal infection unlikely** | Flucoxacillin | Clindamycin |
| **None seen: gonococcal infection likely** | Ceftriaxone | Minor allergy: ceftriaxone Major allergy: meropenem |

**TABLE 75.5** Management of acute arthritis

| Cause of acute arthritis | Management |
| --- | --- |
| **Septic arthritis** | Antibiotic therapy (Table 75.4) Joint drainage Seek advice from orthopedic surgeon/rheumatologist |

*Continued*

| | |
|---|---|
| **Gout** | High-dose NSAID (consider PPI cover) |
| | Colchicine if NSAID contraindicated |
| | Oral corticosteroid (prednisolone 40 mg daily for 1–2 days, then tapered over 7–10 days) if NSAID/colchicine contraindicated or not tolerated |
| | Consider intra-articular corticosteroid in place or oral corticosteroid if only one joint affected |
| **Pseudogout** | Joint drainage |
| | Intra-articular corticosteroid |
| | NSAID (consider PPI cover) |
| | Colchicine if NSAID contraindicated |
| **Flare of rheumatoid arthritis** | Seek advice from rheumatologist |
| **Flare of osteoarthritis** | NSAID (consider PPI cover) |
| | Intra-articular corticosteroid |

NSAID, non-steroidal anti-inflammatory drug; PPI, proton pump inhibitor.

## Further reading

British Society for Rheumatology. Guidelines for management of the hot swollen joint in adults. *Rheumatology* 2006; 45: 1039–41.

Margaretten ME, et al. Does this patient have septic arthritis. *JAMA* 2007; 297: 1478–88.

# 76 Acute vasculitis

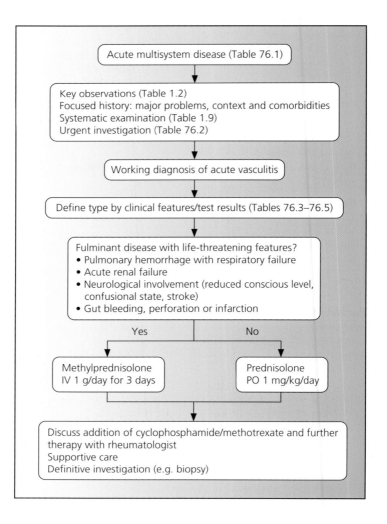

---

**TABLE 76.1** Differential diagnosis of acute multisystem disease*

**Vascular disorder**
- Systemic vasculitis (Tables 76.2, 76.3)
- Multifocal embolism from the heart, e.g. atrial myxoma
- Infective endocarditis (p. 203)
- Aortic atheroembolism
- Aortic dissection with involvement of multiple branch arteries

**Hematological**
- Disseminated intravascular coagulation (Table 78.4)
- Thrombotic thrombocytopenic purpura (Table 78.3)
- Acute leukemia
- Lymphoma

**Infectious disease**
- Sepsis with multiorgan failure
- Tuberculosis
- Falciparum malaria (Table 84.4)
- *Mycoplasma* and *Legionella* infection
- Syphilis, Lyme disease, leptospirosis
- Fungal infection (coccidiodomycosis, histoplasmosis)

**Cancer**
- Metastatic cancer
- Cancer with paraneoplastic syndrome

**Others**
- Poisoning (Table 11.1)
- Drug toxicity
- Pre-eclampsia (Table 85.4)
- Systemic lupus erythematosus
- Antiphospholipid syndrome (recurrent venous or arterial thromboses, fetal loss, mild thrombocytopenia, anticardiolipin antibodies, lupus anticoagulant antibodies)

---

* See also Table 51.3, p. 336.

**Acute vasculitis**

**TABLE 76.2** Investigation in suspected acute vasculitis

### Needed urgently in all patients
- Creatinine, urea, sodium, potassium
- Blood glucose
- Arterial blood gases and pH
- Full blood count
- Coagulation screen if the patient has purpura or jaundice, or the blood film shows hemolysis or a low platelet count
- Blood culture (×2)
- Urine stick test for glucose, blood and protein
- Urine microscopy and culture
- ECG
- Chest X-ray

### For later analysis
- Full biochemical profile
- Erythrocyte sedimentation rate and C-reactive protein
- Serum and urine protein electrophoresis
- Serum complement and other immunological tests (antinuclear antibodies, antineutrophil cytoplasmic antibodies, antiglomerular basement membrane antibodies)
- Echocardiography if clinical cardiac abnormality, major ECG abnormality or suspected endocarditis (p. 203)
- Serology for HIV and hepatitis B and C if clinically indicated or dialysis needed

**TABLE 76.3** Systemic vasculitides

| Vasculitis | Clinical features | Investigation | ANCA result |
|---|---|---|---|
| **Large-vessel vasculitis** | | | |
| Giant-cell arteritis | Age >50 years<br>Headache<br>Temporal artery tenderness<br>or reduced pulsation<br>Scalp tenderness<br>Jaw claudication | ESR >50 mm/h<br>Raised alkaline phosphatase<br>Temporal artery biopsy shows arteritis<br>(positive in 50–80%) | Negative |
| **Medium-sized vessel vasculitis** | | | |
| Polyarteritis nodosa | Weight loss >4 kg<br>Myalgia<br>Neuropathy<br>Hypertension | Hepatitis B serology positive<br>Renal arteriogram shows microaneurysms<br>and abrupt cutoffs of small arteries<br>Biopsy of small- or medium-sized artery<br>shows arteritis | Negative |
| **Small-vessel vasculitis** | | | |
| Wegener<br>granulomatosis | Nasal or oral inflammation<br>(purulent or bloody nasal<br>discharge and oral ulcers) | Nodules, focal shadowing or cavities on<br>chest X-ray<br>Microscopic hematuria or red cell casts<br>Biopsy of involved tissue shows<br>granulomatous arteritis or periarteritis | Positive in ~75% |

*Continued*

**Acute vasculitis**

**Acute vasculitis**

| Vasculitis | Clinical features | Investigation | ANCA result |
|---|---|---|---|
| Microscopic polyarteritis | Pulmonary hemorrhage | Microscopic hematuria or red cell casts Biopsy of involved tissue shows granulomatous arteritis or periarteritis | Positive in ~60% |
| Churg–Strauss arteritis | Asthma Neuropathy | Transient shadowing on chest X-ray Blood eosinophilia Biopsy of involved tissue shows arteritis and extravascular eosinophilia | Positive in ~60% |
| Henoch–Schönlein purpura | Palpable purpura Gastrointestinal bleeding Abdominal pain Hematuria | Raised IgA level in 50–70% Microscopic hematuria, proteinuria Skin biopsy shows vasculitis with IgA-dominant immune deposits | Negative |
| Cryoglobulinemic vasculitis | Palpable purpura Arthralgia | Mixed cryoglobulins Low complement Hepatitis C serology positive Microscopic hematuria or red cell casts | Negative |
| Drug-induced vasculitis | Drug history Palpable purpura Maculopapular rash | Skin biopsy shows leucocytoclastic vasculitis | Negative |

ANCA, antineutrophil cytoplasmic antibodies; ESR, erythrocyte sedimentation rate; IgA, immunoglobulin A.

**TABLE 76.4** Frequency of organ system manifestations in small-vessel vasculitis

| Organ system | Henoch–Schönlein purpura | Cryoglobulinemic vasculitis | Microscopic polyarteritis | Wegener granulomatosis | Churg–Strauss syndrome |
|---|---|---|---|---|---|
| Skin | 90 | 90 | 40 | 40 | 60 |
| Renal | 50 | 55 | 90 | 80 | 45 |
| Pulmonary | <5 | <5 | 50 | 90 | 70 |
| Ear, nose and throat | <5 | <5 | 35 | 90 | 50 |
| Musculoskeletal | 75 | 70 | 60 | 60 | 50 |
| Neurological | 10 | 40 | 30 | 50 | 70 |
| Gastrointestinal | 60 | 30 | 50 | 50 | 50 |

From Jennette, J.C. and Falk, R.J. Small-vessel vasculitis. *N Engl J Med* 1997; **337**: 1512–23.

**Acute vasculitis**

TABLE 76.5 Pulmonary–renal syndromes

| Feature | Goodpasture syndrome | Wegener granulomatosis | Microscopic polyarteritis | Systemic lupus erythematosus |
|---|---|---|---|---|
| **Pulmonary hemorrhage** | Usually present | Common | Common | Uncommon |
| **Glomerulonephritis** | Usually present | Usually present | Usually present | Usually present |
| **Upper airway involvement** | Not seen | Usually present | Uncommon | Uncommon |
| **Rash** | Very rare | Common | Common | Usually present |
| **Arthralgia** | Not seen | Common | Common | Usually present |
| **High ESR** | Very rare | Usually present | Usually present | Usually present |
| **Serology** | Antiglomerular basement membrane antibody | c-ANCA Rarely, p-ANCA | p-ANCA, c-ANCA | Antinuclear antibody Anti-double-stranded DNA antibody Rarely, p-ANCA Low complement |

ANCA, antineutrophil cytoplasmic antibodies; c-ANCA, antibodies with a cytoplasmic pattern of staining; p-ANCA, antibodies with a perinuclear pattern of staining; ESR, erythrocyte sedimentation rate.
From O'Sullivan, B.P. et al. Case records of the Massachusetts General Hospital (Case 30–2002): *N Engl J Med* 2002; **347**: 1009–17.

# Further reading

Bosch X, et al. Antineutrophil cytoplasmic antibodies. *Lancet* 2006; 368: 404–18.

D'Cruz DP, et al. Systemic lupus erythematosus. *Lancet* 2007; 369: 587–96.

Salvarani C, et al. Polymyalgia rheumatica and giant-cell arteritis. *N Engl J Med* 2002; 347: 261–71.

Woywodt A, et al. Wegener's granulomatosis. *Lancet* 2006; 367: 1362–6.

Acute vasculitis

# Hematology/oncology

# 77 Interpretation of full blood count

**TABLE 77.1** Normal values for full blood count

| Variable | Normal range |
|---|---|
| **Hemoglobin** | Male: 13.5–17.5 g/dl<br>Female: 12.0–16.0 g/dl |
| **Hematocrit** | Male: 41–53%<br>Female: 36–46% |
| **Mean corpuscular volume (MCV)** | 80–100 fl |
| **Red cell distribution width (RDW)** | 11.5–14.5% |
| **Reticulocyte count** | 0.5–2.5% red cells |
| **White blood cell count**<br>Neutrophils<br>Lymphocytes<br>Monocytes<br>Eosinophils<br>Basophils | $4.5–11.0 \times 10^9$/L<br>40–70%<br>22–44%<br>4–11%<br>0–8%<br>0–3% |
| **Platelet count** | $150–350 \times 10^9$/L |

From Laboratory reference values. *N Engl J Med* 2004; **351**: 1548–63.

**TABLE 77.2** Clues from the blood film

| Finding | Interpretation/causes |
| --- | --- |
| **Red cells** | |
| Microcytes | See Table 77.3 |
| Macrocytes | See Table 77.5 |
| Red cell aggregration | Rouleaux, seen in:<br>• High polyclonal immunoglobulin<br>• Monoclonal immunoglobulin (paraprotein, e.g. myeloma)<br>• High fibrinogen<br>Agglutination, reflecting the presence of cold agglutinin, seen in:<br>• *Mycoplasma* infection<br>• Infectious mononucleosis<br>• Lymphoproliferative disorder<br>• Idiopathic |
| Fragmented red cells (schistocytes) | Microangiopathic hemolytic anemia, seen in:<br>• Disseminated intravascular coagulation (see Table 78.4)<br>• Thrombotic thrombocytopenic purpura/ hemolytic uremic syndrome (see Table 78.3)<br>• Disseminated cancer<br>• Pre-eclampsia/eclampsia with HELPP syndrome (see Table 85.5)<br>• Malignant phase hypertension<br>Prosthetic heart valve (see Table 30.6)<br>Severe burn |
| 'Bite cells' (keratocytes) | Acute hemolysis induced by oxidant damage (e.g. in glucose-6-phosphate dehydrogenase deficiency) |

*Continued*

| Finding | Interpretation/causes |
|---------|----------------------|
| Target cells | Iron deficiency<br>Thalassemia<br>Liver disease<br>Postsplenectomy |
| Nucleated red cells | Marrow replacement, due to:<br>• Carcinoma (most commonly of breast or prostate origin)<br>• Myelofibrosis<br>• Myeloma<br>• Tuberculosis |
| **White cells** | |
| Blast cells | Leukemias<br>Lymphomas<br>Marrow replacement (see above) |
| **Platelets** | |
| Platelet clumps | EDTA-induced platelet clumping may cause spurious thrombocytopenia |
| **Other findings** | |
| Abnormal cells | Lymphoma cells<br>Myeloma cells |

EDTA, ethylene diaminetetra-acetic acid.
From Bain, B.J. Diagnosis from the blood smear. *N Engl J Med* 2005;
**353**: 498–507; Tefferi, A. et al. How to interpret and pursue an abnormal complete blood cell count in adults. *Mayo Clinic Proc* 2005;
**80**: 923–36.

Interpretation of full blood count

**TABLE 77.3** Microcytic anemia (MCV < 78 fl)

| Cause | Clues from full blood count and film | Other blood results | Causes/comment |
|---|---|---|---|
| **Iron deficiency** | Increased red cell distribution width<br>Anisocytosis<br>Increased platelet count | Low iron<br>Increased transferrin<br>Low ferritin | Commonest cause of microcytic anemia, caused by inadequate dietary intake, malabsorption (e.g. celiac disease) or blood loss |
| **Anemia of chronic disease (ACD)** | Film usually unremarkable | Low iron<br>Low/normal transferrin<br>Normal/increased ferritin | ~20% ACDs are microcytic: causes include Hodgkin disease and renal cell carcinoma |
| **Thalassemia** | Polychromasia<br>Target cells | Normal ferritin<br>Hemoglobin electrophoresis normal in alpha-thalassemia trait and abnormal in beta-thalassemia trait and other thalassemia syndromes | Hematocrit usually >30% and MCV <75 fl in beta-thalassemia trait |

*Continued*

Interpretation of full blood count

| Cause | Clues from full blood count and film | Other blood results | Causes/comment |
|---|---|---|---|
| **Sideroblastic anemia** | Siderocytes may be seen: hypochromic red cells with basophilic stippling that stain positive for iron (Pappenheimer bodies) | Increased ferritin | Rare Hereditary and acquired forms |

MCV, mean corpuscular volume.

Interpretation of full blood count

**TABLE 77.4** Normocytic anemia (MCV 78–100 fl)

| Cause | Clues from full blood count and film | Other blood results | Causes/comment |
|---|---|---|---|
| **Bleeding** | Polychromasia Anisocytosis | Falling hemoglobin without evidence of hemolysis | Occult bleeding may occur from gut or into retroperitoneal space |
| **Hemolysis** | Polychromasia (reflecting increased reticulocyte count) Spherocytes Keratocytes ('bite' cells, due to acute hemolysis induced by oxidant damage, as may occur in G6PD deficiency) Fragmented red cells seen in microangiopathic hemolytic anemia (Table 77.2) | Increased unconjugated bilirubin, increased LDH and reduced serum haptoglobin seen in hemolysis of all causes | Hemolysis is due either to abnormalities of red cells (e.g. G6PD deficiency, sickle cell anemia) or to extrinsic factors (immune and non-immune causes) |

*Continued*

**Interpretation of full blood count**

| Cause | Clues from full blood count and film | Other blood results | Causes/comment |
|---|---|---|---|
| **Anemia of chronic disease** | Film usually unremarkable | Normal/increased ferritin Abnormalities related to underlying cause | Seen in acute and chronic infection, cancer, renal failure, inflammatory disorders (e.g. rheumatoid arthritis, systemic lupus erythematosus), endocrine disorders, and chronic rejection after solid organ transplantation |
| **Bone marrow disorder** | Other cytopenias Leukocytosis Monocytosis Thrombocytosis Blast cells | Paraproteinemia in myeloma | Myelodysplasia, myeloma, leukemia |

G6PD, glucose-6-phosphate dehydrogenase; LDH, lactate dehydrogenase; MCV, mean corpuscular volume.

Interpretation of full blood count

**TABLE 77.5** Macrocytosis (MCV > 100fl)

| Cause | Clues from full blood count and film | Other blood results | Causes/comment |
|---|---|---|---|
| **Drug-induced** | Usually unremarkable | No specific abnormality | Many drugs, e.g. azathioprine, zidovudine |
| **Vitamin B$_{12}$/folate deficiency** | Oval macrocytic red cells, hypersegmented neutrophils, pancytopenia | Low serum B$_{12}$/red cell folate<br><br>Positive intrinsic factor antibodies in pernicious anaemia | B$_{12}$ deficiency: pernicious anemia/malabsorption<br><br>Folate deficiency: inadequate dietary intake/malabsorption |
| **Hemolysis** | See Table 77.4. Hemolytic anemia is usually normocytic but can be macrocytic if there is marked reticulocytosis | | |
| **Primary bone marrow disorder** | MCV usually > 110fl<br>Other cytopenias<br>Leukocytosis<br>Monocytosis<br>Thrombocytosis<br>Blast cells | No specific abnormality | Myelodysplasia, leukemia |

*Continued*

| Cause | Clues from full blood count and film | Other blood results | Causes/comment |
|---|---|---|---|
| **Alcohol** | Alcohol excess may also cause lymphopenia and thrombocytopenia | Abnormal liver function tests, with raised AST (>ALT) and gamma GT | See Tables 63.1, 87.1 and 87.2 |
| **Hypothyroidism** | Usually unremarkable | Raised TSH, low free T4/free T3 | Hypothyroidism may also cause normocytic anemia |
| **Chronic liver disease** | Associated thrombocytopenia may be seen in cirrhosis with portal hypertension and splenomegaly | Abnormal liver function tests/prothrombin time | See p. 394 |

ALT, alanine aminotransferase; AST, aspartate aminotransferase; gamma GT, gamma glutamyl transferase; MCV, mean corpuscular volume; T3, tri-iodothyronine; T4, thyroxine; TSH, thyroid-stimulating hormone.

Interpretation of full blood count

**TABLE 77.6** White blood cell abnormalities

| Finding | Possible causes |
|---|---|
| **Neutrophilia** | Sepsis |
| | Metastatic cancer |
| | Acidosis |
| | Corticosteroid therapy |
| | Trauma, surgery, burn |
| | Myeloproliferative disorders |
| **Neutropenia** | Drugs (e.g. carbimazole) |
| | Infections (e.g. viral, severe bacterial, HIV) |
| | Vitamin $B_{12}$ and folate deficiency |
| | Systemic lupus erythematosus |
| | Felty syndrome |
| | Hematological disorders (e.g. leukemia) |
| **Lymphocytosis** | Infections (e.g. infectious mononucleosis) |
| | Chronic lymphocytic leukemia |
| **Lymphopenia** | Infections (e.g. viral, HIV, severe bacterial) |
| | Immunosuppressive therapy |
| | Systemic lupus erythematosus |
| | Alcohol excess |
| | Chronic renal failure |
| **Monocytosis** | Infections |
| | Myeloproliferative disorders (e.g. chronic myelomonocytic leukemia) |
| | Metastatic cancer |
| **Eosinophilia** | Drug allergy |
| | Parasitic infestation |
| | Hematological disorders (e.g. lymphoma, leukemia) |
| | Churg–Strauss vasculitis |
| | Disorders with eosinophilic involvement of specific organs |
| | Adrenal insufficiency |
| | Atheroembolism |

---

**TABLE 77.7** Causes of pancytopenia

- Aplastic anemia
  - Idiopathic
  - Cytotoxic drugs and radiation
  - Idiosyncratic drug reaction
  - Viral infections
- Acute leukemia
- Marrow replacement
  - Cancer
  - Myelofibrosis
  - Military tuberculosis
- Vitamin $B_{12}$/folate deficiency
- Paroxysmal nocturnal hemoglobinuria
- Myelodysplasia
- HIV

---

**ALERT**
For causes of thrombocytopenia see Tables 78.2 and 85.5.

## Further reading

Bain BJ. Diagnosis from the blood smear. *N Engl J Med* 2005; 353: 498–507.

Tefferi A, et al. How to interpret and pursue an abnormal complete blood count in adults. *Mayo Clin Proc* 2005; 80: 923–36.

Weiss G, Goodnough LT. Anemia of chronic disease. *N Engl J Med* 2005; 352: 1011–23.

Interpretation of full blood count

# 78 Bleeding disorders and thrombocytopenia

**TABLE 78.1** Causes of abnormal bleeding

| Cause | Comment |
|---|---|
| **Inherited disorders of hemostasis** | These are rare in acute medicine |
| | If the patient has had previous surgery, tooth extraction or significant injury without abnormal bleeding, an inherited disorder of hemostasis is unlikely |
| **Acquired disorders of hemostasis** | |
| **Direct effect of drugs** | |
| Warfarin | Inhibits vitamin K-dependent gamma-carboxylation of coagulation factors II, VII, IX and X |
| Heparin | Inhibits thrombin |
| Thrombolytic agents | Activate plasminogen and thus the fibrinolytic system |
| Aspirin, clopidogrel | Inhibit platelet aggregation |
| Platelet glycoprotein IIb/IIIa-receptor antagonists | Inhibit platelet aggregation |
| **Other causes** | |
| Thrombocytopenia | See Table 78.2 |
| | Platelet count $<50 \times 10^9$/L: excessive bleeding after surgery or trauma; $<20 \times 10^9$/L: spontaneous bleeding common; $<10 \times 10^9$/L: spontaneous bleeding usual |

*Continued*

| Cause | Comment |
|---|---|
| Platelet dysfunction | Most often due to drugs, notably aspirin and clopidogrel, but also non-steroidal anti-inflammatory drugs and beta-lactam antibiotics. Also seen in advanced renal failure and myelodysplasia |
| Coagulation factor deficiency or inhibitor | See Table 78.6 |
| | Acquired inhibitors are antibodies to coagulation factors which may be idiopathic or associated with malignancy, autoimmune disorders, pregnancy or clonal proliferative disorders |
| | Typically presents with bleeding into muscles or large ecchymoses |
| Vessel disorder | Corticosteroids, scurvy |

**ALERT**
Drugs, acting directly or indirectly, are the commonest cause of an acquired bleeding disorder.

**TABLE 78.2** Causes of thrombocytopenia

| Setting | Common causes |
|---|---|
| **Acute admission** | Sepsis |
| | Acute alcohol toxicity |
| | Drug-induced thrombocytopenia |
| | Immune thrombocytopenic purpura* |
| | Thrombotic thrombocytopenic purpura (Table 78.3) |
| **Inpatient** | Sepsis |
| | Disseminated intravascular coagulation (Table 78.4) |
| | Drug-induced thrombocytopenia |
| | Dilutional thrombocytopenia from transfusion of plasma-reduced red cells |
| | Post-transfusion purpura |

*Continued*

Bleeding disorders and thrombocytopenia

| Setting | Common causes |
|---|---|
| **Inpatients with cardiac disease** | Use of platelet glycoprotein IIb/IIIa-receptor antagonists<br>Use of adenosine diphosphate-receptor antagonists (e.g. clopidogrel)<br>Heparin-induced thrombocytopenia (Table 78.5)<br>Postcardiopulmonary bypass<br>Use of intra-aortic balloon pump |
| **Pregnancy and peripartum** | See Table 85.5 |
| **Outpatient** | Myelodysplasia<br>Hypersplenism<br>Immune thrombocytopenic purpura*<br>Antiphospholipid antibody syndrome |

\* Immune thrombocytopenic purpura (idiopathic thrombocytopenic purpura, ITP) is diagnosed when there is isolated thrombocytopenia, with no other cause of thrombocytopenia evident (after bone marrow aspiration to rule out myelodysplasia, and HIV testing if indicated).

**TABLE 78.3** Thrombotic thrombocytopenic purpura (TTP)

| Element | Comment |
|---|---|
| **Patient characteristics** | Rare disorder (incidence ~1 per 100,000 per year)<br>Idiopathic TTP most often seen in black women with obesity<br>TTP may be associated with autoimmune disorders (SLE, antiphospholipid antibody syndrome, scleroderma) and with drugs (e.g. quinine, clopidogrel, cancer chemotherapy) |

*Continued*

| Element | Comment |
|---|---|
| **Clinical features** | Weakness |
| | Nausea, vomiting, abdominal pain |
| | Fever |
| | Neurological abnormalities (fits, fluctuating focal deficits) (present in ~50%) |
| | Acute renal failure (uncommon) |
| **Full blood count and film** | Anemia |
| | Thrombocytopenia |
| | No leucopenia |
| | Fragmented red cells (schistocytes) are characteristic |
| | Increased reticulocyte count |
| **Blood results** | Normal prothrombin time and activated partial thromboplastin time |
| | Increased LDH and unconjugated bilirubin (reflecting hemolysis) |
| | Raised creatinine in ~30% |
| **Differential diagnosis** | Disseminated intravascular coagulation |
| | In pregnant women, pre-eclampsia/eclampsia and HELLP syndrome (see Tables 85.4, 85.5) |
| **Management** | Seek advice from a hematologist |
| | Plasma exchange until platelet count normal |
| | Add corticosteroid if no underlying cause found |

LDH, lactate dehydrogenase; SLE, systemic lupus erythematosus.

**TABLE 78.4** Disseminated intravascular coagulation (DIC)

| Element | Comments |
|---|---|
| **Causes** | Sepsis |
| | Trauma (major injury, head injury, fat embolism) |
| | Malignancy |
| | Obstetric complication (amniotic fluid embolism, placental abruption) |

*Continued*

Bleeding disorders and thrombocytopenia

| Element | Comments |
|---|---|
| | Vascular disorder (giant hemangioma, abdominal aortic aneurysm) |
| | Toxin (snake venom, amphetamine poisoning) |
| | Immune-mediated disorder (anaphylaxis, hemolytic transfusion reaction, transplant rejection) |
| | Others (cardiac arrest, drowning, heat stroke) |
| **Clinical features** | Bleeding from skin and mucosae (nose and gums) |
| | Bleeding from surgical incisions, wounds, venepuncture sites |
| | Oliguria/acute renal failure |
| | Jaundice |
| | Acute respiratory distress syndrome (ARDS) due to diffuse alveolar hemorrhage |
| | Confusional state, fits |
| | Adrenal insufficiency (adrenal hemorrhage) |
| | Purpura fulminans |
| **Full blood count and film** | Thrombocytopenia |
| | Fragmented red cells (schistocytes) in ~50% |
| **Blood results** | Prolonged prothrombin time and activated partial thromboplastin time |
| | Low fibrinogen |
| | High fibrin degradation products |
| | High D-dimer |
| **Differential diagnosis** | Thrombotic thrombocytopenic purpura |
| | Chronic DIC (Trousseau syndrome) |
| | Fulminant hepatic failure |
| | HELLP syndrome of pregnancy (see Table 85.5) |
| **Management** | Seek advice from a hematologist |
| | Treat underlying disorder |
| | Consider blood product replacement and heparin therapy |

**TABLE 78.5** Heparin-induced thrombocytopenia

| Element | Comment |
|---|---|
| **Patient characteristics** | Patient receiving unfractionated or low molecular weight heparin (with or without previous exposure to heparin) |
| **Clinical features** | Thrombotic complications in 20–50% (risk of thrombosis persists for up to several weeks after stopping heparin)<br>Venous and arterial thromboses may occur<br>Bleeding complications rare |
| **Full blood count and film** | Falling platelet count (platelet count falls by >50% to $<150 \times 10^9$/L)<br>Platelet count typically recovers within 4–14 days after stopping heparin |
| **Blood results** | Positive test for heparin-dependent antibodies |
| **Differential diagnosis** | Sepsis<br>Thrombocytopenia due to other drugs |
| **Management** | Seek advice from a hematologist<br>Stop heparin<br>Use alternative anticoagulant therapy with direct-acting thrombin inhibitor (e.g. bivalirudin) or heparinoid (danaparoid) |

**TABLE 78.6** Acquired causes of prolonged prothrombin time (PT) and activated partial thromboplastin time (APTT)

**Test result**

| PT | APTT | Cause |
|---|---|---|
| Prolonged | Normal | Warfarin therapy<br>Vitamin K deficiency<br>Liver disease<br>Acquired factor VII deficiency<br>Inhibitor of factor VII |

*Continued*

| Test result | | |
| --- | --- | --- |
| **PT** | **APTT** | **Cause** |
| Normal | Prolonged | Heparin therapy |
| | | Inhibitor of factors VIII, IX, XI or XII |
| | | Acquired von Willebrand disease (usually associated with autoimmune or clonal proliferative disorders) |
| | | Lupus anticoagulant (associated with thrombosis) |
| Prolonged | Prolonged | Liver disease |
| | | Disseminated intravascular coagulation (Table 78.4) |
| | | Excess heparin |
| | | Excess warfarin |
| | | Heparin + warfarin therapy |
| | | Primary amyloidosis-associated factor X deficiency |
| | | Inhibitor of prothrombin, fibrinogen or factors V or X |

## Further reading

Arepally GM, Ortel TL. Heparin-induced thrombocytopenia. *N Engl J Med* 2006; 355: 809–17.

Dahlback B. Blood coagulation. *Lancet* 2000; 355: 1627–32.

George JN. Thrombotic thrombocytopenic purpura. *N Engl J Med* 2006; 354: 1927–35.

Moake JL. Thrombotic microangiopathies. *N Engl J Med* 2002; 347: 589–600.

Toh CH, Dennis M. Disseminated intravascular coagulation: old disease, new hope. *BMJ* 2003; 327: 974–7.

Warkentin TE. Drug-induced immune-mediated thrombocytopenia – from purpura to thrombosis. *N Engl J Med* 2007; 36: 891–3.

# 79 Management of anticoagulation

---

**TABLE 79.1** Indications for unfractionated heparin (UFH)* or low molecular weight heparin (LMWH)†

- Prevention of deep vein thrombosis (UFH and LMWH)
- Treatment of deep vein thrombosis or pulmonary embolism (UFH and LMWH) (pp. 224, 231)
- Treatment of non-ST elevation acute coronary syndrome (UFH and LMWH) (p. 169)
- As adjunct to thrombolytic therapy with alteplase (UFH) (p. 163)
- Treatment of acute peripheral arterial occlusion (UFH)

---

* Unfractionated heparin for treatment is best given by continuous IV infusion; the infusion rate is adjusted to maintain the activated partial thromboplastin time (APTT) at 1.5–2.5 × control (see Table 79.2).
† Low molecular weight heparins are given by SC injection; monitoring of the APTT is not required.

---

**TABLE 79.2** Unfractionated heparin by infusion

---

### Loading dose
- 5000–10,000 units (100 units/kg) IV over 5 min

### Infusion
- 25,000 units made up in saline to 50 ml (500 units/ml)
- Start the infusion at 1400 units/h (2.8 ml/h) using a syringe pump
- Check the activated partial thromboplastin time (APTT) at 6 h
- Adjust the dose as follows:

---

| APTT time* | Action |
|---|---|
| >7.0 | Stop infusion for 30–60 min and then reduce infusion rate by 500 units/h. Recheck APTT in 4 h |

*Continued*

| APTT time* | Action |
|---|---|
| **5.1–7.0** | Reduce infusion rate by 500 units/h. Recheck APTT in 4h |
| **4.1–5.0** | Reduce infusion rate by 300 units/h. Recheck APTT in 10h |
| **3.1–4.0** | Reduce infusion rate by 100 units/h. Recheck APTT in 10h |
| **2.6–3.0** | Reduce infusion rate by 50 units/h. Recheck APTT in 10h |
| **1.5–2.5** | No change in infusion rate. Recheck APTT in 10h |
| **1.2–2.4** | Increase infusion rate by 200 units/h. Recheck APTT in 10h |
| **<1.2** | Increase infusion rate by 400 units/h |

- Heparin can cause an immune-mediated thrombocytopenia, which may be complicated by thrombosis: check the platelet count daily if given for longer than 5 days and stop heparin immediately if this falls

\* Target 1.5–2.5 × control; target in pregnancy 1.5–2.0 × control.
From *Drug and Therapeutics Bulletin* 1992; **30**: 77–80.

**TABLE 79.3** Indications for warfarin anticoagulation

| Indication | Target INR |
|---|---|
| Treatment of DVT or pulmonary embolism | 2.5 |
| Treatment of recurrent DVT or pulmonary embolism on warfarin | 3.5 |
| Atrial fibrillation: prevention of thromboembolism | 2.5 |
| Atrial flutter or fibrillation: in preparation for cardioversion | 2.5 |
| Rheumatic mitral stenosis (in sinus rhythm or atrial fibrillation) | 2.5 |

*Continued*

| Indication | Target INR |
|---|---|
| Bioprosthetic heart valve* | 2.5 |
| Mechanical prosthetic heart valve[†] | 2.5–4.0 |
| Acute myocardial infarction: treatment of left ventricular mural thrombus | 2.5 |

DVT, deep vein thrombosis; INR, international normalized ratio.

* Patients with bioprosthetic heart valves are generally given warfarin for 3 months after surgery until endothelialization occurs, and aspirin thereafter; in patients with chronic atrial fibrillation, warfarin should be continued indefinitely.

[†] The target depends on the exact type of mechanical prosthetic heart valve and its location (aortic or mitral), and the presence of other risk factors for thromboembolism.

**TABLE 79.4** Clinical conditions affecting response to warfarin

### Increased anticoagulation
- Impaired liver function
- Congestive heart failure
- Renal failure
- Malabsorptive states
- Hyperthyroidism
- Age over 70 years
- Low body weight

### Decreased anticoagulation
- Hypothyroidism
- Transfusion of whole blood or fresh frozen plasma
- Diet high in vitamin K (green vegetables)
- Hereditary resistance to warfarin

### ALERT
Drug interactions with warfarin are common and can be serious. When starting or stopping a treatment in a patient taking warfarin, check the list in the *British National Formulary* (www.bnf. org) for an interaction.

Management of anticoagulation

**TABLE 79.5** Starting warfarin: general points

- Check the INR first: if this is over 1.4, do not start warfarin before discussion with a hematologist
- A regimen for starting warfarin is given in Table 79.6. This is suitable for patients under 70 who are not known to be abnormally sensitive to the anticoagulant effect of warfarin (Table 79.4)
- Patients over 70, or those with comorbidities which increase their sensitivity to warfarin (Table 79.4), should start with 2–5 mg doses
- Overlap warfarin with low molecular weight heparin for at least 6 days. Continue overlap until INR is in therapeutic range for 2 days
- Heparin by IV infusion will increase the INR if the APTT is above the therapeutic range

APTT, activated partial thromboplastin time; INR, international normalized ratio.

**TABLE 79.6** Starting warfarin: dosage regimen for patients aged <70 years with normal sensitivity to warfarin (see Table 79.4), and target INR 2.5

| Day | International normalized ratio (INR) (best checked 09.00–10.00) | Dose of wafarin (mg) to be given that evening (17.00–18.00) |
|---|---|---|
| 1 | 1.4 or above | Establish cause of coagulation disorder |
| | | Do not start warfarin before discussion with a hematologist |
| | <1.4 | 10 |
| 2 | <1.8 | 10 |
| | 1.8 | 1 |
| | >1.8 | 0.5 |
| 3 | <2.0 | 10 |
| | 2.0–2.1 | 5 |
| | 2.2–2.3 | 4.5 |
| | 2.4–2.5 | 4 |
| | 2.6–2.7 | 3.5 |

*Continued*

| Day | International normalized ratio (INR) (best checked 09.00–10.00) | Dose of wafarin (mg) to be given that evening (17.00–18.00) |
|---|---|---|
| | 2.8–2.9 | 3 |
| | 3.0–3.1 | 2.5 |
| | 3.2–3.3 | 2 |
| | 3.4 | 1.5 |
| | 3.5 | 1 |
| | 3.6–4.0 | 0.5 |
| | >4.0 | Give none |
| **4** | <1.4 | Ask advice from a hematologist |
| | 1.4 | 8 |
| | 1.5 | 7.5 |
| | 1.6–1.7 | 7 |
| | 1.8 | 6.5 |
| | 1.9 | 6 |
| | 2.0–2.1 | 5.5 |
| | 2.2–2.3 | 5 |
| | 2.4–2.6 | 4.5 |
| | 2.7–3.0 | 4 |
| | 3.1–3.5 | 3.5 |
| | 3.6–4.0 | 3 |
| | 4.1–4.5 | Miss 1 day then give 2 mg |
| | >4.5 | Miss 2 days then give 1 mg |

From Fennerty, A., et al. Anticoagulants in venous thromboembolism. *BMJ* 1988; **297**:1285–8.

Management of anticoagulation

**Management of anticoagulation**

**TABLE 79.7** Management of over-anticoagulation or bleeding in a patient taking warfarin

| International normalized ratio (INR) | Clinical condition | Action |
|---|---|---|
| **>1.5** | Major bleeding or rapid reversal for surgery needed | Stop warfarin<br>Give vitamin K 5 mg IV<br>If there is life-threatening bleeding (e.g. intracranial hemorrhage), give vitamin K 10 mg IV plus prothrombin complex concentrate 50 IU/kg IV<br>Recheck INR after 4 h<br>In other circumstances, give fresh frozen plasma 1 L (15 ml/kg) IV; repeat 6-hourly until INR is <1.5 and bleeding has stopped<br>Discuss management with a hematologist |
| **>8** | No bleeding or minor bleeding | Stop warfarin; restart when INR is <5<br>If there is minor bleeding or if INR is >15 (>12 in patients over 70), and there is no mechanical prosthetic valve give vitamin K 0.5 mg IV plus fresh frozen plasma 1 L IV<br>If the patient is at increased risk of bleeding or if INR is 12–15 in patients under 70, give vitamin K 0.5 mg IV |

*Continued*

| International normalized ratio (INR) | Clinical condition | Action |
|---|---|---|
| | | Repeat dose of vitamin K if INR remains >5 after 24 h Discuss management with a hematologist |
| **6–8** | No bleeding or minor bleeding | Stop warfarin; restart when INR is <5 |
| **<6 but >0.5 units above target value** | No bleeding | Reduce dose or stop warfarin; restart when INR is <5 |

**ALERT**
Full reversal of anticoagulation in a patient with a mechanical prosthetic heart valve carries a risk of valve thrombosis; discuss management with a hematologist.

**ALERT**
If there is unexpected bleeding at therapeutic INR, a structural lesion (e.g. carcinoma of bladder or large bowel) must be excluded.

Management of anticoagulation

## Further reading

Aguilar MI, et al. Treatment of warfarin-associated intracerebral hemorrhage: literature review and expert opinion. *Mayo Clin Proc* 2007; 82: 82–92.

British Society for Haematology. Guidelines on oral anticoagulation (warfarin): third edition – 2005 update. *Br J Haematol* 2005; 132: 277–85.

Hirsh J, et al. AHA/ACC foundation guide to warfarin therapy. *J Am Coll Cardiol* 2003; 41: 1633–52.

Vahanian A. et al. Guidelines on the management of valvular heart disease. *Eur Heart J* 2007; 28: 230–68.

# 80 Sickle cell crisis

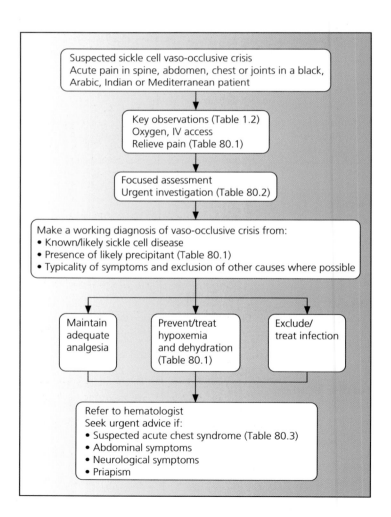

Suspected sickle cell vaso-occlusive crisis
Acute pain in spine, abdomen, chest or joints in a black, Arabic, Indian or Mediterranean patient

↓

Key observations (Table 1.2)
Oxygen, IV access
Relieve pain (Table 80.1)

↓

Focused assessment
Urgent investigation (Table 80.2)

↓

Make a working diagnosis of vaso-occlusive crisis from:
• Known/likely sickle cell disease
• Presence of likely precipitant (Table 80.1)
• Typicality of symptoms and exclusion of other causes where possible

↓

| Maintain adequate analgesia | Prevent/treat hypoxemia and dehydration (Table 80.1) | Exclude/ treat infection |

↓

Refer to hematologist
Seek urgent advice if:
• Suspected acute chest syndrome (Table 80.3)
• Abdominal symptoms
• Neurological symptoms
• Priapism

**TABLE 80.1** Management of sickle cell vaso-occlusive crisis

| Action | Comment |
|---|---|
| **Make the diagnosis** | Known sickle cell disease (or likely sickle cell disease based on the sickle solubility test and blood film)? Acute pain in the spine, abdomen, chest or joints? Presence of a likely precipitant (infection, dehydration, strenuous exercise, exposure to cold and psychological stress)? Exclusion of other causes where possible |
| **Relieve pain** | If the pain is severe and oral analgesia not effective, give morphine 0.1 mg/kg IV or SC, repeated every 20 min until pain is controlled, then 0.05–0.1 mg/kg every 2–4 h IV or SC. Consider using PCA Give adjuvant non-opioid analgesia (paracetamol + NSAID) Prescribe laxative (e.g. lactulose) routinely and other medications (antipruritic, antiemetic, anxiolytic) as needed Monitor pain score, conscious level, respiratory rate, arterial oxygen saturation, heart rate and blood pressure every 30 min until pain is controlled and stable, and then every 2 h Give additional doses of morphine (50% of maintenance dose) every 30 min for breakthrough pain If respiratory rate <10/min, omit maintenance analgesia If severe respiratory depression (<8/min) or sedation, give naloxone 100 µg IV, repeated every 2 min as needed Consider reducing analgesia after 2–3 days and replacing parenteral with oral opioid Discharge when pain is controlled and improving without analgesia or requiring only paracetamol/NSAID/codeine |

*Continued*

Sickle cell crisis

| Action | Comment |
|---|---|
| **Prevent/treat hypoxemia** | Give oxygen by nasal cannulae or mask (see Table 15.4) if arterial oxygen saturation is <95% |
| **Prevent/treat dehydration** | Ensure a fluid intake of 60 ml/kg/day (oral or IV) Unless symptoms are very mild, start fluid replacement with IV glucose or saline Monitor fluid balance, electrolytes and creatinine |
| **Exclude/treat infection** | Assess the patient for evidence of infection. Investigations required urgently are given in Table 80.2 Fever (usually <38°C) may occur without infection (reflecting tissue necrosis). Suspect infection if the temperature is >38°C Adults with sickle cell disease are effectively splenectomized and thus at particular risk of infection with capsulate bacteria: *Pneumococcus*, *Meningococcus* and *Haemophilus influenzae* type B Suspect *Salmonella* gastroenteritis if there is diarrhea and vomiting Antibiotic therapy should be started after taking blood for culture. If there is no clinical focus of infection, give cefuroxime (+ macrolide if there are chest signs) |
| **Physiotherapy** | Incentive spirometry, performed regularly every 2 h, is beneficial in patients with chest pain, back pain, respiratory infection or hypoxia, reducing the risk of acute chest syndrome and atelectasis |
| **Blood transfusion** | Blood transfusion should be considered if hemoglobin falls >2 g/dl; discuss with a hematologist Exchange transfusion is indicated for severe acute chest syndrome (Table 80.3) |

NSAID, non-steroidal anti-inflammatory drug; PCA, patient controlled analgesia.
From Guidelines for the management of the acute painful crisis in sickle cell disease. *Br J Haematol* 2003; **120**: 744–52.

Sickle cell crisis

**TABLE 80.2** Urgent investigation in suspected vaso-occlusive crisis of sickle cell disease

- Sickle solubility test and hemoglobin (Hb) electrophoresis (if diagnosis not previously established)*
- Steady-state hemoglobin and Hb electrophoresis (from clinic card if diagnosis is established)
- Full blood count, reticulocyte count and film[†]
- Blood group and antibody screen
- Blood culture (×2)
- Urine microscopy and culture
- Chest X-ray
- Arterial blood gases (if arterial oxygen saturation <90%, chest X-ray shadowing, or respiratory symptoms)
- Creatinine, sodium and potassium
- Liver function tests if abdominal pain or jaundice

* Solubility test indicates the presence of HbS, and is therefore positive in both homozygotes (SS) and heterozygotes (AS, sickle cell trait) and also in double heterozygotes (S beta Thal, HbSC).
[†] Blood film in sickle cell disease (homozygous SS): normochromic normocytic anemia; raised reticulocyte count; Howell–Jolly bodies (reflecting hyposplenism) in adults, usually sickle cells. Numerous target cells indicate HbSC.

Sickle cell crisis

**ALERT**
Sickle cell crises causing increased anemia are much less common than vaso-occlusive crises:

- Sequestration crisis (in the sinuses of the enlarged spleen in children)
- Aplastic crisis (reduced marrow erythropoiesis, e.g. after parvovirus infection)
- Increased hemolysis crisis (following infections).

The clue is the rapid fall in hemoglobin. These crises must be recognized early because transfusion can be life-saving. Seek advice from a hematologist.

| **TABLE 80.3** Acute chest syndrome in sickle cell disease | |
|---|---|
| **Element** | **Comment** |
| **Precipitants** | Infection (viral, bacterial, mycoplasmal and chlamydial)<br>Bone marrow infarction with fat embolism<br>Pulmonary thromboembolism (p. 231)<br>Hypoventilation/atelectasis |
| **Diagnostic criteria** | Breathlessness, chest pain<br>Focal chest signs, fever<br>Hypoxia<br>Chest X-ray shows new shadowing involving at least one complete lung segment |
| **Management** | Contact a hematologist and intensive care physician for advice if you suspect the diagnosis<br>Give oxygen 28–60% by mask and monitor oxygen saturation by pulse oximetry, aiming to maintain $SaO_2$ >92%. Check arterial blood gases (recheck after 4h or if deterioration occurs)<br>Ensure optimum pain control and fluid balance (Table 80.1)<br>Start empirical antibiotic therapy with cefuroxime + macrolide IV<br>Mechanical ventilation and exchange transfusion are needed if $PaO_2$ cannot be maintained above 9kPa (70mmHg) with 60% oxygen by mask |

## Further reading

British Society for Haematology. Guidelines for the management of the acute painful crisis in sickle cell disease. *Br J Haematol* 2003; 120: 744–52.

Stuart MJ, Nagel RL. Sickle-cell disease. *Lancet* 2004; 364: 1343–60.

# 81 Anaphylaxis and anaphylactic shock

Suspected anaphylactic shock
Hypotension, breathlessness, wheeze, skin and mucosal urticaria, erythema and angioedema, following exposure to potential allergen (Table 81.1)
See Table 81.2 for differential diagnosis

↓

Remove allergen
Call resuscitation team
Oxygen, ECG monitor, IV access
Lie patient flat and raise foot of bed

↓

Give epinephrine 500 µg IM (0.5 ml of 1 in 1000 solution) in mid anterolateral thigh, repeated as necessary at 5 min intervals

**Airway/breathing**
Nebulized salbutamol for wheeze
If there is respiratory distress due to upper airway obstruction: endotracheal intubation or tracheotomy

**Circulation**
Give saline IV 1 L over 30 min
If systolic BP remains <90 mmHg, give further saline 1 L over 30 min
If systolic BP remains <90 mmHg after 2 L or more of fluid, start an infusion of epinephrine via a central line and give further fluid guided by central venous pressure

**Drug therapy**
Give chlorphenamine 20 mg IV over 1 min and hydrocortisone 300 mg IV
Then give chlorphenamine 8 mg 8-hourly PO for 48 h and hydrocortisone 300 mg 6-hourly IV for 24 h

**Management of mild to moderate anaphylaxis:**
Table 81.3

**Patient education and follow-up after anaphylaxis:**
Table 81.4

**TABLE 81.1** Causes of anaphylactic and anaphylactoid reaction*

**Drugs**
- Antibiotics, most commonly beta-lactam class
- Non-steroidal anti-inflammatory drugs
- Radiographic contrast media
- Chemotherapeutic agents for cancer
- Streptokinase
- Neuromuscular blocking agents
- Thiopental
- Vitamin K

**Others**
- Blood products
- Allergen extracts
- Insect stings/bites
- Foods (e.g. nuts, seafood)
- Latex

* Anaphylactic and anaphylactoid reactions to drugs are clinically indistinguishable. Anaphylactoid reactions are due to direct triggering of the release of mediators by the drug itself and may therefore occur after the first dose.

**TABLE 81.2** Differential diagnosis of anaphylaxis*

| Disorder | Comment |
|---|---|
| **Hereditary angioedema** | No urticaria<br>Treat with C1-esterase inhibitor replacement concentrate or fresh frozen plasma |
| **ACE inhibitor angioedema** | No urticaria<br>May develop days to years after starting ACE inhibitor |
| **Severe asthma** | No urticaria or angioedema |

*Continued*

| Disorder | Comment |
|----------|---------|
| **Panic disorder** | No urticaria, angioedema, hypoxia or hypotension<br>Functional stridor may develop in acute panic disorder as a result of forced adduction of vocal cords |
| **Vasovagal reaction** | No urticaria or angioedema |
| **Scombroid poisoning** | Scombroid contamination is caused by bacterial overgrowth in improperly stored dark-meat fish (e.g. tuna, mackerel)<br>Symptoms appear within 30 min of eating spoiled fish: urticaria, nausea, vomiting, diarrhea, headache<br>Treat with antihistamine |

ACE, angiotensin-converting enzyme.
* Anaphylaxis is associated with the release of histamine and tryptase from mast cells. Check the serum tryptase level (within 6 h of the attack) if there is doubt as to the diagnosis of anaphylaxis.

---

**TABLE 81.3** Management of mild to moderate anaphylaxis

- Admit patients with a history of life-threatening reactions or severe asthma
- Observe for a minimum of 4 h after resolution of symptoms and signs (time course of reaction may be uniphasic, protracted or biphasic)
- Give chlorphenamine 8 mg 8-hourly PO for 24–48 h

---

**TABLE 81.4** Patient education and follow-up after anaphylaxis

- If anaphylaxis was due to medication, inform patient of the drug responsible for the reaction, and record this in the 'Alert' section of the medical record.
- A bracelet engraved with this information may be obtained from Medic-Alert Foundation International
- Patients at high risk of anaphylaxis should carry epinephrine for self-injection in the event of further exposure to allergen. Consult the *British National Formulary* for a suitable device
- Refer patients with moderate or severe reactions to a clinical immunologist for follow-up
- Specific allergen immunotherapy (desensitization) may be indicated in the case of severe anaphylactic reaction to bee or wasp stings

---

## Further reading

Brown SGA. Anaphylaxis: clinical concepts and research priorities. *Emerg Med Australasia* 2006; 18: 155–69.

# 82 Complications of cancer

| **TABLE 82.1** Complications of cancer | |
|---|---|
| **Complication** | **Reference** |
| **Breathlessness** | Table 82.2 |
| **Confusional state** | Table 82.3 |
| **Vomiting** | Table 82.4 |
| **Pain** | Tables 82.5, 82.6 |
| **Acute superior vena cava obstruction** | Table 82.7 |
| **Upper airway obstruction** | See p. 245 |
| **Pleural effusion** | See p. 283 |
| **Cardiac tamponade** | See p. 216 |
| **Hyponatremia** | See p. 439 |
| **Hypercalcemia** | See p. 451 |
| **Raised intracranial pressure** | See p. 360 |
| **Spinal cord compression** | See p. 339 |
| **Deep vein thrombosis** | See p. 224 |
| **Pulmonary embolism** | See p. 231 |

Complications of cancer

**TABLE 82.2** Causes of breathlessness in the patient with cancer (see also Chapter 14)

| Cause | Onset and progression | Associated clinical features | Investigation | Management options |
|---|---|---|---|---|
| **Upper airway obstruction (p. 245)** | Relentless progression May rapidly progress to complete occlusion of airway | Stridor, wheeze | Flow–volume loop Flexible laryngoscopy Computed tomography (CT) | Corticosteroids Debulking of intraluminal lesions Stenting of extrinsic compression Radiotherapy |
| **Acute superior vena cava obstruction** | Rapid onset and progression of dyspnea | Facial swelling Distension of the neck veins Prominent chest wall veins | CT | See Table 82.7 |
| **Pulmonary embolism** | Acute dyspnea | Hypoxemia | $\dot{V}/\dot{Q}$ scan CT pulmonary angiography | See p. 231 |

Continued

| Cause | Onset and progression | Associated clinical features | Investigation | Management options |
|---|---|---|---|---|
| **Bronchial obstruction causing lung collapse/ consolidation** | Gradual onset Progression over days | Reduced chest movements, percussion note dull, breath sounds reduced on affected side | Chest X-ray Bronchoscopy | Laser therapy Stenting |
| **Pleural effusion (p. 283)** | Insidious onset Slow progression over days to weeks | Reduced chest wall movements and stony dull percussion note on affected side | Chest X-ray Ultrasound | Aspiration Pleurodesis |
| **Cardiac tamponade (p. 216)** | Insidious onset Progression over days to weeks | Raised jugular venous pressure Pulsus paradoxus | Echocardiography | Pericardiocentesis Pericardial window |
| **Lymphangitis carcinomatosa** | Insidious onset Relentless progression | Basal crackles | Chest X-ray CT | Corticosteroids Chemotherapy for sensitive tumors |

---

**TABLE 82.3** Causes of a confusional state in the patient with cancer

As well as other causes of confusional state (see Table 20.3), consider in particular:
- Opioid-induced neurotoxicity (may present with agitated confusion: reduce dose of opioid, ensure adequate hydration, and use haloperidol if needed to treat agitation)
- Brain/meningeal metastases
- Hyponatremia
- Hypercalcemia
- Paraneoplastic syndromes

---

**TABLE 82.4** Causes of vomiting in the patient with cancer

| Syndrome | Causes | Management | |
| --- | --- | --- | --- |
| | | **First-line** | **Second-line** |
| **Meningeal irritation or stretch** | Intracranial tumor causing raised intracranial pressure | Dexamethasone | Add cyclizine or levomepromazine |
| | Meningeal infiltration by tumor | Radiotherapy | |
| | Skull metastases | | |
| **Abdominal and pelvic tumor** | Mesenteric metastases | Cyclizine | Levomepromazine |
| | Liver metastases | | |
| | Ureteric obstruction | | |
| | Retroperitoneal cancer | | |

*Continued*

| Syndrome | Causes | Management | |
| --- | --- | --- | --- |
| | | **First-line** | **Second-line** |
| **Malignant bowel obstruction** | Mechanical obstruction: intrinsic or extrinsic by tumor Functional obstruction: intestinal motility disorder caused by malignant involvement of blood supply, bowel muscle or nerves, or paraneoplastic neuropathy | Haloperidol or cyclizine | Reduce gastric secretions: ranitidine or octreotide |
| **Gastric stasis** | Opioids and anticholinergic drugs Mechanical resistance to emptying: ascites, hepatomegaly, peptic ulcer, gastritis, tumor Paraneoplastic autonomic failure causing gastroparesis | If starting opioids: metoclopramide or haloperidol | Levomepromazine |

*Continued*

| Syndrome | Causes | Management First-line | Second-line |
|----------|--------|------------|-------------|
| **Chemically/ metabolically induced** | Drugs: opioids, antiepileptics, cytotoxics, antibiotics, digoxin<br>Metabolic: e.g. hypercalcemia<br>Toxins: e.g. bacterial exotoxins, tumor necrosis | Treat underlying cause<br>Haloperidol | Cyclizine |
| **Movement-related nausea and vomiting** | Abdominal tumors | Levomepromazine | Hyoscine hydrobromide (transdermal patch is an alternative route of administration) |

**TABLE 82.5** Causes of pain in the patient with cancer due to the cancer

| Tissue affected | Mechanism of pain | Characteristics of pain/comments |
|-----------------|-------------------|----------------------------------|
| **Bone** | Tumor in bone, stretching the periosteum | Continuous, dull, poorly localized pain, worsened by weight bearing or by straining the bone |
| | Pathological fracture caused by lysis of bone by tumor | Severe pain worsened by the slightest passive movement |

*Continued*

| Tissue affected | Mechanism of pain | Characteristics of pain/comments |
|---|---|---|
| **Pleura and peritoneum** | Infiltration of pleura or peritoneum by tumor | Well-localized sharp pain provoked by inspiration<br>Non-malignant causes are common (e.g. pulmonary embolism and pneumonia) |
| **Visceral pain** | Pain from deep structures of chest, abdomen or pelvis | Pain poorly localized to the affected viscera and may refer to other sites. May be tender to palpation over affected organ<br>Non-malignant causes are common |
| **Nerve compression pain** | Compression of nerve by tumor or bone | Pain may be continuous (e.g. tumor compression) or intermittent (e.g. skeletal instability), but only investigation will differentiate the cause<br>Reduced sensation or paresthesiae are common |
| **Neuropathic pain** | Altered spinal and central neurotransmitter levels caused by nerve damage | Unpleasant sensory change (e.g. burning, cold, numb, stabbing) in the distribution of a peripheral nerve or nerve root. Often accompanied by hypersensitivity or allodynia (pain on light touch)<br>May involve the sympathetic system and have a vascular distribution accompanied by sympathetic changes (pallor or flushing, sweating or absence of sweating) |

*Continued*

| Tissue affected | Mechanism of pain | Characteristics of pain/comments |
|---|---|---|
| **Central nervous system** | Spinal cord compression (p. 339) | Spinal pain is usually first feature<br>Motor and sensory signs occur later<br>Sphincter disturbance is a late sign |
| | Cerebral metastases | Headache on lying flat, vomiting, drowsiness, focal neurological deficit |

**TABLE 82.6** Other causes of pain in the patient with cancer

| Mechanism | Comment |
|---|---|
| **Chemotherapy** | Pain may be associated with the infusion of chemotherapy. Peripheral neuropathy and severe mucositis can also occur although these take longer to develop |
| **Radiotherapy** | Can cause inflammation and ulceration of exposed mucous membranes (e.g. gut, vagina, bladder)<br>Myelopathy may occur following radiation of the cervical and thoracic spinal cord (tends to develop weeks after treatment and may take up to 6 months to resolve) |
| **Hormonal therapy** | Tumor flare may occur transiently with initiation of luteinizing hormone releasing hormone (LHRH) therapy in patients with prostate cancer<br>Tumor flare may also occur following hormonal treatment of breast cancer |

*Continued*

| Mechanism | Comment |
|---|---|
| **Indirectly related to cancer** | E.g. pulmonary embolism, peptic ulceration, constipation, infection, pressure sores |
| **Other causes** | E.g. pre-existing arthritis |

**TABLE 82.7** Acute superior vena cava obstruction

| Element | Comment |
|---|---|
| **Causes** | Two-thirds of cases due to cancer: lung cancer (72%); lymphoma (12%); other cancers (16%) One-third of cases due to non-malignant causes, most often thrombosis associated with intravenous catheter or leads of pacemaker/ICD |
| **Clinical features** | Swelling of the face or neck (80%), often with cyanosis or plethora Swelling of the arm (70%) Breathlessness ( 65%) Cough (50%) Distended neck veins and prominent chest wall collateral veins |
| **Diagnosis** | Chest X-ray usually abnormal in cancer-related SVC obstruction, with mediastinal widening (in two-thirds) and pleural effusion (in one-quarter). CT with contrast for definitive diagnosis, or MRI if contrast administration contraindicated |
| **Management of SVC obstruction due to cancer** | Seek expert advice Obtain tissue for histological/cytological diagnosis Corticosteroids if suspected lymphoma or thymoma (as steroid-responsive) Radiotherapy/chemotherapy as appropriate to cancer type Stent placement if severe symptoms requiring urgent relief of obstruction |

CT, computed tomography; ICD, implantable cardioverter-defibrillator; MRI, magnetic resonance imaging; SVC, superior vena cava.

## Further reading

Halfdanarson TR, et al. Oncologic emergencies: diagnosis and treatement. *Mayo Clinic Proc* 2006; 81: 835–48.

Wilson LD, et al. Superior vena cava syndrome with malignant causes. *N Engl J Med* 2007; 356: 1862–9.

See also links in Symptom Management, Cancer Specialist Library, NHS National Library for Health (http://www.library.nhs.uk/cancer/SearchResults.aspx?catID=12286).

Complications of cancer

# Miscellaneous

# 83 Acute medical problems in HIV-positive patients

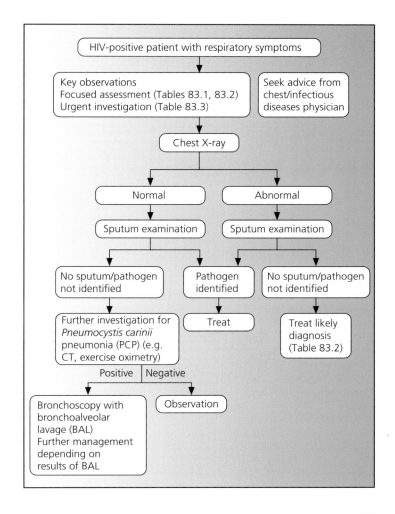

**TABLE 83.1** Respiratory symptoms in the HIV-positive patient

| CD4 T cell count ($\times 10^6$/L) | | |
|---|---|---|
| >500 | 200–500 | <200 |
| Usual causes | Usual causes | Usual causes |
| *Mycobacterium tuberculosis* infection | *M. tuberculosis* infection | *Pneumocystis carinii (jiroveci)* pneumonia |
| | | *M. tuberculosis* infection |
| | | *M. avium intracellulare* infection |
| | | Cytomegalovirus pneumonitis |
| | | Fungal pneumonia |
| | | Kaposi sarcoma |

**ALERT**
Seek expert advice from an infectious diseases physician on the management of acute medical problems in the HIV-positive patient.

**TABLE 83.2** Diagnostic clues in the HIV-positive patient with respiratory symptoms.

| Diagnosis | Clinical features | Chest X-ray features |
|---|---|---|
| **Pneumocystis carinii (jiroveci) pneumonia (PCP)** | Dyspnea<br>Dry cough<br>Lungs clear, or sparse basal crackles<br>Fever<br>See Table 83.4 | Diffuse bilateral interstitial or alveolar shadowing<br>Lobar consolidation rare<br>Pleural effusion rare<br>Pneumothorax may occur<br>See Table 83.4 |

*Continued*

| Diagnosis | Clinical features | Chest X-ray features |
|---|---|---|
| *Mycobacterium tuberculosis* infection | Cough<br>Hemoptysis<br>Fever | More often typical of tuberculosis if CD4 count is >200: multiple areas of consolidation, often with cavitation, in one or both upper lobes |
| *Mycobacterium avium intracellulare* infection | Cough<br>Dyspnea<br>Fever | Often normal |
| Bacterial pneumonia (p. 268) | Commoner in smokers<br>Productive cough<br>Focal signs<br>Fever | Focal consolidation |
| Cytomegalovirus pneumonitis | Clinically indistinguishable from PCP (dual infection may occur) | Diffuse bilateral interstitial shadowing |
| Fungal pneumonia | Fever<br>Cough<br>Weight loss<br>Systemic features of fungal infection may be present (skin lesions, lymphadenopathy, hepatosplenomegaly) | Diffuse bilateral interstitial shadowing in ~50%<br>Focal shadowing, nodules, cavities, pleural effusion and hilar adenopathy may be seen |

*Continued*

| Diagnosis | Clinical features | Chest X-ray features |
|---|---|---|
| **Kaposi sarcoma** | No fever<br>Dyspnea<br>More common in homosexual men and Africans than IV drug users<br>May be associated with cutaneous Kaposi sarcoma | Diffuse bilateral interstitial shadowing, more nodular than PCP<br>May be unilateral and associated with hilar adenopathy<br>Pleural effusion strongly suggestive |

**TABLE 83.3** Urgent investigation of the HIV-positive patient with respiratory symptoms

- Chest X-ray
- Arterial blood gases
- Full blood count and film
- CD4 T cell count and viral load
- Blood culture (positive in most patients with *Mycobacterium avium intracellulare* infection: use specific myobacterial culture bottles)
- Blood glucose
- Creatinine, sodium and potassium
- Liver function tests
- Lactate dehydrogenase (raised in *Pneumocystis carinii* (*jiroveci*) pneumonia)
- Expectorated sputum if available for Gram and Ziehl–Nielsen stain and culture
- Induced sputum (using hypertonic saline via nebulizer) for staining for *P. carinii* (*jiroveci*)

**TABLE 83.4** *Pneumocystis carinii* (*jiroveci*) pneumonia (PCP): diagnosis and management

| Element | Comment |
|---|---|
| **Patients at risk** | Newly diagnosed HIV infection with advanced disease (CD4 count <200)<br>Patients with previous PCP or CD4 count <200 who are not taking prophylaxis |
| **Clinical features** | Subacute onset<br>Fever (~90%)<br>Cough (~95%), usually non-productive<br>Progressive breathlessness (~95%)<br>Tachypnea (~60%)<br>Chest examination normal in ~50% |
| **Chest X-ray features** | Initially normal in up to 25%<br>Commonest abnormalities are diffuse bilateral interstitial or alveolar shadowing<br>Lobar consolidation rare<br>Pleural effusion rare<br>Pneumothorax may occur |
| **Induced sputum** | Staining of induced sputum for *P. carinii* (*jiroveci*) trophic forms and cysts<br>Specificity ~100%, sensitivity 50–90% |
| **Bronchoscopy with bronchoalveolar lavage** | Indicated if PCP is suspected but induced sputum is non-diagnostic or cannot be done<br>Specificity ~100%, sensitivity ~80–90% |
| **Antimicrobial therapy** | First choice: co-trimoxazole PO or IV for 21 days. Causes hemolysis in glucose-6-phosphate dehydrogenase-deficient patients (African/Mediterranean). Other side effects include nausea, vomiting, fever, rash, marrow suppression and raised transaminases<br>Alternative regimens: primaquine + clindamycin; atovaquone; pentamidine |

*Continued*

| Element | Comment |
|---|---|
| **Adjuvant steroid therapy** | Start immediately if severe PCP (breathless at rest; $PaO_2$ breathing air <8 kPa; extensive interstitial shadowing on chest X-ray)<br>Give prednisolone 40 mg twice daily PO for 5 days, followed by prednisolone 40 mg daily PO for 5 days, then prednisolone 20 mg daily PO for 11 days |

**TABLE 83.5** Headache/confusion/focal neurological signs in the HIV-positive patient

| CD4 T cell count ($\times 10^6$/L) | | |
|---|---|---|
| **>500** | **200–500** | **<200** |
| Usual causes | Usual causes<br>HIV encephalopathy | Usual causes<br>Cerebral lymphoma<br>Toxoplasmosis<br>Cryptococcal meningitis (p. 332)<br>Tuberculous meningitis (p. 331)<br>Progressive multifocal leucoencephalopathy |

- Arrange urgent cranial CT or MRI
- Perform a lumbar puncture if the scan is normal (p. 627). Send cerebrospinal fluid for: cell count; protein concentration; glucose (fluoride tube); Gram, Ziehl–Nielson and India ink stains; and serological tests for *Cryptococcus* and *Toxoplasma gondii*.
- If no diagnosis can be made, give empirical treatment for toxoplasmosis with sulfadiazine and pyrimethamine, and repeat CT/MRI after 2–3 weeks.
- Seek expert advice from an infectious diseases physician or neurologist.

| TABLE 83.6 Acute diarrhea in the HIV-positive patient* | | |
| --- | --- | --- |
| **Cause** | **Clinical features** | **Diagnosis/treatment** |
| **Cryptosporidiosis (*Cryptosporidium* species)** | Subacute onset Associated abdominal pain Severe diarrhea | Identification of oocysts in stool Seek expert advice on treatment |
| **Isosporiasis (*Isospora belli*)** | Incubation period 1 week Associated fever, abdominal pain, diarrhea with fatty stools | Identification of oocysts in stool, duodenal aspirate or jejunal biopsy Seek expert advice on treatment |
| **Cytomegalovirus** | Diarrhea may be accompanied by systemic illness and hepatitis | Serological tests for cytomegalovirus Seek expert advice on treatment |

*In addition to the causes of acute diarrhea in Tables 59.3–59.5, other pathogens may be responsible as listed in table above.

*Acute medical problems in HIV-positive patients*

## Further reading

Hammer SM. Management of newly diagnosed HIV infection. *N Engl J Med* 2005; 353: 1702–10.

Huang L, et al. Intensive care of patients with HIV infection. *N Engl J Med* 2006; 355: 173–81.

Simon V, et al. HIV/AIDS epidemiology, pathogenesis, prevention, and treatment. *Lancet* 206; 368: 489–504.

Thomas CF Jr, Limper AH. Pneumocystis pneumonia. *N Engl J Med* 2004; 35: 2487–98.

# 84 Fever on return from abroad

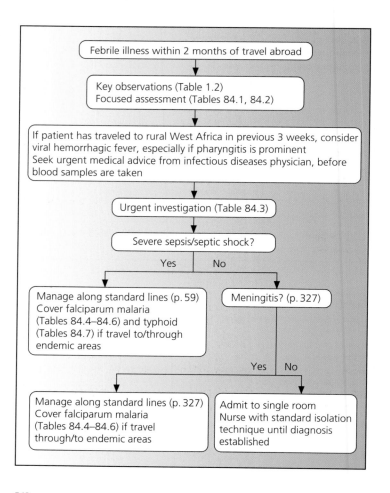

Febrile illness within 2 months of travel abroad

↓

Key observations (Table 1.2)
Focused assessment (Tables 84.1, 84.2)

↓

If patient has traveled to rural West Africa in previous 3 weeks, consider viral hemorrhagic fever, especially if pharyngitis is prominent
Seek urgent medical advice from infectious diseases physician, before blood samples are taken

↓

Urgent investigation (Table 84.3)

↓

Severe sepsis/septic shock?

Yes — No

**Yes:**
Manage along standard lines (p. 59)
Cover falciparum malaria
(Tables 84.4–84.6) and typhoid
(Tables 84.7) if travel to/through endemic areas

**No:**
Meningitis? (p. 327)

Yes — No

**Yes:**
Manage along standard lines (p. 327)
Cover falciparum malaria
(Tables 84.4–84.6) if travel through/to endemic areas

**No:**
Admit to single room
Nurse with standard isolation technique until diagnosis established

**TABLE 84.1** Focused assessment of the patient with a febrile illness after travel abroad

**History**
- Which countries traveled to and through? Travel in urban or rural areas or both?
- Immunizations before travel
- Malaria prophylaxis taken as prescribed?
- When did symptoms first appear (Table 84.2)?
- Treatments taken?
- Known or possible exposure to infection (including sexually transmitted diseases)?

| Exposure | Potential infection or disease |
|---|---|
| **Raw or undercooked foods** | Enteric infections, hepatitis A, trichinosis |
| **Drinking untreated water; milk, cheese** | Salmonellosis, shigellosis, hepatitis A, brucellosis |
| **Fresh water swimming** | Schistosomiasis, leptospirosis |
| **Sexual contact** | HIV, syphilis, hepatitis B, gonococcemia |
| **Insect bites** | Malaria, dengue fever (mosquitoes); typhus, Crimean-Congo hemorrhagic fever, borreliosis, tularemia (ticks); Chagas disease (triatomine bugs); African trypanosomiasis (tse tse flies) |
| **Animal exposure or bites** | Rabies, Q fever, tularemia, borreliosis, viral hemorrhagic fevers, plague |
| **Exposure to infected persons** | Lassa, Marburg or Ebola viruses; hepatitis; typhoid; meningococcemia |

*Continued*

**Fever on return from abroad**

| Examination | |
|---|---|
| **Sign** | **Potential infection or disease** |
| **Rash** | Dengue fever, typhoid, typhus, syphilis, gonorrhea, Ebola virus, brucellosis |
| **Jaundice** | Hepatitis A and B (patients afebrile when jaundice appears), malaria, yellow fever, leptospirosis, relapsing fever, cytomegalovirus and Epstein–Barr virus infection |
| **Lymphadenopathy** | Rickettsial infections, brucellosis, dengue fever, HIV, Lassa fever, visceral leishmaniasis |
| **Hepatomegaly** | Amoebiasis, malaria, typhoid, hepatitis, leptospirosis |
| **Splenomegaly** | Malaria, relapsing fever, trypanosomiasis, typhoid, brucellosis, kala-azar, typhus, dengue fever |
| **Eschar (painless ulcer with black center and erythematous margin)** | Typhus, borreliosis, Crimean-Congo hemorrhagic fever |
| **Hemorrhage** | Lassa, Marburg or Ebola viruses; Crimean-Congo hemorrhagic fever; Rift valley fever; dengue; yellow fever; meninococcemia; epidemic louse borne typhus; Rocky Mountain spotted fever |

**ALERT**
Exclude malaria in any patient with a febrile illness presenting within 1 year (especially within the first 3 months) of return from an endemic area (most of Africa, Asia, Central and South America).

**ALERT**
Chemoprophylaxis does not ensure full protection and may
prolong the incubation period.

---

**TABLE 84.2** Typical incubation periods for selected tropical infections

**Short (<10 days)**
- Arboviral infections (including dengue fever)
- Enteric bacterial infections
- Typhus (louse-borne, flea-borne)
- Plague
- Paratyphoid
- Viral hemorrhagic fever (Lassa, Marburg, Ebola)

**Medium (10–21 days)**
- Malaria
- Typhoid fever
- Scrub typhus, Q fever, spotted fever group
- African trypanosomiasis
- Brucellosis
- Leptospirosis

**Long (>21 days)**
- Viral hepatitis
- Malaria
- Tuberculosis
- HIV
- Schistosomiasis (Katayama fever)
- Amoebic liver abscess
- Visceral leishmaniasis
- Filariasis

Fever on return from abroad

**ALERT**
In patients who have traveled to rural West Africa within the
previous 3 weeks, a viral hemorrhagic fever must be considered,
particularly if pharyngitis is a prominent symptom. Seek advice
from an infectious diseases physician on management, before
blood samples are taken.

**TABLE 84.3** Urgent investigation of the patient with a febrile illness after travel abroad

- Full blood count
- Blood film for malarial parasites if travel to or through an endemic area; the intensity of the parasitemia is variable in malaria. If the diagnosis is suspected but the film is negative, repeat blood films every 8 h for 2–3 days
- Blood glucose
- Creatinine, sodium and potassium
- Liver function tests
- Blood culture ×2
- Throat swab
- Urine stick test, microscopy and culture
- Stool microscopy and culture
- Serology as appropriate (e.g. for suspected viral hepatitis, *Legionella* pneumonia, typhoid, amoebic liver abscess, leptospirosis)
- Chest X-ray
- Lumbar puncture if neck stiffness present

**TABLE 84.4** Falciparum malaria

| Element | Comment |
|---|---|
| **Clinical features** | Prodromal symptoms of malaise, headache, myalgia, anorexia and mild fever |
| | Paroxysms of fever lasting 8–12 h |
| | Dry cough, abdominal discomfort, diarrhea and vomiting common |
| | Moderate tender hepatosplenomegaly (without lymphadenopathy) |
| | Jaundice may occur |
| **Cerebral malaria** | Reduced conscious level |
| | Focal or generalized fits common |

*Continued*

| Element | Comment |
|---|---|
| | Abnormal neurological signs may be present (including opisthotonos, extensor posturing of decorticate or decerebrate pattern, sustained posturing of limbs, conjugate deviation of the eyes, nystagmus, dysconjugate eye movements, bruxism, extensor plantar responses, generalized flaccidity) |
| | Retinal hemorrhages common (papilledema may be present but is unusual) |
| | Abnormal patterns of breathing common (including irregular periods of apnea and hyperventilation) |
| **Blood results** | Neutropenia<br>Thrombocytopenia |
| **Diagnosis** | Microscopy of Giemsa-stained thick and thin blood films. The thick film is more sensitive in diagnosing malaria. The thin film allows species identification and quantification of the percentage of parasitized red cells |
| **Treatment** | Supportive management as for severe sepsis (p. 59)<br>Chemotherapy (Table 84.5)<br>Management of complications (Table 84.6)<br>Seek advice from infectious diseases physician |

**TABLE 84.5** Falciparum malaria: chemotherapy

- In most parts of the world, *Plasmodium falciparum* is now resistant to chloroquine and so this should not be used

**Patient seriously ill or unable to take tablets**
- Quinine should be given by IV infusion
- Loading dose: 20 mg/kg (up to a maximum of 1.4 g) of quinine salt given over 4 h by IV infusion (omit if quinine, quinidine or mefloquine given within the previous 24 h), followed after 8 h by maintenance dose

*Continued*

- Maintenance dose: 10 mg/kg (up to a maximum of 700 mg) of quinine salt given over 4h by IV infusion 8-hourly, until the patient can swallow tablets to complete the 7 day course. Reduce the maintenance dose to 5–7 mg/kg of quinine salt if IV treatment is needed for more than 48h
- The course of quinine should be followed by either a single dose of three tablets of Fansidar (each tablet contains pyrimethamine 25 mg and sulfadoxine 500 mg), or (if Fansidar resistant) doxycycline 200 mg daily PO for 7 days when renal function has returned to normal or clindamycin 450 mg 8-hourly PO for 5 days

**Patient not seriously ill and able to swallow tablets**
- Quinine 600 mg of quinine salt 8-hourly PO for 7 days, followed by either a single dose of three tablets of Fansidar, or (if Fansidar resistant) doxycycline 200 mg daily PO for 7 days, or clindamycin 450 mg 8-hourly PO for 7 days

*Or*
- Malarone (proguanil with atovaquone) four tablets once daily for 3 days

*Or*
- Riamet (artemether with lumefantrine): if weight is over 35 kg, give four tablets initially, followed by five further doses of four tablets at 8, 24, 36, 48 and 60h (total 24 tablets over 60h)
- It is not necessary to give Fansidar, doxycycline or clindamycin after treatment with Malarone or Riamet

**TABLE 84.6** Falciparum malaria: management of complications

| Complication | Comment/management |
|---|---|
| **Hypotension** | Give colloid (or blood if PCV <20% and hemoglobin <7 g/dl) to maintain CVP at +5 cmH$_2$O (avoid higher levels because of the risk of pulmonary edema) Start inotropic vasopressor therapy if systolic BP remains <90 mmHg despite fluids (Table 9.5) *Continued* |

| Complication | Comment/management |
|---|---|
| | Start antibiotic therapy for possible coexistent Gram-negative sepsis after taking blood cultures (Table 10.5) |
| **Hypoglycemia** | This is a common complication: blood glucose should be checked 4-hourly, or if conscious level deteriorates or if fits occur |
| | If blood glucose is <3.5 mmol/L, give 50 ml of glucose 50% IV and start an IV infusion of glucose 10% (initially 1 L 12-hourly) via a large peripheral or central vein |
| **Fits** | Recheck blood glucose |
| | Manage along standard lines (p. 349) |
| | Exclude coexistent bacterial meningitis by CSF examination (NB lumbar puncture should not be done within 1 h of a major seizure) |
| **Pulmonary edema** | May occur from excessive IV fluid or ARDS (p. 185) |
| | Manage along standard lines (p. 185) |

ARDS, acute respiratory distress syndrome; CSF, cerebrospinal fluid; CVP, central venous pressure; PCV, packed cell volume.

**Fever on return from abroad**

| **TABLE 84.7** Typhoid | |
|---|---|
| **Element** | **Comment** |
| **Clinical features** | Insidious onset with malaise, headache, myalgia, dry cough, anorexia and fever |
| | Abdominal pain, distension and tenderness |
| | Initial constipation followed later by diarrhea |
| | Ileal perforation (due to necrosis of Peyer patch in bowel wall) resulting in peritonitis in ~2% |
| | Gastrointestinal bleeding (due to erosion of Peyer patch into vessel) in ~15% |

*Continued*

| Element | Comment |
|---|---|
| | Encephalopathy in ~10% |
| | Liver and spleen often palpable after first week |
| | Erythematous macular rash (rose spots) on upper abdomen and anterior chest (may occur during second week) in ~25% |
| **Blood results** | Raised white cell count |
| | Abnormal liver function tests |
| **Diagnosis** | Blood culture positive in 40–80% |
| | Stool and urine culture positive after first week |
| | Widal test positive in 50–75% |
| **Treatment** | Supportive management as for severe sepsis (p. 59) |
| | Antibiotic therapy with quinolone or ceftriaxone |
| | Seek advice from infectious diseases physician |

## Further reading

Bhan MK, et al. Typhoid and paratyphoid fever. *Lancet* 2005; 366: 749–62.

British Infection Society (2007). Algorithm for the initial assessment and management of malaria in adults. British Infection Society website (http://www.britishinfectionsociety. org/malaria.html).

Freedman DO. Spectrum of disease and relation to place of exposure among ill returned travellers. *N Engl J Med* 2006; 354: 119–30.

Ryan ET, et al. Illness after international travel. *N Engl J Med* 2002; 347: 505–16.

Whitty CJM, et al. Malaria: an update on treatment of adults in non-endemic countries. *BMJ* 2006; 333: 241–5.

Wilders-Smith A, Schwartz E. Dengue in travellers. *N Engl Med* 2005; 353: 924–32.

# 85 Acute medical problems in pregnancy and peripartum

---

**TABLE 85.1** Breathlessness/respiratory failure in peripartum period

- Pre-eclampsia/eclampsia (Table 85.4)
- Pulmonary edema due to pre-existing cardiac disease (e.g. mitral stenosis, aortic stenosis)
- Pulmonary edema due to peripartum cardiomyopathy
- Tocolytic-induced (terbutaline, ritodrine, salbutamol) pulmonary edema
- Amniotic fluid embolism
- Venous air embolism
- Aspiration of gastric contents during labor or soon after delivery
- Pneumonia
- Pulmonary embolism

---

**TABLE 85.2** Chest pain/hypotension/cardiac arrest in peripartum period

- Pulmonary embolism
- Coronary dissection
- Acute coronary syndrome due to atherosclerosis
- Aortic dissection
- Peripartum cardiomyopathy
- Amniotic fluid embolism
- Septic shock
- Anaphylactic shock

---

**TABLE 85.3** Headache in pregnancy/peripartum period

- Pre-eclampsia/eclampsia (Table 85.4)
- Hemorrhagic stroke
- Cerebral venous sinus thrombosis
- Migraine

**TABLE 85.4** Pre-eclampsia and eclampsia

| Element | Comment |
|---|---|
| **Recognition** | Hypertension (systolic BP >140 mmHg or diastolic BP >90 mmHg) and proteinuria (1+ or more on dipstick or >300 mg/day) detected for the first time after 20 weeks' gestation (may present postpartum) |
| | Eclampsia is pre-eclampsia complicated by fits |
| **Complications** | Fits (eclampsia) (<1%) |
| | Intracerebral hemorrhage (rare) |
| | Pulmonary edema/aspiration (2–5%) |
| | Renal failure (acute tubular necrosis/renal cortical necrosis) (1–5%) |
| | Disseminated intravascular coagulopation/HELPP syndrome (hemolysis, elevated liver enzymes, low platelet count) (10–20%) |
| | Liver failure or hemorrhage (<1%) |
| | Placental abruption (1–4%) |
| | Preterm delivery/fetal growth restriction/perinatal death |
| **Management** | If pre-eclampsia is suspected, seek urgent advice from an obstetrician |
| | Management includes: |
| | • Control of severe hypertension (with labetalol or nifedipine) |
| | • Magnesium to prevent/treat fits |
| | • Delivery of fetus |

From Sibai, B. et al. Pre-eclampsia. *Lancet* 2005; **365**: 785–99.

**TABLE 85.5** Thrombocytopenia in pregnancy/postpartum

| Cause | Comment |
|---|---|
| **Gestational thrombocytopenia** | Incidence is ~5% of pregnancies<br>May be mild form of ITP<br>Diagnosed when there is:<br>• Mild thrombocytopenia (platelet count typically >70 × 10$^9$/L)<br>• No past history of thrombocytopenia (except during a previous pregnancy)<br>• No other cause for thrombocytopenia is evident<br>• Spontaneous resolution after delivery |
| **Immune thrombocytopenic purpura (ITP)** | ITP is more likely than gestational thrombocytopenia if thrombocytopenia occurs during early pregnancy or if the platelet count is <50 × 10$^9$/L<br>Exclude other causes of thrombocytopenia<br>Discuss management with a hematologist |
| **HELPP syndrome (hemolysis, elevated liver enzymes, low platelet count)** | Usually complicates severe pre-eclampsia (Table 85.4), although 15–20% of patients do not have antecedent hypertension or proteinuria<br>Features are:<br>• Microangiopathic hemolytic anemia<br>• Serum LDH >600 units/L<br>• Serum AST >70 units/L<br>• Platelet count <100 × 10$^9$/L<br>Management is as for pre-eclampsia<br>*Continued* |

Acute medical problems in pregnancy and peripartum

| Cause | Comment |
|---|---|
| **Thrombotic thrombocytopenic purpura (TTP, p. 502)** | Rare disorder characterized by thrombocytopenia and microangiopathic hemolytic anemia<br>Usually occurs in late pregnancy or in the postpartum period<br>Features supporting diagnosis of TTP rather than HELPP syndrome:<br>• Absence of preceding hypertension/proteinuria<br>• Severe thrombocytopenia<br>• Absence of liver function abnormalities<br>• Normal prothrombin and activated partial thromboplastin times<br>Treatment is with plasma exchange<br>TTP is not improved by delivery of fetus |
| **Disseminated intravascular coagulation (DIC, p. 503)** | May be caused by amniotic fluid embolism, placental abruption or sepsis<br>Seek advice from a hematologist<br>Treat underlying disorder<br>Consider blood product replacement and coagulation inhibitor therapy |

AST, aspartate aminotransferase; LDH, lactate dehydrogenase.

## Further reading

Davies S. Amniotic fluid embolus: a review of the literature. *Can J Anaesth* 2001; 48: 88–98.

Duley L, et al. Management of pre-eclampsia. *BMJ* 2006; 332: 463–8.

James PR, Nelson-Piercy C. Management of hypertension before, during, and after pregnancy. *Heart* 2004; 90: 1499–504.

Moore J, Baldisseri MR. Amniotic fluid embolism. *Crit Care Med* 2005; 33(suppl 10): S279–85.

Scarsbrook AF, Gleeson FV. Investigating suspected pulmonary embolism in pregnancy. *BMJ* 2007; 334: 418–19.

Sibai B, et al. Pre-eclampsia. *Lancet* 2005; 365: 785–99.

# 86 Psychiatric problems in acute medicine

**TABLE 86.1** Clinical features of acute confusional state, dementia and acute functional psychosis

| Characteristic | Acute confusional state | Dementia | Acute functional psychosis |
|---|---|---|---|
| **Onset** | Sudden | Insidious | Sudden |
| **Course over 24 h** | Fluctuating, nocturnal exacerbation | Stable | Stable |
| **Consciousness** | Reduced | Clear | Clear |
| **Attention** | Globally disordered | Normal, except in severe cases | May be disordered |
| **Orientation** | Usually impaired | Often impaired | May be impaired |
| **Cognition** | Globally impaired | Globally impaired | May be selectively impaired |
| **Hallucinations** | Usually visual, or visual and auditory | Often absent | Predominantly auditory |
| **Delusions** | Fleeting, poorly systematized | Often absent | Sustained, systematized |

*Continued*

| Characteristic | Acute confusional state | Dementia | Acute functional psychosis |
|---|---|---|---|
| Psychomotor activity | Increased, reduced, or shifting unpredictably | Often normal | Varies from psychomotor retardation to severe hyperactivity |
| Speech | Often incoherent, slow or rapid | Difficulty finding words, perseveration | Normal, slow or rapid |
| Involuntary movements | Often asterixis or coarse tremor | Often absent | Usually absent |
| Physical illness or drug toxicity | One or both present (see Table 20.3) | Often absent | Usually absent |

From Lipowski, Z.J. Delirium in the elderly patient. *N Engl J Med* 1989; **320**: 578–82.

**TABLE 86.2** Management of agitated or aggressive behavior

| Action | Comment |
|---|---|
| Assessment of patient | Obtain background information: age, psychiatric and medical diagnoses, current medication<br>Exclude/treat hypoglycemia (p. 423)<br>If restraint of the patient may be needed, for the safety of the patient and other patients/staff, call for help from trained staff |

*Continued*

| Action | Comment |
|---|---|
| **Behavioral measures and oral therapy** | Behavioral measures should be tried first: 'talking down', reassurance, distraction, seclusion<br>Consider starting/increasing regular oral medication, e.g. lorazepam 1 mg 8-hourly |
| **Drug therapy for rapid tranquillization** | If the patient will not take oral medication, and rapid tranquillization is needed:<br>• Give lorazepam 1 mg IM + haloperidol 5 mg IM (do not mix in the same syringe). Repeat after 30 min if necessary<br>Or<br>• Give diazepam 10 mg IV + haloperidol 5 mg IV (lower doses in frail or elderly patients), over 5 min. Repeat after 10 min if necessary<br>Before administering drugs, make sure the patient is securely restrained to avoid inadvertent injury. Continue restraint until the patient is sedated |
| **Maximum doses in 24 h** | Lorazepam: 4 mg IM or PO<br>Diazepam: 40 mg IV<br>Haloperidol: 18 mg IM/IV or 30 mg PO |
| **Side effects** | Benzodiazepines: hypotension and respiratory depression<br>Haloperidol: confusion, extrapyramidal side effects |
| **Monitoring** | Nurse the patient in the recovery position<br>Ensure the airway is patent (p. 245)<br>Monitor heart rate, blood pressure, respiratory rate and arterial oxygen saturation<br>Give supplemental oxygen if oxygen saturation is <92% (p. 98)<br>Reverse respiratory depression with flumazenil (p. 119) if needed |
| **Further management** | Consider regular oral medication, e.g. haloperidol 2.5–5 mg 8-hourly and/or lorazepam 1 mg 8-hourly<br>Exclude/treat underlying medical problems<br>Seek advice from a psychiatrist |

Psychiatric problems in acute medicine

**TABLE 86.3** Psychiatric assessment of a patient after self-poisoning or deliberate self-harm

- This should be done when the patient has recovered from the physical effects of the poisoning
- Patients at increased risk of suicide and those with overt psychiatric illness should be discussed with a psychiatrist
- Follow-up by the general practitioner or psychiatric services should be arranged before discharge

**Points to be covered in the assessment**
- Circumstances of the overdose: carefully planned, indecisive or impulsive; taken alone or in the presence of another person; action taken to avoid intervention or discovery; suicidal intent admitted?
- Past history of self-poisoning or self-injury; psychiatric history or contact with psychiatric services; alcohol or substance abuse?
- Family history of depression or suicide?
- Social circumstances
- Mental state: evidence of depression or psychosis?

**Characteristics of patients at increased risk of suicide after self-poisoning**
- Middle-aged or elderly male
- Widowed/divorced/separated
- Unemployed
- Living alone
- Chronic physical illness
- Psychiatric illness, especially depression
- Alcohol or substance abuse
- Circumstances of poisoning: massive; planned; taken alone; timed so that intervention or discovery unlikely
- Suicide note written or suicidal intent admitted

Psychiatric problems in acute medicine

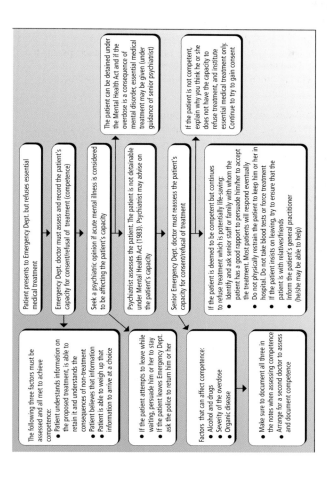

Patient presents to Emergency Dept. but refuses essential medical treatment

Emergency Dept. doctor must assess and record the patient's capacity for consent/refusal of treatment (competence)

Seek a psychiatric opinion if acute mental illness is considered to be affecting the patient's capacity

Psychiatrist assesses the patient. The patient is not detainable under Mental Health Act (1983). Psychiatrist may advise on the patient's capacity

Senior Emergency Dept. doctor must reassess the patient's capacity for consent/refusal of treatment

The patient can be detained under the Mental Health Act and if the overdose is a consequence of mental disorder, essential medical treatment may be given (under guidance of senior psychiatrist)

If the patient is not competent, explain why you think he or she does not have the capacity to refuse treatment, and institute essential medical treatment only. Continue to try to gain consent

The following three factors must be assessed and all met to achieve competence:
- Patient understands information on the proposed treatment, is able to retain it and understands the consequences of non-treatment
- Patient believes that information
- Patient is able to weigh up that information to arrive at a choice

- If the patient attempts to leave while waiting, persuade him or her to stay
- If the patient leaves Emergency Dept. ask the police to return him or her

Factors that can affect competence:
- Alcohol and drugs
- Severity of the overdose
- Organic disease

- Make sure to document all three in the notes when assessing competence
- Arrange for a second doctor to assess and document competence

If the patient is deemed to be competent but continues to refuse treatment which is potentially life-saving:
- Identify and ask senior staff or family with whom the patient has a good rapport to persuade him/her to accept the treatment. Most patients will respond eventually
- Do not physically restrain the patient to keep him or her in hospital. Do not take blood tests or force treatment
- If the patient insists on leaving, try to ensure that the patient is with relatives/friends
- Inform the patient's general practitioner (he/she may be able to help)

FIGURE 86.1 Algorithm for the management of a patient admitted with self poisoning or deliberate self harm who refuses treatment and is at risk of harm. From Hassan, T.B. et al. *BMJ* 1999; **319**: 107–9.

## Further reading

American College of Emergency Physicians. Clinical policy: critical issues in the diagnosis and management of the adult psychiatric patient in the emergency department. *Ann Emerg Med* 2006; 47: 79–99.

Butler C, Zeman AZJ. Neurological syndromes which can be mistaken for psychiatric conditions. *J Neurol Neurosurg Psychiatry* 2005; 76 (suppl I): i31–i38.

Hassan TB, et al. Managing patients with deliberate self harm who refuse treatment in the accident and emergency department. *BMJ* 1999; 319: 107–9.

Skegg K. Self-harm. *Lancet* 2005; 366: 1471–83.

Psychiatric problems in acute medicine

# 87 Alcohol-related problems in acute medicine

**TABLE 87.1** Taking an alcohol history

| Information needed | Questions to ask |
|---|---|
| **Average weekly alcohol consumption and pattern of drinking**<br>• One unit of alcohol equals 10 ml by volume (8 g by weight) of pure alcohol<br>• The percentage alcohol by volume (abv) of any drink equals the number of units in 1 L of that drink (e.g. a bottle (750 ml) of wine (12% abv) contains 9 units)<br>• Hazardous drinking is defined as >4 units/day for men and >2 units/day for women | Do you ever drink alcohol?<br>What do you usually drink?<br>How many times each week do you drink? How much do you have on these occasions?<br>Are there times when you drink more heavily than this? |
| **Is there alcohol dependence?** | Do you drink every day? What time of day is your first drink?<br>If you do not drink for a day or miss your first drink of the day, how do you feel?<br>How would you rate alcohol as one of your priorities? Is it sometimes hard to think of anything else?<br>Have you ever needed medication to stop drinking? |

*Continued*

| Information needed | Questions to ask |
|---|---|
| **Has alcohol caused medical, psychiatric or social problems?** | Has alcohol ever caused you any problems in the past? What were these? |
| | Has anyone close to you expressed worries about your drinking? Did this cause difficulties between you? |
| | Are you concerned about your alcohol use? |
| | Has alcohol ever affected your work or ability to sort things out at home? |
| | Has alcohol ever got you into trouble with the police (e.g. drink-driving offence)? |
| | Is your alcohol use leaving you short of money? |

From McIntosh, C. and Chick, J. Alcohol and the nervous system. *J Neurol Neurosurg Psych* 2004; **75** (III): 16–21.

**TABLE 87.2** Common acute medical problems in the patient who drinks heavily

| System | Problems |
|---|---|
| **Neuropsychiatric** | Alcohol withdrawal syndrome |
| | Major seizures related to alcohol withdrawal |
| | Wernicke encephalopathy (thiamine deficiency) |
| | Polyneuropathy |
| | Depression anxiety |
| | Self-poisoning |
| **Respiratory** | Pneumonia (including aspiration pneumonia) |
| | Smoking-related disorders (~80% of patients with alcohol dependence smoke) |

*Continued*

| System | Problems |
|---|---|
| **Cardiovascular** | Acute atrial fibrillation |
| | Alcoholic cardiomyopathy |
| **Liver and pancreas** | Alcoholic hepatitis (p. 404) |
| | Acute pancreatitis (p. 406) |
| | Cirrhosis |
| **Alimentary tract** | Variceal bleeding |
| | Alcoholic gastritis |
| | Poor diet with consequent vitamin deficiencies |
| **Musculoskeletal** | Myopathy |
| | Fractures |
| **Hematological** | Macrocytosis |
| | Anemia |
| | Thrombocytopenia |
| | Leucopenia |

**TABLE 87.3** Management of alcohol withdrawal syndrome and Wernicke encephalopathy

| Problem | Features | Management |
|---|---|---|
| **Alcohol withdrawal syndrome** | Signs of autonomic hyperactivity (appear within hours of the last drink, usually peaking within 24–48h): tremor, sweating, nausea, vomiting, anxiety, agitation | Manage severe alcohol withdrawal syndrome on the high-dependency unit |
| | Alcohol withdrawal delirium (delirium tremens): acute confusional state, auditory and visual hallucinations, marked autonomic hyperactivity | General supportive measures: fluid replacement if needed; exclusion of hypoglycemia; treatment of intercurrent illness (e.g. pneumonia, alcoholic hepatitis); vitamin supplements (vitamin B compound, strong, two tablets daily, thiamine 100 mg 12-hourly PO, |

*Continued*

Alcohol-related problems in acute medicine

| Problem | Features | Management |
|---|---|---|
| | Delirium tremens may be complicated by hyperthermia, hypovolemia, electrolyte derangement and respiratory infection | and vitamin C 50 mg 12-hourly PO)<br>Mild or moderate withdrawal symptoms: treat with reducing doses of oral chlordiazepoxide<br>Severe withdrawal symptoms: treat initially with IV benzodiazepine (monitor respiratory rate and oxygen saturation) |
| **Seizures related to alcohol withdrawal** | One to six tonic-clonic seizures without focal features which begin within 48 h of stopping drinking<br>May occur up to 7 days after stopping drinking if the patient has been taking benzodiazepines | Usually brief and self-limiting and do not require specific treatment<br>If frequent or prolonged, manage as status epilepticus (p. 349)<br>Exclude/treat hypoglycemia |
| **Wernicke encephalopathy** | Confusional state<br>Nystagmus<br>Sixth nerve palsy (unable to abduct the eye)<br>Ataxia with wide-based gait; may be unable to stand or walk | Treat with IV thiamine (Pabrinex IV high-potency injection, containing thiamine 250 mg per 10 ml (2 ampoules): one pair of ampoules 12-hourly for 5–7 days, given slowly over 10 min (may cause anaphylaxis), followed by oral thiamine |

## Further reading

Brathen G, et al. European Federation of Neurological Societies guideline on the diagnosis and management of alcohol-related seizures (2005). European Federation of Neurological Societies website (http://www.efns.org/content.php?pid=145).

Kosten TR, O'Connor PG. Management of drug and alcohol withdrawal. *N Engl J Med* 2003; 348: 1786–95.

McIntosh C, Chick J. Alcohol and the nervous system. *J Neurol Neurosurg Psychiatry* 2004; 75 (suppl III): iii16–iii21.

Moss M, Burnham EL. Alcohol abuse in the critically ill patient. *Lancet* 2006; 368: 231–42.

Alcohol-related problems in acute medicine

# 88 Hypothermia

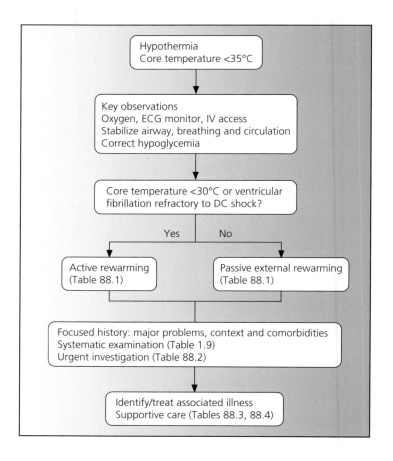

Hypothermia
Core temperature <35°C

↓

Key observations
Oxygen, ECG monitor, IV access
Stabilize airway, breathing and circulation
Correct hypoglycemia

↓

Core temperature <30°C or ventricular
fibrillation refractory to DC shock?

Yes          No

Active rewarming          Passive external rewarming
(Table 88.1)              (Table 88.1)

Focused history: major problems, context and comorbidities
Systematic examination (Table 1.9)
Urgent investigation (Table 88.2)

↓

Identify/treat associated illness
Supportive care (Tables 88.3, 88.4)

**TABLE 88.1** Rewarming methods

| Method | Comment |
|---|---|
| **Passive external rewarming** | Indicated for mild hypothermia (core temperature 32.2–35°C<br><br>Nurse in a side room heated to 20–30°C on a ripple mattress with the blankets supported by a bed cage<br><br>Give warmed, humidified oxygen by facemask<br><br>IV fluids can be warmed (42–44°C)<br><br>Aim for a slow rise in core temperature around 0.5°C per hour |
| **Active rewarming methods** | Indicated for moderate (<32.2–28°C) and severe (<28°C) hypothermia |
| Forced air warming blanket (Bair–Hugger) | Rewarms by blowing air of up to 43°C into a blanket that lies on or surrounds the patient; may be available in theater suite<br><br>Rate of rewarming faster than with passive external rewarming; may result in hypotension |
| Inhalation of warmed oxygen via endotracheal tube | Oxygen is warmed in a waterbath humidifier<br><br>Monitor the gas temperature at the mouth and maintain it around 44°C: this will require modification of most ventilators |
| Other methods of active rewarming | Peritoneal dialysis<br>Esophageal thermal probe<br>Cardiopulmonary bypass |

Hypothermia

---

**TABLE 88.2** Urgent investigation in hypothermia

- Blood glucose (raised blood glucose (10–20 mmol/L) is common (due to insulin resistance) and should not be treated with insulin because of the risk of hypoglycemia on rewarming)
- Sodium, potassium and creatinine (renal failure may be due to hypovolemia/hypotension and rhabdomyolysis)
- Liver function tests
- Full blood count
- C-reactive protein
- Arterial pH and gases (severe hypothermia results in metabolic acidosis)
- Blood culture
- Thyroid function (if age >50 or suspected thyroid disease, p. 464) (for later analysis)
- Blood and urine for toxicology screen if no other cause for hypothermia is evident
- ECG (Fig. 88.1)
- Chest X-ray
- X-ray pelvis and hips if history of a fall or clinical signs of fractured neck of femur

---

**ALERT**
Hypothermia is most often seen in the elderly (usually as a consequence of acute illness) and in those living rough (due to the combination of alcohol and cold exposure).

---

**TABLE 88.3** Management of hypothermia

| Problem | Comment/management |
|---|---|
| **Deranged blood glucose** | Treat hypoglycemia<br>Raised blood glucose (10–20 mmol/L) is common (due to insulin resistance) and should not be treated with insulin because of the risk of hypoglycemia on rewarming |

*Continued*

| Problem | Comment/management |
|---|---|
| **Arrhythmias** | Ventricular fibrillation may occur at core temperatures below 28–30°C. Precipitants include central vein cannulation, chest compression, endotracheal intubation and IV injection of epinephrine. DC countershock may not be effective until core temperature is >30°C. Continue cardiopulmonary resuscitation for longer than usual (as hypothermia protects the brain from ischemic injury)<br><br>Sinus bradycardia does not need treatment: temporary pacing is only indicated for complete heart block<br><br>Atrial fibrillation and other supraventricular arrhythmias are common and usually resolve as core temperature returns to normal |
| **Hypovolemia/hypotension** | Most hypothermic patients are volume depleted (due in part to cold-induced diuresis)<br><br>If chest X-ray does not show pulmonary edema, start an IV infusion of normal saline 1 L over 4 h via a warming coil: further fluid therapy should be guided by the blood pressure, central venous pressure and urine output |
| **Acute renal failure** | Bladder catheter to monitor urine output |
| **Sepsis** | Pneumonia is a common cause and complication of hypothermia: give co-amoxiclav 1.2 g IV or cefotaxime 1 g IV once blood cultures have been taken. Further doses need not be given until the core temperature is >32°C |
| **Cause of hypothermia** | Hypothermia in the elderly is often the consequence of acute illness (e.g. pneumonia, stroke, myocardial infarction, fractured neck of femur)<br><br>Consider poisoning with alcohol or psychotropic drugs if no other cause of hypothermia is evident |

Hypothermia

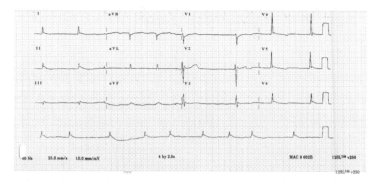

**FIGURE 88.1** ECG in hypothermia (core temperature 30°C) showing bradycardia, prolongation of ECG intervals, and elevation of the J point in the chest leads giving a J or Osborne wave.

**Hypothermia**

---

**TABLE 88.4** Monitoring in hypothermia

**Continuous display**
- ECG
- Arterial oxygen saturation by pulse oximeter

**Check hourly**
- Conscious level (e.g. Glasgow coma scale, p. 297) until fully conscious
- Rectal temperature
- Respiratory rate
- Blood pressure: if systolic BP falls below 100 mmHg reduce the rate of rewarming and give further IV fluid
- Central venous pressure (NB do not put in a central line until core temperature is >30°C as it may precipitate ventricular fibrillation)
- Urine output

**Check 4-hourly**
- Blood glucose

---

## Further reading

Epstein E, Anna K. Accidental hypothermia. *BMJ* 2006; 332: 706–9.

# 89 Drowning and electrical injury

---

**TABLE 89.1** Assessment after drowning

**History**
- Circumstances of drowning
- Time of rescue
- Time of initiation of cardiopulmonary resuscitation
- Time to return of spontaneous circulation
- Time to first spontaneous gasp
- How long in the water?
- Temperature of the water
- Quality of water: clean/contaminated; salt/fresh
- Known illness?

**Examination**
- Key observations (see Table 1.2) and systematic examination (see Table 1.9)
- Head or cervical spine injury?
- Other injuries?

---

**ALERT**
The lungs bear the brunt of injury after drowning.

**ALERT**
Alcohol and substance use may be the cause of ~50% of adult drowning deaths.

---

**TABLE 89.2** Investigation after drowning

- Arterial blood gases and pH
- Chest X-ray
- Blood glucose
- Creatinine and electrolytes
- Urine stick test (?myoglobinuria)
- Full blood count
- Blood alcohol level and toxicology screen (serum (10 ml), urine (50 ml) and gastric aspirate (50 ml)) if cause of drowning is unclear
- X-ray cervical spine if there is neck pain, reduced conscious level or cause of drowning is unclear
- CT head if there are signs of head injury, reduced conscious level or cause of drowning is unclear
- ECG

---

**TABLE 89.3** Management after drowning: degree of immersion injury

| Degree of immersion injury | Features | Management |
|---|---|---|
| **Minor** | Normal conscious level No respiratory symptoms, normal respiratory examination, normal arterial oxygen saturation and blood gases | Observe for 6–8 h, then discharge if remains well |
| **Moderate** | Normal conscious level Hypoxemia corrected by oxygen 35–60% | Admit to high-dependency unit See Table 89.4 |
| **Severe** | Reduced conscious level Hypoxemia not corrected by oxygen 60% | Admit to intensive therapy unit See Table 89.4 |

**TABLE 89.4** Management after drowning: complications of drowning

| Complication of drowning | Comment/management |
|---|---|
| **Respiratory failure**<br>This may be due to:<br>• Airway obstruction (p. 245)<br>• Brain injury<br>• Acute respiratory distress syndrome (ARDS, see Table 29.7)<br>• Pneumonia | If conscious level reduced, check airway for inhaled foreign material and vomitus: bronchoscopy may be needed to clear the airway<br>Endotracheal intubation to protect airway if Glasgow Coma Scale score is 8 or less<br>Give oxygen initially 100%<br>Ventilatory support with non-invasive ventilation (continuous positive airways pressure) or mechanical ventilation with positive end-expiratory pressure may be needed<br>If drowning occurred in contaminated water, start antibiotic therapy with co-amoxiclav 1.2 g IV or cefotaxime 1 g IV (further doses need not be given until the core temperature is >32°C) |
| **Hypoxic-ischemic brain injury** | See Table 56.3 and 56.4 for management of raised intracranial pressure |
| **Hypothermia** | Check core temperature with low-reading rectal thermometer<br>Manage mild hypothermia (core temperature 32.2–35°C) with passive external rewarming, and moderate ( < 32.2–28°C) and severe ( < 28°C) hypothermia with active rewarming (see Table 88.1)<br>*Continued* |

| Complication of drowning | Comment/management |
|---|---|
| Arrhythmias | See Table 88.3 for management of arrhythmias in hypothermia |
| Ingestion of water | If conscious level reduced, place a nasogastric tube to drain the stomach |
| Acute renal failure | Acute tubular necrosis may occur due to hypoxemia, hypotension, or rhabdomyolysis with hemoglobinuria or myoglobinuria See p. 410 for management of acute renal failure |
| Injuries to head, trunk and limbs | Request orthopedic review if there are musculoskeletal injuries |
| Consider underlying disease | Alcohol/substance use Epilepsy Acute coronary syndrome Primary arrhythmia (e.g. congenital long QT syndrome) Diabetes with hypoglycemia Attempted suicide |

**TABLE 89.5** Effects of electrical injury

| Feature | Lightning | High voltage | Low voltage |
|---|---|---|---|
| Voltage, V | >30 × 106 | >1000 | <600 |
| Current, A | >200,000 | <1000 | <240 |
| Duration | Instantaneous | Brief | Prolonged |
| Type of current | DC | DC or AC | Mostly AC |
| Cardiac arrest | Asystole | Ventricular fibrillation | Ventricular fibrillation |

*Continued*

| Feature | Lightning | High voltage | Low voltage |
|---|---|---|---|
| **Respiratory arrest** | Direct CNS injury | Indirect trauma or tetanic contraction of respiratory muscles | Tetanic contraction of respiratory muscles |
| **Muscle contraction** | Single | Single (DC), tetanic (AC) | Tetanic |
| **Burns** | Rare, superficial | Common, deep | Usually superficial |
| **Rhabdomyolysis** | Uncommon | Very common | Common |
| **Blunt injury (cause)** | Blast effect (shock wave) | Fall (muscle contraction) | Fall (uncommon) |
| **Acute mortality** | Very high | Moderate | Low |

AC, alternating current; CNS, central nervous system; DC, direct current.
From Koumbourlis, A.C. Electrical injuries. *Crit Care Med* 2002; **30**: S424–30.

**TABLE 89.6** Investigation after electrical injury

- Blood glucose
- Creatinine and electrolytes
- Creatine kinase (?rhabdomyolysis)
- Troponin
- Urine stick test (?myoglobinuria)
- Full blood count
- Arterial blood gases and pH
- ECG
- Chest X-ray

Drowning and electrical injury

**TABLE 89.7** Management after electrical injury

| Complication of electrical injury | Comment/management |
| --- | --- |
| **Burns** | Seek advice on management from burns unit<br>Patients with burns above the neck may have associated airway/lung injury with respiratory failure |
| **Musculoskeletal injuries** | Refer to orthopedic surgeon<br>Periosteal burns, destruction of bone matrix and osteonecrosis may occur<br>Deep electrothermal tissue injury may result in edema and compartment syndrome |
| **Neurological and ocular injury** | Manifestations of electrical injury include paralysis, autonomic dysfunction, secondary complications such as head or spinal injury, ruptured eardrum, hyphema and vitreous hemorrhage<br>Arrange CT/MRI if there is evidence of neurological injury |
| **Cardiac injury** | Cardiac contusion may occur<br>Incidence of arrhythmia following electrical injury is ~15%, most benign and transient (atrial arrhythmias, first- and second-degree atrioventricular block and bundle branch block)<br>Monitor ECG. Request echocardiography if plasma troponin is raised or if there is significant arrhythmia |
| **Acute renal failure** | May occur due to hypovolemia (from extravasation of fluid) and rhabdomyolysis (from muscle injury)<br>Fluid resuscitation<br>See p. 410 for management of acute renal failure |
| **Injury to abdominal viscera** | Damage is uncommon<br>Refer to general surgeon if suspected |

> **ALERT**
> Vigorous fluid resuscitation is the key to improving the outcome
> after major electrical injury.

## Further reading

Koumbourlis AC. Electrical injuries. *Crit Care Med* 2002; 30: S424–30.
Salomez F, Vincent J-L. Drowning: a review of epidemiology, pathophysiology, treatment
and prevention. *Resuscitation* 2004; 63: 261–8.

# 90 Palliative care

See also Chapter 82.

---

**TABLE 90.1** Goals of care for patients who are dying

**Comfort measures**
*Goal 1* Current medication assessed and non-essentials discontinued
*Goal 2* As required subcutaneous drugs, written up according to protocol
(for pain, agitation, respiratory tract secretions, nausea, vomiting)
*Goal 3* Discontinue inappropriate interventions (e.g. blood tests,
antibiotics, IV fluids or drugs, turning regimens, observations); document
not for cardiopulmonary resuscitation; ICD if present programed off

**Psychological and insight issues**
*Goal 4* Ability to communicate in English assessed as adequate
(translator not needed)
*Goal 5* Insight into condition assessed

**Religious and spiritual support**
*Goal 6* Religious and spiritual needs assessed with patient and family

**Communication with family or others**
*Goal 7* Identify how family or other people involved are to be informed
of patient's impending death
*Goal 8* Family or other people involved should be given relevant
hospital information

**Communication with primary healthcare team**
*Goal 9* General practitioner is aware of patient's condition

**Summary**
*Goal 10* Plan of care explained and discussed with patient and family
*Goal 11* Family or other people involved express understanding of plan
of care

---

ICD, implantable cardioverter-defibrillator.
Adapted from the Liverpool care pathway for the dying patient; from
Ellershaw, J. and Ward, C. Care of the dying patient: the last hours or
days of life. *BMJ* 2003; **326**: 30–4.

**TABLE 90.2** Management of cancer pain: analgesia

- Diagnose the cause (see Tables 82.5, 82.6) and consider specific treatment
- Treat pain symptomatically using the WHO analgesic ladder (see below), combined with adjuvant therapy if indicated (Table 90.3)
- Seek advice from a palliative care physician

| Severity of pain | Management |
|---|---|
| **Mild** | Paracetamol 1 g 6-hourly PO and/or NSAID (e.g. diclofenac SR 75 mg 12-hourly PO)<br>Add an adjuvant if indicated (Table 90.3) |
| **Moderate** | Add an opioid, e.g. codeine 30–60 mg 6-hourly PO<br>Continue paracetamol (e.g. combined with codeine as co-codamol) and/or NSAID<br>Add an adjuvant if indicated (Table 90.3) |
| **Severe** | Substitute a more potent opioid, e.g. morphine:<br>• Give regular 4-hourly doses of 5–10 mg morphine (lower if the patient is elderly, frail, has liver disease or renal impairment) with an extra dose of the same size for breakthrough pain as needed<br>• Review daily requirements after 24–48 h and adjust the regular/breakthrough doses as needed<br>• Once a stable daily dose is established, maintenance should be with controlled release morphine (once or twice daily preparations are available)<br>Continue paracetamol and/or NSAID<br>Add an adjuvant if indicated (Table 90.3)<br>*Continued* |

Palliative care

| Severity of pain | Management |
|---|---|
| **Acute severe pain** | If not taking opioid: give morphine 5–15 mg (5 mg if the patient is small or elderly, 15 mg if large build) IM/SC, repeated 4-hourly and for breakthrough pain as needed<br>If taking opioid: calculate the 4-hourly dose and give the equivalent IM/SC dose (for morphine, one-half the oral dose; for diamorphine, one-third of the oral morphine dose), repeated 4-hourly and for breakthrough pain as needed<br>An antiemetic should also be given (e.g. prochlorperazine or metoclopramide, p. 148) |

NSAID, non-steroidal anti-inflammatory drug; WHO, World Health Organization.

**TABLE 90.3** Management of cancer pain: adjuvant therapies

| Drug | Indication | Dose | Adverse effects |
|---|---|---|---|
| **Non-steroidal anti-inflammatory drugs (NSAIDs)** | Bone metastases<br>Soft tissue infiltration<br>Liver pain<br>Inflammatory pain | E.g. diclofenac 50 mg 8-hourly PO or SR, 75 mg 12-hourly PO, or 100 mg suppository once daily | Gastric irritation and bleeding, fluid retention, headache, renal impairment |

*Continued*

| Drug | Indication | Dose | Adverse effects |
|---|---|---|---|
| **Corticosteroid** | Raised intracranial pressure Nerve compression Soft tissue infiltration Pain from liver metastases | Dexamethasone 8–16 mg daily as single morning dose. Titrate down to lowest dose that controls pain | Gastric irritation if used together with NSAID, fluid retention, confusion, Cushingoid appearance, candidiasis, diabetes |
| **Gabapentin** | Nerve pain of any etiology | 100 mg at night (starting dose) | Mild sedation, tremor, confusion |
| **Amitriptyline** | Nerve pain of any etiology | 10–25 mg at night (starting | Sedation, dizziness, confusion, dry mouth, constipation, urinary retention |
| **Carbamazepine** | Nerve pain of any etiology | 100–200 mg at night (starting dose) | Vertigo, sedation, constipation, rash |
| **Bisphosphonate** | Painful bone metastases | Various regimens | Hypocalcemia, flu-like symptoms |

Palliative care

**Palliative care**

**TABLE 90.4** Management of breathlessness

| Element | Comment |
|---|---|
| **General measures** | Sit the patient up (increases vital capacity and reduces abdominal splinting)<br>Arrange cool airflow over the patient's face with a fan or by opening a window<br>Give oxygen if oxygen saturation is <92%<br>Identify and treat the underlying cause (p. 524) if appropriate<br>Maintain a calm empathic approach and presence |
| **Controlled breathing technique** | Sit the patient up<br>Control the breathing rate<br>Use the lower chest breathing technique<br>Relax the shoulders and upper chest. Massage by a carer from behind can help this, and provides psychological support |
| **Treat anxiety if present** | Lorazepam 0.5–1 mg sublingually can be given acutely |
| **Morphine therapy** | Start with oral morphine 2.5 mg regularly every 4 h, and as required (give 5–10 mg regularly every 4 h and as required, if there has been previous treatment with codeine)<br>After 1–2 days, calculate the total dose given over 24 h, and use this to recalculate the 4-hourly dose: the new 4-hourly and 'as required' dose is one-sixth of the new total daily dose<br>Repeat this process every 1–2 days until breathlessness is controlled<br>Once a stable dose has been reached, this can be converted to once- or twice-daily modified-release morphine |

*Continued*

| Element | Comment |
|---------|---------|
| | If the patient is already on regular (analgesic) morphine: increase the dose of regular morphine by 30–50% every 2–3 days until symptoms are controlled, or adverse effects prevent further dose increases |

**TABLE 90.5** Medication by syringe driver to control symptoms in terminal phase

| Drug | Administration |
|------|----------------|
| **Opioid for control of pain/ breathlessness** | Diamorphine is the opioid of choice for SC infusion<br>Parenteral diamorphine is approximately three times as potent as oral morphine, so the total daily dose of oral morphine should be divided by three to obtain the 24 h dose of diamorphine SC<br>Morphine can be used if diamorphine is not available: total daily dose of oral morphine should be halved to obtain the 24 h dose of morphine SC |
| **Corticosteroid** | Dexamethasone can be given as a single SC dose in the morning, or as a 24 h SC infusion (compatible with diamorphine)<br>1 mg of oral dexamethasone is equivalent to 1.2 mg dexamethasone phosphate or 1.3 mg dexamethasone sodium phosphate<br>The dose should be adjusted to the nearest volume that can be easily measured |

*Continued*

| Drug | Administration |
|------|----------------|
| **Benzodiazepine as anxiolytic** | Midazolam is the anxiolytic of choice for SC infusion<br>Start with 10–20 mg SC over 24 h (compatible with diamorphine) |
| **Other medications as needed, e.g. antiemetic** | Discuss route of administration and compatibility with diamorphine with pharmacist |

## Further reading

Ellershaw J, Ward C. Care of the dying patient: the last hours or days of life. *BMJ* 2003; 326: 30–4.

Morrison RS, Meier DE. Palliative care. *N Engl J Med* 2004; 350: 2582–90.

Murray SA, et al. Illness trajectories and palliative care. *BMJ* 2005; 330: 1007–11.

See also links in Symptom Management, Cancer Specialist Library, NHS National Library for Health (http://www.library.nhs.uk/cancer/SearchResults.aspx?catID=12286).

Palliative care

# Procedures in acute medicine

# 91 Arterial blood gas sampling

---

**TABLE 91.1** Indications for arterial blood gas sampling

**Suspected respiratory failure**
- Arterial oxygen saturation by oximetry <92%
- Respiratory rate <8 or >30/min
- Other clinical features suggesting respiratory failure (see Table 16.1)

**Other cardiopulmonary syndromes and disorders**
- Acute chest pain
- Acute breathlessness
- Hypotension
- Acute pulmonary edema
- Pulmonary embolism
- Pneumonia
- Severe asthma (with $SaO_2$ <92%)
- Exacerbation of chronic obstructive pulmonary disease

**Metabolic disorders**
- Reduced conscious level or coma
- Severe poisoning
- Sepsis
- Diabetic ketoacidosis and hyperosmolar non-ketotic hyperglycemia
- Renal failure
- Liver failure

---

## Technique

**1** Samples may be taken from the radial, brachial or femoral arteries. The radial artery of the non-dominant hand is the preferred site. If you use the brachial artery, the elbow should be fully extended over a pillow to prevent movement of the artery during sampling.

**2** Confirm the indications for the procedure. Explain the procedure to the patient and obtain consent.

**3** Put on gloves. Inject 1 ml of lidocaine 1% into the skin and around the artery using an orange (25 G) needle: pain leads to hyperventilation which will acutely lower arterial $PCO_2$. Sampling should be done with a blue (23 G) needle and a heparinized 5 ml syringe (draw up 1 ml of heparin 1000 units/ml to heparinize the barrel, then expel the excess) or a commercially available preheparinized syringe (again having expelled the excess).

**4** Locate the artery with your index and middle fingers to establish its course. Advance the needle, angled at about 45°, into the segment between your fingers. Sample 3 ml of blood. After removing the needle, put a folded gauze swab over the puncture site; you or an assistant should maintain pressure over the site for 10 min to achieve hemostasis.

**5** Expel any bubbles from the syringe. Remove the needle directly into a disposal bin and cap the syringe. Invert the syringe several times to ensure good mixing of blood and heparin. Analyse the sample within 5 min or transport in a mixture of ice and water for analysis within 30 min. The inspired oxygen concentration should be stated to allow interpretation of arterial $PO_2$.

## Interpreting the results

See Chapters 15–17 for interpretation of arterial blood gases and pH.

## Further reading

Tegtmeyer K, et al. Placement of an arterial line. *N Engl J Med* 2006; 354: e13.

# 92 Central vein cannulation

> **ALERT**
> You should only do central vein cannulation if you are trained in the procedure or are being supervised by someone who is trained. Whenever possible, ultrasound should be used to guide central vein cannulation.

---

**TABLE 92.1** Central vein cannulation: indications, contraindications and potential complications

---

**Indications**
- Measurement of central venous pressure (CVP):
  - Transfusion of large volumes of fluid required (the fluid itself can be given faster via a large-bore peripheral IV cannula)
  - Fluid challenge in patients with oliguria or hypotension
  - To exclude hypovolemia when clinical evidence is equivocal
- Insertion of a temporary pacing lead (see Chapter 93) or pulmonary artery catheter
- Administration of some drugs (e.g. epinephrine, norepinephrine and dopamine) and IV feeding solutions which have to be given via a central vein
- Renal replacement therapy and plasmapheresis
- No suitable peripheral veins for IV infusion

**Contraindications**
- Bleeding disorder (including platelet count $< 50 \times 10^9$/L, INR $> 1.5$, receiving anticoagulant-dose heparin, during or after thrombolytic therapy): discuss management with a hematologist. If central venous access is needed urgently, before the bleeding disorder can be corrected, use the femoral vein in preference to the internal jugular vein

*Continued*

---

**Potential complications**

*During placement*

- Arterial puncture or laceration, which in the case of the carotid artery may lead to hematoma formation in the neck with compromise of the airway
- Pneumothorax (via internal jugular or subclavian vein) or tension pneumothorax
- Hemothorax
- Cardiac tamponade (can be caused by central venous catheter introduced by any route, if its tip lies below the pericardial reflection and it perforates the vessel wall; least likely via internal jugular vein)
- Injury to adjacent nerves
- Air embolism

*After placement*

- Infection
- Venous thrombosis

---

INR, international normalized ratio.

---

**ALERT**

The use of ultrasound to guide central venous cannulation increases the success rate of the procedure from 60% to >90% and reduces the overall complication rate from 30% to less than 10%.

## Assistance/equipment

- One assistant to help with the procedure.
- Ultrasound machine.
- Sterile sheath for ultrasound probe and sterile ultrasound gel.
- Central venous catheter set.

## Choosing the approach

- Cannulation of the internal jugular vein is generally associated with fewer complications than with the subclavian vein, and is the recommended approach in patients with bleeding tendency (because of the risk of uncontrollable bleeding from inadvertent puncture of the subclavian artery) or respiratory disease (because of the greater risk of pneumothorax with subclavian access). The right internal jugular vein is preferable to the left as it is contralateral to the thoracic duct and the circulation of the dominant cerebral hemisphere.

- The femoral vein is a safe route if rapid access is required (e.g. for placement of temporary pacing lead in a hemodynamically unstable patient). Its drawbacks are an increased risk of infection and venous thrombosis.
- An antecubital fossa vein can be used to place a central line for infusions, but manipulation of a pacing lead via this route can be very difficult.
- Use ultrasound to guide central vein cannulation if available and especially if previous access has been difficult or the patient is at risk of complications (e.g. bleeding disorder).

## Ultrasound-guided technique for cannulation of internal jugular vein
### Preparation

1 Confirm the indications for the procedure. Explain the procedure to the patient and obtain consent.

2 Prepare the surroundings: clear the bedside and remove the bed head; ensure adequate lighting; position your trolley, clinical waste bowl and ultrasound device.

3 Prepare the patient: connect an ECG monitor and oxygen saturation monitor; give oxygen via a mask (which will lift the drape off the face); lie the patient flat with the pillow removed, and an absorbent pad under the neck and shoulder.

4 Visualize the internal jugular vein with ultrasound. The vein can be distinguished from the artery by its compressibility and phasic change with respiration (Figs 92.1, 92.2). If the internal jugular vein is relatively flat (i.e. central venous pressure is low), consider either head-down tilt or peripheral IV administration of fluid to increase its size.

5 Open the procedure pack onto the trolley by the bedside. Put on mask, gown and gloves. Prepare the skin with chlorhexidine or povidone-iodine and apply drapes. Put the windowed drape over the target area, and additional drapes to cover the end of the bed and to bridge from the bed to the procedure trolley.

6 Open the sterile sheath for the ultrasound probe. Identify the open (distal) end and place sterile ultrasound gel inside it. Your assistant

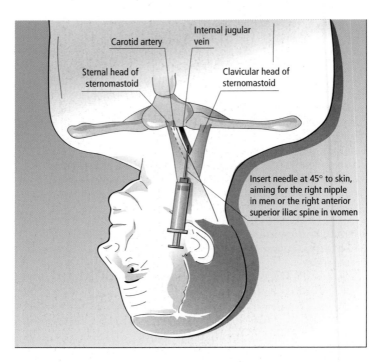

**FIGURE 92.1** Relations of the right internal jugular vein: landmark approach to venepuncture.

**FIGURE 92.2** The appearance of the right internal jugular vein with ultrasound, before (a) and after (b) compression by the ultrasound probe. The vein can be distinguished from the artery by its compressibility. The depth from the skin to the anterior wall of the vein averages 11 mm (range 6–18 mm). The vein is usually 10 mm in diameter, but is narrower in volume-depletion. Head-down tilt or volume loading increases the diameter of the vein and facilitates venepuncture.

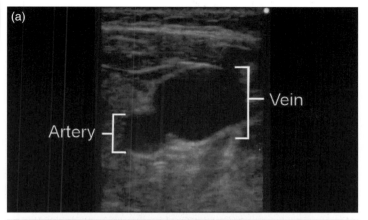

(a)

Vein

Artery

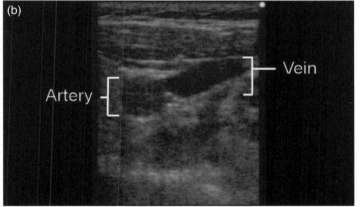

(b)

Vein

Artery

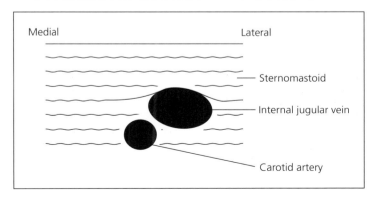

Medial             Lateral

Sternomastoid

Internal jugular vein

Carotid artery

should hold the probe vertically by its cable and lower it into the open end of the sheath. Then unfurl the sheath along the probe and secure the open end over the probe with an elastic band, ensuring that the sheath is flush with the probe face.

**7** Reconfirm the location of the internal jugular vein with the sheathed probe. Assess the distance from the skin to the vein. Plan your vein puncture site and 'upstream' skin puncture site.

**8** Anesthetize the skin with 2 ml of lidocaine 1% using a 25 G (orange) needle. Ensure that the skin bleb will cover the area needed for sutures. Then infiltrate a further 2–3 ml of lidocaine along the planned needle path.

**9** While the local anesthetic is taking effect, prepare the venous catheter. Flush all lumens with normal saline. Leave the central lumen open for passage of the guidewire but cap the other ports. Flush the dilator with normal saline. Ensure the guidewire flows freely from its coil. Prepare a site adjacent to the patient where you can conveniently put the guidewire with the straightener for the J tip in place. Have the skin blade and dilator close to hand.

### Venepuncture

**10** Mount the needle for the central vein puncture on a 10 ml syringe containing 5 ml of normal saline and flush it. Ensure that the needle is not put on too tightly. Taking the probe in your left hand, visualize the vein at the target puncture site.

**11** With the syringe and needle in your right hand, puncture the skin upstream of the probe and then stop. Angle the probe towards the needle and identify the needle artefact. Adjust the needle angle to ensure the artefact is in line with the center of the vein. Slowly advance the needle with continuous gentle aspiration. Monitor and adjust the probe angle to track the needle tip if feasible. Venepuncture is indicated by aspiration of venous blood or visualized puncture of the vein. Stop advancing the needle and re-aspirate to confirm you are in the vein.

**12** Hold the needle steady in position and carefully place the ultrasound probe on a sterile surface. Then use your left hand to stabilize the needle at the skin. Check again by aspiration that the needle is still in the vein. Remove the syringe while supporting the needle. Blood should drip from the needle. If it does not, then cover the hub of the needle with your thumb and use a clean syringe to aspirate venous blood. If blood cannot be aspirated, leave the needle in place and rescan the vein.

## Placing the catheter

**13** Having confirmed you are still in the vein, pick up the guidewire and gently advance it (J end leading) into the needle and vein. Take care not to displace the needle while you are doing this. If resistance is felt, withdraw the guidewire slightly, depress the needle hub to reduce the angle into the vein and try again to pass the wire. If it still will not pass, remove the guidewire and and re-aspirate to check the needle is indeed in the vein. Pass the guidewire to just beyond the 20 cm marking. Withdraw the needle over the guidewire and cover the puncture site with a piece of gauze, held in place with your left hand.

**14** Use the blade to make a short incision along the guidewire at the site of skin puncture to allow passage of the dilator and catheter.

**15** Mount the dilator on the guidewire and advance it with gentle rotation and forward pressure to insert it to a depth of 3–4 cm. There is no need to insert the whole length of the dilator, indeed this may cause complications.

**16** Remove the dilator and again cover the puncture site with gauze. Mount the catheter onto the guidewire and advance it with gentle rotation and forward pressure to insert it to a depth of around 12 cm. Remove the guidewire. Aspirate the central lumen to confirm venous blood and then flush with normal saline. Close the port with a sterile bung. Confirm satisfactory placement of the catheter with ultrasound.

**17** Apply suture wings to the catheter as it exits the skin and suture through each wing hole, taking care that the sutures are placed deeply and not tied too tightly.

**18** Remove the sterile drape from around the catheter and clean the skin with wet gauze to remove any blood. Blot with dry sterile gauze. Use an alcohol swab to clean the skin and the line and when the alcohol has dried, cover the skin puncture site with a bio-occlusive dressing. A second dressing should be used to support the upper part of the catheter.

## Final points

**19** Remove all drapes and sit the patient up. Check that the dressings are satisfactory. Clear up and dispose of sharps safely. Arrange a chest X-ray to confirm the position of the catheter. The tip of the catheter should be at or above the carina to ensure that it lies above the pericardial reflection. Write a note of the procedure in the patient's record, documenting technique (i.e. ultrasound-guided or not), vein

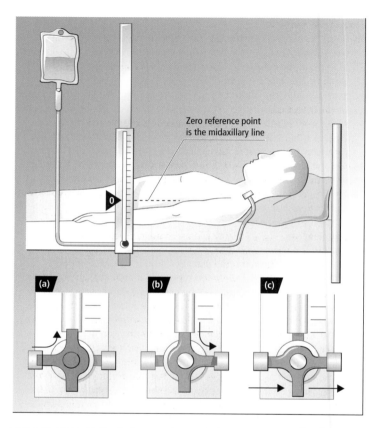

**FIGURE 92.3** Method of measuring central venous pressure (CVP). CVP line with the position of the three-way tap for: (a) priming the manometer; (b) reading the CVP; and (c) fluid infusion. (Redrawn from Davidson, T.I. *Fluid Balance*. Oxford: Blackwell Scientific Publications, 1987.)

used, any complications and postprocedure chest X-ray findings. If the catheter needs to be used immediately, use pressure monitoring to confirm the location is venous and not arterial before any infusion is started (Fig. 92.3).

## Troubleshooting
### Frequent ventricular extrasystoles or ventricular tachycardia during procedure
• May indicate that the tip of the guidewire has passed across the tricuspid valve into the right ventricle: draw it back.

### Catheter infection
• *Staphylococcus aureus* and *Staph. epidermidis* are the commonest pathogens, but infection with Gram-negative rods and fungi may occur in immunocompromised patients.
• If the catheter is obviously infected (tenderness, erythema and purulent discharge at the skin exit site), the catheter must be removed and the tip sent for culture. If the patient is febrile or has other signs of sepsis, take blood cultures (one via the catheter and one from the peripheral vein) and start antibiotic therapy.
• Initial treatment should be with IV vancomycin or teicoplanin (to cover meticillin-resistant *Staph. aureus* (MRSA) plus gentamicin if Gram-negative infection is possible.
• If cultures show *Staph. aureus* infection with bacteremia, IV antistaphylococcal therapy should be given for 2 weeks. For *Staph. epidermidis* and Gram-negative infection, give IV therapy until the patient has been afebrile for 24–48 h. For *Pseudomonas* infection, give IV therapy for 7–10 days. Seek advice from a microbiologist.
• If the catheter is possibly infected (fever or other systemic signs of sepsis, but the skin exit site is clean), take blood cultures (one via the catheter and one from the peripheral vein). The decision to remove the catheter before culture results are back depends on the likelihood of it being infected, how long the catheter has been in and if there is another source of infection. If both blood cultures grow the same organism, the catheter must be removed and antibiotic therapy given as above.

## Landmark-guided technique for cannulation of the femoral vein
**1** Lie the patient flat. The leg should be slightly abducted and externally rotated. Identify the femoral artery below the inguinal ligament: the femoral vein usually lies medially (Fig. 92.4). Shave the groin. Prepare with skin with chlorhexidine or povidone-iodine and apply drapes.
**2** Infiltrate the skin and subcutaneous tissues with 5–10 ml of lidocaine 1%. Nick the skin with a small scalpel blade. Place two fingers of your

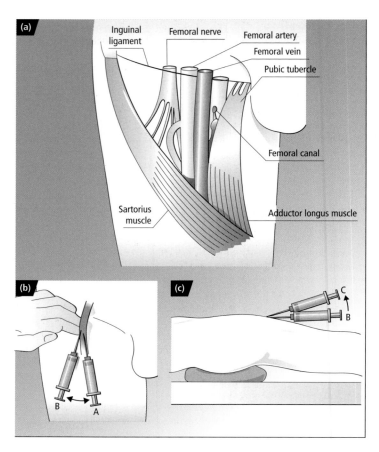

**FIGURE 92.4** Right femoral vein puncture: (a) anatomy of the femoral vein; and (b, c) technique. (From Rosen, M. et al. *Handbook of Percutaneous Central Venous Catheterization*, 2nd edn. London: W.B. Saunders, 1993.)

left hand on the femoral artery to define its position. Holding the syringe in your right hand, place the tip of the needle at the entry site on the skin. Move the syringe slightly laterally, and advance the needle at an angle of around 30° to the skin whilst aspirating for blood. The vein is usually reached 2–4 cm from the skin surface.

**3** If the vein is not found, withdraw slowly whilst aspirating. Flush the needle to make sure it is not blocked. Try again, aiming slightly to the left or right of your initial pass.

## Further reading

Chapman GA, et al. Visualisation of the needle position using ultrasonography. *Anaesthesia* 2006; 61: 148–58.

Higgs ZCJ. The Seldinger technique: 50 years on. *Lancet* 2005; 366: 1407–9.

McGee DC, Gould MK. Preventing complications of central venous catheterization. *N Engl J Med* 2003; 348: 1123–33.

Pittiruti M, et al. Which is the easiest and safest technique for central venous access? A retrospective survey of more than 5,400 cases. *J Vasc Access* 2000; 1: 100–7.

Stonelake PA, Bodenham AR. The carina as a radiological landmark for central venous catheter tip position. *Br J Anaesth* 2006; 96: 335–40.

# 93 Temporary cardiac pacing

**ALERT**
You should only do transvenous cardiac pacing if you are trained in the procedure or are being supervised by someone who is trained. In some cases the risks of temporary pacing outweigh its benefits, and management with a standby external pacing system may be preferable to transvenous pacing.

---

**TABLE 93.1** Temporary cardiac pacing: indications, contraindications and potential complications

**Indications**
- Bradycardia/asystole (sinus or junctional bradycardia or second/third degree atrioventricular (AV) block) associated with hemodynamic compromise and unresponsive to atropine (p. 47)
- After cardiac arrest due to bradycardia/asystole
- To prevent perioperative bradycardia. Temporary pacing is indicated in:
  - Second degree Mobitz type 2 AV block or complete heart block
  - Sinus/junctional bradycardia or second degree Mobitz type I (Wenckebach) AV block or bundle branch block (including bifascicular and trifascicular block) only if there is a history of syncope or presyncope
- Atrial or ventricular overdrive pacing to prevent recurrent monomorphic ventricular tachycardia (p. 22) or polymorphic ventricular tachycardia with preceding QT prolongation (torsade de pointes) (p. 28)

*Continued*

### Contraindications

- Risks of temporary pacing outweigh benefits: e.g. rare symptomatic sinus pauses, or complete heart block with a stable escape rhythm and no hemodynamic compromise. Discuss management with a cardiologist. Consider using standby external pacing system instead of transvenous pacing
- Prosthetic tricuspid valve

### Complications

- Complications of central vein cannulation (p. 589), especially bleeding in patients with acute coronary syndromes treated with thrombolytic therapy (reduced with ultrasound-guided approach, p. 591)
- Cardiac perforation by pacing lead (may rarely result in cardiac tamponade)
- Arrhythmias (including ventricular fibrillation) during placement of pacing lead
- Infection of pacing lead

## Assistance/equipment

- One assistant to help with the procedure and a radiographer to set up and operate the X-ray screening equipment.
- Temporary pacing lead (a 6 French lead is easier to manipulate than a 5 French one but its greater stiffness increases the risk of cardiac perforation).
- Pacing box and connecting lead.
- Central vein cannulation pack, central venous catheter (one French size larger than the pacing lead to be used) and ultrasound device for central vein imaging.
- X-ray screening equipment.

## Technique

### Preparation

1 Confirm the indications for the procedure. Check there is no major contraindication to central vein cannulation. Decide on the route of venous access. Choose the femoral vein in preference to the internal jugular vein if the patient is hemodynamically unstable (especially if you

have limited experience, as placement of the lead via the femoral vein is usually easier) or has received thrombolysis. Ensure that a defibrillator and other resuscitation equipment are to hand.

**2** Explain the procedure to the patient, and obtain consent. Check that the bed is suitable for X-ray screening and that the screening equipment can obtain satisfactory access to the patient.

**3** Connect an ECG monitor (making sure the leads are off the chest, so that they are not confused with the pacing lead when screening) and put in a peripheral venous cannula. Give supplemental oxygen via nasal cannulae or a mask, with continuous monitoring of oxygen saturation by oximetry. If sedation is needed, give midazolam 2 mg (1 mg in the elderly) IV over 30 s, followed after 2 min by increments of 0.5–1 mg if needed (usual range 2.5–7.5 mg).

**4** Put on mask, gown and gloves. Prepare the skin with chlorhexidine or povidone-iodine and apply drapes to a wide area. Unpack the pacing lead and check that it will pass down the central venous catheter.

### Cannulation of a central vein

**5** See Chapter 92.

### Placement of the lead (Figs 93.1–93.3)

**6** Advance the lead into the right atrium and direct it towards the apex of the right ventricle (just medial to the lateral border of the cardiac silhouette): it may cross the tricuspid valve easily.

**7** If you have difficulty, form a loop of lead in the right atrium. With slight rotation and advancement of the wire, the loop should prolapse across the tricuspid valve.

**8** Manipulate the lead so that the tip curves downwards at the apex of the right ventricle and lies in a gentle S-shape within the right atrium and ventricle. Displacement of the lead may occur if there is too much or not enough slack.

**9** Ask your assistant to attach the terminal pins of the pacing lead to the connecting lead and pacing box.

### Checking the threshold

**10** Set the box to 'demand' mode with a pacing rate faster than the intrinsic heart rate. Set the output at 3 V. This should result in a paced rhythm. If it does not, you need to find a better position. Before moving from a position that may have taken a long while to achieve, make sure the problem is not due to loose contacts: check these are all secure.

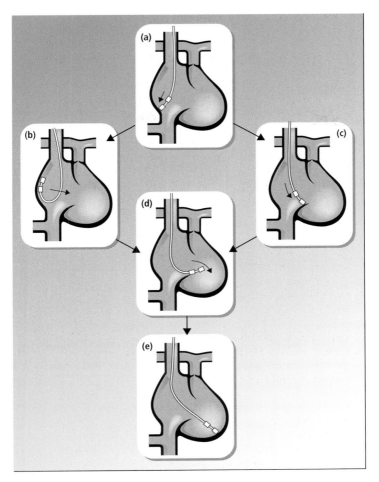

**FIGURE 93.1** Placement of a ventricular pacing lead from the superior vena cava (via the internal jugular or subclavian veins). (a) The lead is advanced to the low right atrium. (b) Further advancement produces a loop or bend in the distal lead, which is then rotated medially. (c) Alternatively, the lead in low right atrium deflects off the tricuspid annulus directly into the right ventricle. (d) Superior orientation of the lead tip in the ventricle requires clockwise torque during advancement to avoid the interventricular septum. (e) Final lead position in the right ventricular apex. The catheter position in (b) is suitable for atrial pacing. From Ellenbogen, K.A. (ed.) *Cardiac Pacing*. Boston: Blackwell Scientific Publications, 1992; 178–9.

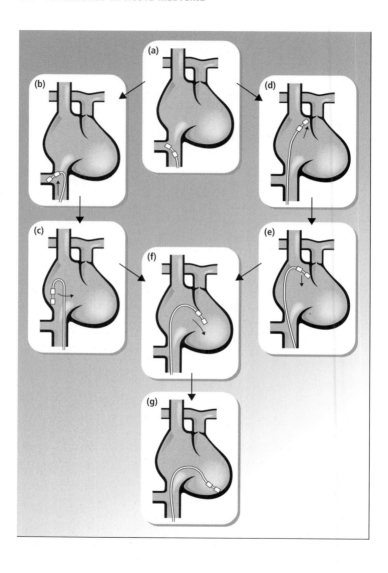

**11** Progressively reduce the output until there is failure to capture: the heart rate drops abruptly and pacing spikes are seen but not followed by paced beats. A threshold of <1 V is ideal. A threshold a little above this is acceptable if the lead position is stable.

**12** Check the stability of the lead position. Set the box at a rate faster than the intrinsic heart rate, with an output of 1 V (or just above threshold). Ask the patient to cough forcefully and breathe deeply. Watch the monitor for loss of capture.

### Final points

**13** Set the output at more than three times the threshold or 3 V, whichever is higher. Set the mode to 'demand'. If the patient is now in sinus rhythm at a rate of >50/min, set a back-up rate of 50/min. If there is atrioventricular block or bradycardia, set at 70–80/min (90–100/min if there is cardiogenic shock).

**14** Remove the insertion sheath, with screening of the lead and counter-advancement if needed to prevent displacement. If the sheath has a hemostatic valve, it can be left in place.

**15** Suture the lead (or sheath if left in place) to the skin close to the point of insertion and cover it with a dressing. The rest of the lead should be looped and fixed to the skin with adhesive tape.

**16** Clear up and dispose of sharps safely. Arrange a chest X-ray to confirm a satisfactory position of the lead and exclude a pneumothorax. Write a procedure note in the patient's record documenting: indications/access/

Temporary cardiac pacing

---

**FIGURE 93.2** Placement of a ventricular pacing lead from the inferior vena cava (via the femoral vein). (a) The lead is advanced to the hepatic vein. (b) The lead tip engages in the proximal hepatic vein and is advanced further. (c) A loop or bend is formed in the distal lead, which is then rotated medially. (d) Alternatively, the lead is advanced to the high medial right atrium. (e) With advancement, a bend is formed in the lead, which is then quickly withdrawn or 'snapped' back to the level of the tricuspid orifice. (f) After crossing the tricuspid valve, the lead is advanced with counterclockwise torque to avoid the interventricular septum. (g) Final lead position in the right ventricular apex. The lead positions in (c) and (d) can be used for atrial pacing. From Ellenbogen, K.A. (ed.) *Cardiac Pacing.* Boston: Blackwell Scientific Publications, 1992; 178–9.

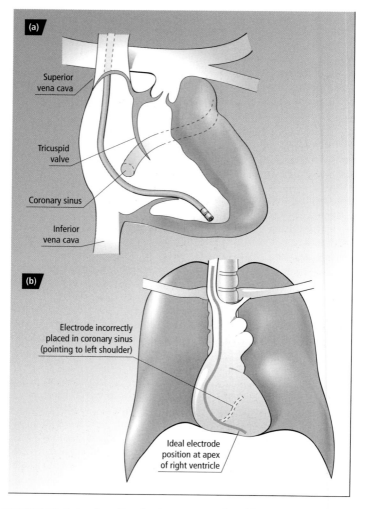

**(a)**

Superior
vena cava

Tricuspid
valve

Coronary sinus

Inferior
vena cava

**(b)**

Electrode incorrectly
placed in coronary sinus
(pointing to left shoulder)

Ideal electrode
position at apex
of right ventricle

**FIGURE 93.3** Lead position for temporary pacing: (a) anatomy; and (b)
screening.

threshold/final pacemaker box settings/any complications/postprocedure chest X-ray findings/plan of management.

## Aftercare

**17** Check the pacing threshold daily. The threshold usually rises to 2–3 times its initial value over the first few days after insertion because of endocardial edema. The commonest reason for failure to capture and/or sense after the procedure is lead displacement.

**18** If infection related to the lead is suspected, see p. 597.

## Troubleshooting
### The pacing lead cannot be advanced into the heart

- This can happen if you have cannulated the carotid artery rather than the internal jugular vein: the pacing lead bounces off the aortic valve. Ask advice from a senior colleague or cardiologist. If inadvertent arterial cannulation is confirmed, withdraw the lead and sheath and apply pressure over the vessel to achieve hemostasis.
- A pacing lead placed via the femoral vein will usually pass easily up the iliac veins and inferior vena cava, with a little manipulation, but may keep diving into other veins. Reducing the curve on the end of the lead may make this less likely to happen.

### Tachyarrhythmias

- Ventricular extrasystoles and non-sustained ventricular tachycardia are common as the lead crosses the tricuspid valve and do not require treatment.
- If there is sustained ventricular tachycardia, withdraw the pacing lead and it will usually terminate.
- Ventricular fibrillation may occur with manipulation of the lead in the right ventricle, especially in patients with acute coronary syndromes, and requires defibrillation and other standard measures (p. 13).
- If ventricular tachycardia recurs after placement, check that the position of the lead is still satisfactory and that excess slack has not formed in the area of the tricuspid valve.

### Causes of failure to capture

- Contacts are not secure: check these.
- Pacing lead not in right ventricle: it may be in the right atrium, in the coronary sinus (a lead in the coronary sinus points towards the left

shoulder) or in the splenic vein (with femoral vein access). Ask advice from a senior colleague or cardiologist.

• Pacing lead has perforated the right ventricle. This may cause pericardial chest pain and diaphragmatic pacing at low output (3V or less). Withdraw the lead and reposition it. Be aware that cardiac tamponade may occur following cardiac perforation but is rare.

## Further reading

Gammage MD. Temporary cardiac pacing. *Heart* 2000; 83: 715–20.

# 94 Pericardial aspiration

**ALERT**
You should only do pericardial aspiraton if you are trained in the
procedure or are being supervised by someone who is trained.

---

**TABLE 94.1** Pericardial aspiration: indications, contraindications and
potential complications

**Indications**
- Cardiac tamponade (p. 216). Echocardiography must be done first to
  confirm the presence of a pericardial effusion unless there is cardiac
  arrest from presumed tamponade
- Pericardial effusion due to suspected bacterial pericarditis (p. 214)
- To establish the cause of a moderate or large pericardial effusion
  when other investigations have failed to do so

**Contraindications**
- Pericardial effusion of less than 2 cm width: discuss management
  with a cardiologist
- Bleeding disorder (including platelet count $<50 \times 10^9$/L, INR >1.5, or
  receiving anticoagulant-dose heparin): discuss management with a
  hematologist

**Potential complications (incidence in patients without
contraindications <5%)**
- Penetration of a cardiac chamber (usually right ventricle) (may result
  in acute tamponade)
- Laceration of a coronary artery (may result in acute tamponade)
- Pneumothorax
- Perforation of stomach or colon (with subcostal approach)

INR, international normalized ratio.

## Assistance/equipment

- One assistant to monitor the patient during the procedure and assist with equipment.
- Echocardiography device (to image pericardial effusion and, if necessary, the guidewire) and echocardiographer.
- Long needle (e.g. 10 cm, 18 G).
- Guidewire (e.g. 80 cm, 0.035" diameter, with J end).
- Dilator (7 French).
- Pigtail catheter (e.g. 40 cm long, 7 French diameter, multiple side holes).
- Drainage bag and connector.
- Sets containing the required kit are commercially available.

## Technique using echocardiography
### Preparation

1 Confirm the indications for the procedure. Check there is no uncorrected bleeding disorder. Blood should be sent for group and save. Ensure that a defibrillator and other resuscitation equipment are to hand.

2 Explain the procedure to the patient and obtain consent. The patient should be propped up so the pericardial effusion pools anteriorly and inferiorly. The two approaches are subcostal and anterior (Fig. 94.1). Choose the approach with the larger width of effusion (should be 2 cm wide or greater, whichever approach is used), and decide on the optimum needle trajectory, avoiding the liver or lung. With the subcostal approach, an entry point in the angle between the xiphisternum and the left costal margin is usually satisfactory, with the needle directed cranially towards the suprasternal notch. With the anterior approach, the entry point should be 3–5 cm from the lateral border of the sternum (avoiding the internal mammary artery) and close to the superior margin of one of the ribs (avoiding the vascular bundle running along the inferior margin of the rib). Measure the depth from the skin surface to the pericardial effusion and mark the planned puncture site with an indelible marker.

3 Connect an ECG monitor and put in a peripheral venous cannula. Give supplemental oxygen via nasal cannulae or a mask, with continous monitoring of oxygen saturation by oximetry. Give sedation with midazolam (2 mg (1 mg in the elderly) IV over 30 s, followed after 2 min by increments of 0.5–1 mg if sedation is not adequate; usual range 2.5–7.5 mg).

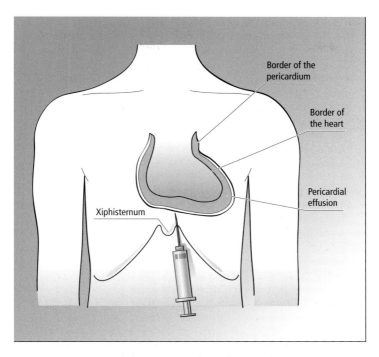

Border of the
pericardium

Border of
the heart

Pericardial
effusion

Xiphisternum

**FIGURE 94.1** Pericardial aspiration: subcostal approach.

4 Put on mask, gown and gloves. Prepare the skin from mid-chest to mid-abdomen with chlorhexidine or povidone-iodine and apply drapes to a wide area.

### Pericardiocentesis
5 Anesthetize the skin at the planned puncture site with a 25 G (orange) needle, and then use a 21 G (green) needle to infiltrate local anesthetic along the intended needle track towards the effusion (Fig. 94.1). With the anterior approach, a green needle is usually long enough to enter the effusion. Allow the local anesthetic time to work and then make a small skin incision at the puncture site.

**6** *Subcostal approach* (Fig. 94.1): attach the long needle to a 10 ml syringe containing lidocaine 1% and advance it slowly along the anesthetized track aiming for the suprasternal notch. Angle it at about 30° so that it passes just under the costal margin. Every centimeter or so, inject some lidocaine and aspirate. *Anterior approach*: attach the long needle to a 10 ml syringe containing saline and advance it slowly towards the effusion, aspirating as you go.

**7** When you aspirate pericardial fluid, advance the needle a couple of millimeters further, then remove the syringe and introduce about 20 cm of the guidewire (J end leading). See section on troubleshooting below if you are not sure whether the fluid is hemorrhagic pericardial effusion or blood.

**8** Pass the dilator over the guidewire to dilate the subcutaneous track and pericardium (taking care not to advance it further into the effusion) and then remove the dilator.

**9** Put the pigtail catheter on the guidewire and advance it over the guidewire and into the pericardial space, so that around 20 cm of the catheter is within the pericardium. It helps to keep the guidewire fairly taut.

**10** Remove the guidewire and aspirate 50 ml or more via the catheter. Take specimens for microscopy, culture and cytology. Attach the connector and drainage bag to the catheter via a three-way tap. If the indication for pericardiocentesis was cardiac tamponade, aspirate as much fluid as possible.

**11** Insert a skin suture and loop it over the catheter several times tying it each time, or use a device to anchor and support the catheter as it exits the skin.

**Final points**

**12** Clear up and dispose of sharps safely. Arrange a chest X-ray to exclude pneumothorax. Check with echocardiography the size of the residual effusion. Write a note of the procedure in the patient's record, documenting: indications/approach/appearance of pericardial fluid/ samples sent/any complications/postprocedure chest X-ray findings/ postprocedure echocardiographic findings/plan of management.

**Aftercare**

**13** Leave the catheter on free drainage. Analgesia may be needed to relieve pericardial pain. Remove the catheter within 72 h to prevent infection.

**14** Further management depends on the etiology of the effusion.

## Troubleshooting
### You cannot enter the effusion
- Check that the diagnosis is correct and that the effusion does not look solid or loculated.
- Consider using an alternative approach (subcostal or anterior), provided the effusion is >2 cm thickness.

### The pigtail catheter will not pass over the guidewire into the pericardial space
- Check that the guidewire is correctly positioned within the cardiac shadow (it can be imaged by echocardiography).
- Check that the guidewire is held taut and not looped.
- Repeat the dilatation of the subcutaneous track.

### You aspirate heavily bloodstained fluid
- The possibilities are: hemorrhagic effusion (common in malignancy or Dressler syndrome); venous puncture; right heart puncture; or laceration of a coronary artery with hemopericardium.
- Keep hold of the needle, but remove the syringe and empty it into a clean pot. Blood will clot, but even heavily blood-stained effusion will not.
- Remove 5 ml more fluid and reinject whilst imaging using echocardiography. The cavity containing the needle tip will be marked by microbubbles.
- If you are still in doubt, compare the hematocrit of the fluid with that of a venous sample (both sent in ethylene diaminetetra-acetic acid (EDTA) tubes), or connect to a pressure monitor: right ventricular penetration is shown by a characteristic waveform.

## Further reading
Tsang TSM, et al. Echocardiographically guided pericardiocentesis: evolution and state-of-the-art technique. *Mayo Clin Proc* 1998; 73: 647–52.

Vayre F, et al. Subxiphoid pericardiocentesis guided by contrast two-dimensional echocardiography in cardiac tamponade: experience of 110 consecutive patients. *Eur J Echocardiography* 2000; 1: 66–71.

Pericardial aspiration

# 95 DC cardioversion

> **ALERT**
> You should only do DC cardioversion if you are trained in the procedure or are being supervised by someone who is trained.

The management of cardiac arrest and tachyarrhythmias is summarized in Chapters 2–7.

---

**TABLE 95.1** DC cardioversion: indications, contraindications and potential complications

**Indications**
- Conversion of ventricular and supraventricular tachyarrhythmias

**Contraindications**
- When another treatment is better (e.g. pharmacological cardioversion) or there is acceptance of supraventricular arrhythmia with rate control. Seek advice from a cardiologist about the management of hemodynamically stable tachyarrhythmias before cardioversion.
- Digoxin toxicity
- Hypokalemia
- Thyrotoxicosis if in atrial fibrillation (cardioversion unlikely to be successful without correction of thyrotoxicosis)

**Potential complications**
- Ventricular fibrillation if the shock is delivered during the vulnerable phase of the cardiac cycle: its delivery should be synchronized with the QRS complex to avoid this
- Bradyarrhythmias postcardioversion
- Interference with settings of permanent pacemakers and implantable cardioverter-defibrillators (these should be checked postcardioversion)
- Embolism of thrombus from the left atrium after cardioversion of atrial fibrillation or flutter
- Complications of general anesthesia
- Skin burns from shocks

---

## Assistance/equipment
- An anesthetist and anesthetic equipment.
- Defibrillator and resuscitation equipment.
- One assistant to monitor the patient and help with equipment.

## Technique in hemodynamically stable patients
### Preparation
**1** Attach an ECG monitor and record a 12-lead ECG. Check the arrhythmia. General aspects of the preparation of the patient before cardioversion of atrial fibrillation or flutter are summarized in Table 95.2. Contact an anesthetist to discuss the anesthetic management and timing of the procedure. Discuss the procedure with the patient and obtain consent.

DC cardioversion

**TABLE 95.2** Checklist before DC cardioversion of hemodynamically stable atrial fibrillation or flutter

| Check | Action |
| --- | --- |
| **Anticoagulation** | Arrythmia reliably known to be of less than 2 days' duration, no structural heart disease and low risk of thromboembolism (see Table 7.3, p. 45):<br>• Anticoagulation with heparin/warfarin is not needed<br>• Consider aspirin 300 mg PO before and for 2 weeks after cardioversion<br>Arrhythmia reliably known to be of less than 2 days' duration, but structural heart disease or moderate/high risk of thromboembolism (Table 7.3, p. 45):<br>• Either postpone cardioversion until fully anticoagulated (as for arrhythmia of >2 days' duration, see below) or<br><br>*Continued* |

| Check | Action |
|---|---|
| | • Consider transesophageal echocardiography to exclude left and right atrial thrombus. If no atrial thrombus is found, cardioversion can be done. Give low molecular weight heparin before and after cardioversion, and continue heparin until warfarin anticoagulation is established with an INR >2.0 *Arrhythmia of uncertain duration or more than 2 days' duration*: <br> • Warfarin anticoagulation should be given with an INR >2.0 for at least 3 weeks before the procedure and on the day of the procedure, and continued for at least 1 month after cardioversion |
| **Plasma potassium** | Check this is >3.5 mmol/L. Correct hypokalemia before cardioversion (p. 447) |
| **Digoxin** | Check that there are no features to suggest toxicity (nausea, slow ventricular response, frequent ventricular extrasystoles) and that if the dose is high (>0.25 mg/day), renal function is normal |
| **Thyroid function** | Check that thyroid function is normal: cardioversion of atrial fibrillation due to thyrotoxicosis (which may be otherwise occult) is unlikely to be successful |
| **Tachybrady syndrome** | Consider placing a temporary pacing lead or having an external pacing system on stand-by, as asystole or severe bradycardia may follow DC cardioversion |
| **Nil by mouth** | Water or clear fluids up to 2 h before anesthesia Food and other drinks up to 6 h before anesthesia |

INR, international normalized ratio.

**2** Put in a peripheral venous cannula, give supplemental oxygen via nasal cannulae or a facemask, and monitor arterial oxygen saturation by oximetry. Check the blood pressure. Check that the defibrillator, resuscitation equipment and drugs are to hand.

**3** Lie the patient down and change the ECG leads from the bedside monitor to the defibrillator. Adjust the leads until the R waves are significantly higher than the T waves and check that the synchronizing marker falls consistently on the QRS complex and not the T wave. Place self-adhesive defibrillator pads or gel pads (for use with hand-held paddle electrodes) on the sternum and over the cardiac apex.

**4** The anesthetist administers general anesthesia or deep sedation.

### Countershock

**5** When the patient is anesthetized, charge the defibrillator and deliver an appropriate charge to cardiovert the arrhythmia (Table 95.3). If the first shock fails to restore a sinus rhythm, deliver a second and if needed a third shock, at higher energy. The operator should call to all staff that

**TABLE 95.3** Cardioversion of arrhythmias: charges

| Arrhythmia | First shock (J) | | Second and third shocks (J) | |
|---|---|---|---|---|
| | **Monophasic** | **Biphasic** | **Monophasic** | **Biphasic** |
| **Ventricular fibrillation or pulseless ventricular tachycardia** | 360 | 200 | 360 | 200 |
| **Other ventricular tachycardias** | 200 | 120–150 | 360 | 200 |
| **Atrial fibrillation** | 200 | 120–150 | 360 | 200 |
| **Atrial flutter** | 100 | 70–120 | 200 | 150 |
| **Other supraventricular arrhythmias** | 100 | 70–120 | 200 | 150 |

the defibrillator is being charged and again before delivering the shock, and should look to make sure that no one is in contact directly or indirectly with the patient before the shock is delivered.

### Aftercare

**6** Record a 12-lead ECG. Consider prophylactic antiarrhythmic therapy to maintain the sinus rhythm. Write a note of the procedure in the patient's record, documenting: indications/anesthetic technique/shocks delivered/any complications/postprocedure rhythm/plan of management.

**7** Continue heparin/warfarin anticoagulation for at least 1 month (or indefinitely if indicated) after successful cardioversion of atrial fibrillation or flutter of more than 48h duration.

## Further reading

Klein AL, et al. Use of transesophageal echocardiography to guide cardioversion in patients with atrial fibrillation. *N Engl J Med* 2001; 344: 1411–20.

Stellbrink C, et al. Safety and efficacy of enoxaparin compared with unfractionated heparin and oral anticoagulants for prevention of thromboembolic complications in cardioversion of nonvalvular atrial fibrillation: the Anticoagulation in Cardioversion using Enoxaparin (ACE) trial. *Circulation* 2004; 109: 997–1003.

See also Resuscitation Council (UK) website (http://www.resus.org.uk/pages/faqDefib. htm).

# 96 Insertion of a chest drain

**ALERT**
You should only insert a chest drain if you are trained in the procedure or are being supervised by someone who is trained. Whenever possible, the decision to place a chest drain, and the type of drain to be used, should be discussed with a thoracic surgeon or chest physician.

---

**TABLE 96.1** Insertion of a chest drain: indications, contraindications and potential complications

**Indications**
- Drainage of a large symptomatic pneumothorax (p. 280)
- Drainage of a pneumothorax of any size in a patient receiving mechanical ventilation
- Drainage of a large pleural effusion causing dyspnea
- Drainage of a complicated parapneumonic effusion or empyema

**Contraindications**
- Bleeding disorder (including platelet count $< 50 \times 10^9$/L, INR > 1.5, receiving anticoagulant-dose heparin, during or after thrombolytic therapy): discuss management with a hematologist before insertion
- Uncertain diagnosis: confirm that you have not misdiagnosed an emphysematous bulla for a pneumothorax, or lung collapse for a pleural effusion
- Lung adherent to chest wall

*Continued*

**Potential complications**
*During the procedure (<5%)*
- Vasovagal reaction
- Perforation of the lung parenchyma or diaphragm
- Malposition of the chest tube including subcutaneous placement
- Bleeding from a lacerated intercostal artery

*After the procedure (<10%)*
- Clotting, kinking or dislodgement of the chest tube
- Infection at the insertion site and in the pleural space
- Re-expansion pulmonary edema, usually after rapid drainage of large pleural effusion; rare after drainage of pneumothorax

INR, international normalized ratio.

## Assistance/equipment
- One assistant is needed to monitor the patient and assist with the equipment.
- Chest tube of appropriate size (choose a small-bore tube, 10–14 French, for pneumothorax or uncomplicated pleural effusion).
- Pack with appropriate surgical instruments for standard technique, or Seldinger kit.
- Underwater seal.

## Technique
### Preparation
1 Confirm the indications for the procedure. Check the position of the pneumothorax or effusion by examination and inspection of the chest X-ray. Ultrasound can be used to define the location and anatomy of a pleural effusion. Explain the procedure to the patient and obtain consent.
2 Assemble the underwater seal (Fig. 96.1) and check that the connections fit. Choose an appropriate drain, e.g. 10–14 French for a pneumothorax and low viscosity pleural effusions.
3 Connect an ECG monitor and put in a peripheral venous cannula. Give supplemental oxygen via nasal cannulae or a mask, with continous monitoring of oxygen saturation by oximetry. Give sedation with

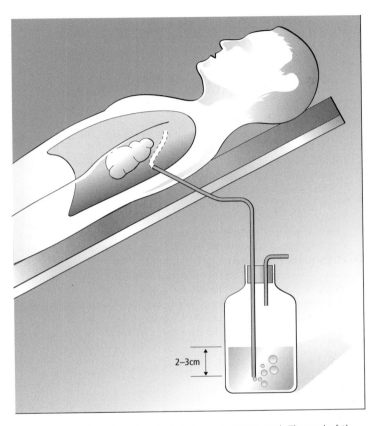

**FIGURE 96.1** Insertion of a chest drain: underwater seal. The end of the tube is 2–3 cm below the level of the water in the bottle. If intrapleural pressure rises above 2–3 cmH$_2$O, air will bubble out. If intrapleural pressure becomes negative, water rises up the tube only to fall again when the intrapleural pressure falls towards atmospheric. The system operates as a simple one-way valve. When the pneumothorax has resolved, the water level will generally be slightly negative throughout the respiratory cycle and reflect the normal fluctuation in intrapleural pressure, and when the patient coughs air will no longer bubble out. (From Brewis, R.A.L. *Lecture Notes on Respiratory Diseases*, 3rd edn. Oxford: Blackwell Scientific Publications, 1985; 290.)

Insertion of a chest drain

2–3 cm

midazolam (2 mg (1 mg in the elderly) IV over 30 s, followed after 2 min by increments of 0.5–1 mg if sedation is not adequate (usual range 2.5–7.5 mg), or opioid premedication IM 1 h before the procedure.

4  Position the patient semirecumbent with the hand resting behind his or her neck (Fig. 96.2). Identify the 5th interspace in the midaxillary line (level with the nipple in a man and the root of the breast in a woman): this is the safest site of insertion. Mark the site with a ballpoint pen.

5  Put on a mask, gown and gloves. Prepare with skin with chlorhexidine or povidone-iodine and apply drapes.

6  Draw up 10 ml of lidocaine 1%. Infiltrate the skin with 2–3 ml using a 25 G (orange) needle, then change to a 21 G (green) needle to infiltrate subcutaneous tissues. Advance the needle into the thorax until air (or effusion) is aspirated, then withdraw slightly and infiltrate about 5 ml around the pleura, leaving a further 2–3 ml in the needle track as you withdraw. If you cannot freely aspirate air or fluid from the pleural space, do not proceed further at this site, and ask advice from a senior colleague.

7  Make a 1–1.5 cm incision with a scalpel in line with and just above the edge of the lower rib of the intercostal space.

8  Place two interrupted 3/0 non-absorbable sutures across the incision. These should be left loose so the tube can pass, and will be tied when

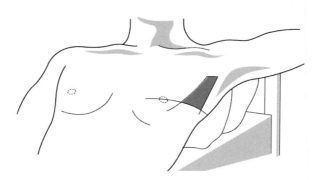

**FIGURE 96.2** The 'safe triangle' for the insertion of a chest drain. (From BTS guidelines for the insertion of a chest drain. *Thorax* 2003; **58** (Suppl. II): ii53–9.)

the tube is removed. Place a 1/0 non-absorbable suture above the incision, which will be used to anchor the tube (Fig. 96.3).

### Standard technique

9  Using a Spencer Wells or similar forceps, enlarge the track down to and through the pleura, so that the tube will pass with a snug fit.

10  Take the tube off the trocar (which should not enter the thoracic cavity) and holding the tip of the tube with the forceps, pass it into the pleural cavity. To drain a pneumothorax, direct the tube towards the apex of the thoracic cavity, until about 25 cm of drain are within the chest. The side holes on the tube must be well within the chest or subcutaneous emphysema will result. To drain an effusion, direct the tube posterobasally.

11  Attach the underwater seal bottle to the chest tube.

12  Anchor the tube with the 1/0 suture wrapped and tied several times around it. Place a pad of gauze between the skin and the tube, and tape the tube to the side of the chest.

Insertion of a chest drain

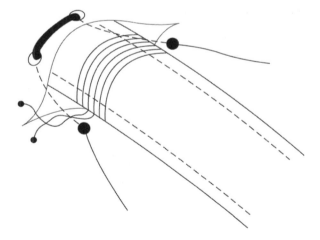

**FIGURE 96.3** Stay and closing sutures for a chest drain. (From BTS guidelines for the insertion of a chest drain. *Thorax* 2003; **58** (Suppl. II): ii53–9.)

### Seldinger technique

**9a** Advance the introducer needle mounted on a 10 ml syringe into the pleural space, and confirm free aspiration of air or effusion. Pass the guidewire, J end first, through the needle into the pleural space, directing it apically for a pneumothorax or posterobasally for an effusion. Remove the needle and then pass the graduated-size dilators in turn over the guidewire to dilate a track for the chest tube.

**10a** Pass the chest tube with its dilator over the guidewire into the pleural space. To drain a pneumothorax, direct the tube towards the apex of the thoracic cavity, until about 25 cm of drain are within the chest. The side holes on the tube must be well within the chest or subcutaneous emphysema will result. To drain an effusion, direct the tube posterobasally. Then remove the guidewire and dilator, leaving the chest tube in place.

**11a** Attach the underwater seal bottle to the chest tube

**12a** Anchor the tube with the 1/0 suture wrapped and tied several times around it. Place a pad of gauze between the skin and the tube, and tape the tube to the side of the chest.

### Final points

**13** Remove the drapes and sit the patient up. Check that the tube is securely anchored and the dressings are satisfactory. Clear up and dispose of sharps safely. Arrange a chest X-ray to check the position of the tube. Write a note of the procedure in the patient's record, documenting: indications/approach/chest tube size/technique/any complications/postprocedure chest X-ray findings/plan of management.

### Aftercare of chest drain placed for pneumothorax

**14** The chest drain should not be clamped unless the underwater seal bottle is being changed or has to be elevated above the patient.

**15** If the lung has not re-expanded on the postprocedure chest X-ray, apply 2.5 kPa suction to the outlet from the underwater seal bottle using a high volume, low pressure pump (e.g. Vernon Thompson pump).

**16** Repeat the chest X-ray the following morning. If the lung is fully re-expanded, and the underwater seal bottle has stopped bubbling:
- Stop suction.
- Wait 24 h and then repeat the chest X-ray.

- If the lung remains fully re-expanded, and there is no bubbling in the underwater seal bottle when the patient coughs, remove the drain.
**17** Consider premedication with morphine/cyclizine IM 1 h before removal of the drain. Take down the dressing. Cut and remove the suture which has anchored the drain. The drain should be briskly withdrawn while the patient performs a Valsalva maneuver or during expiration. An assistant should hold a gauze swab over the incision while you tie the two interrupted 3/0 sutures (to be removed after 5 days). Cover the incision with an adhesive dressing.
**18** The patient can be discharged. Arrange follow-up in the chest clinic in 7–10 days, with a repeat chest X-ray taken prior to the appointment.

## Troubleshooting
### Pain
- Pain around the chest incision may occur. Non-steroidal anti-inflammatory drugs (NSAIDs) are usually effective, but initially opioids may be necessary.
- If the pain is distant from the incision, you should check the position of the cannula tip. If it is curled against the interior of the thoracic cavity, withdraw it slightly. There should be about 25 cm of intrathoracic tube in an adult of normal size.

### Fluid level does not swing with breathing
- Tube kinked: this usually occurs because of angulation over the ribs and may be corrected by releasing the dressing. Occasionally it is necessary to withdraw the drain slightly.
- Tube blocked: if the tube is too small, which is the commonest fault, it can easily become blocked by secretions. It should be replaced by a larger one.
- Wrong position: if the drainage holes are wholly or partially extrapleural, which can be diagnosed from the chest film, the tube needs to be removed and another replaced.

### Surgical emphysema
- A little localized subcutaneous air is usual.
- Increasing surgical emphysema may indicate malposition of the tube with a drainage hole in a subcutaneous position; if so, a new tube must be inserted.

Insertion of a chest drain

### Pneumothorax does not resolve
- If the tube is well positioned, of adequate size (the largest that can be comfortably inserted) and not blocked, this indicates a persisting bronchopleural fistula.
- Seek expert advice from a chest physician or thoracic surgeon. Some will resolve with increased suction.

## Further reading
Laws D, et al. British Thoracic Society guidelines for the insertion of a chest drain. *Thorax* 2003; 58 (suppl II): ii53–ii59.

# 97 Lumbar puncture

> **TABLE 97.1** Lumbar puncture: indications, contraindications and potential complications
>
> **Indications**
> - Suspected meningitis (p. 327). If you suspect bacterial meningitis, take blood cultures and start antibiotic therapy immediately (p. 329), before performing lumbar puncture
> - Suspected subarachnoid hemorrhage (p. 321)
> - Suspected Guillain–Barré syndrome (p. 342)
>
> **Contraindications**
> - Reduced level of consciousness
> - Focal neurological signs (long tract or posterior fossa)
> - Papilledema
> - Generalized tonic-clonic seizure in the preceding hour
> - Bleeding disorder (including platelet count $<50 \times 10^9$/L, INR >1.5, or receiving anticoagulant-dose heparin)
>
> **Potential complications** (other than post-lumbar puncture headache, these are rare in patients without contraindications to lumbar puncture)
> - Post-lumbar puncture headache (around 20% patients will experience this)
> - Cerebral herniation in patients with raised intracranial pressure
> - Injury to nerve roots, causing radicular pain/sensory loss
> - Bleeding causing spinal cord injury
> - Meningitis due to introduction of infection
>
> INR, international normalized ratio.

**ALERT**
Lumbar puncture may be performed in patients with contraindications, but not before you have obtained expert advice from a neurologist or neurosurgeon.

## Assistance/equipment
- One assistant to monitor the patient during the procedure and assist with equipment.
- Spinal needle: choose a 20 or 22 G needle (for accurate measurement of opening pressure).
- Manometer and three-way tap.
- Three plain sterile containers (numbered) and a fluoride tube for glucose (to be sent with a blood glucose sample, taken before the lumbar puncture).

## Technique
### Preparation

**1** Confirm the indications for the procedure and check there are no contraindications. Explain the procedure to the patient and obtain consent. If sedation is needed, give midazolam 2 mg (1 mg in the elderly) IV over 30 s, followed after 2 min by increments of 0.5–1 mg if needed (usual range 2.5–7.5 mg). If sedation is given, the patient should receive supplemental oxygen via nasal cannulae or a mask, and arterial oxygen saturation should be monitored by pulse oximetry.

**2** Move the patient to the edge of the bed on the left side if you are right handed (Fig. 97.1). The thoracolumbar spine should be maximally flexed. It does not matter if the neck is not flexed. Place a pillow between the knees to prevent torsion of the spine.

**3** Define the plane of the iliac crests which runs through L3/L4. The spinal cord in the adult ends at the level of L1/L2. Choose either the L3/L4 or L4/L5 spaces. Mark the space using your thumbnail or an indelible marker.

**4** Put on gloves. Prepare the skin with chlorhexidine or povidone-iodine over the intended puncture site and surrounding area, and apply a drape. It helps to place an additional drape on top of the patient so that you can recheck the position of the iliac crest if necessary.

**5** Draw up lidocaine 1%, assemble the manometer and undo the tops of the bottles. Check that the stylet of the needle moves freely. Place everything within easy reach.

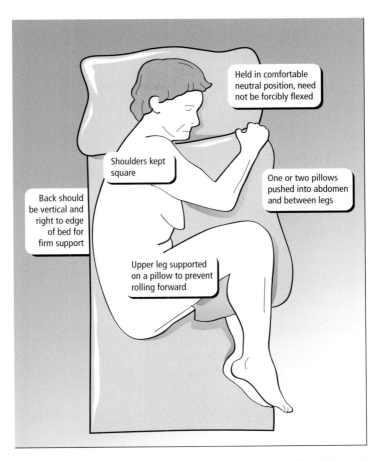

**FIGURE 97.1** Positioning the patient for lumbar puncture. (From Patten, J. *Neurological Differential Diagnosis*. London: Harold Starke, 1977; 262.)

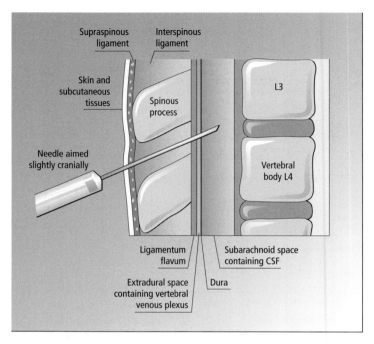

**FIGURE 97.2** Anatomy of lumbar puncture.

### Lumbar puncture

**6** Stretch the skin over the chosen space with the finger and thumb of your left hand, placed on the spinous processes of the adjacent vertebrae (Fig. 97.2). Put 1–2 ml of lidocaine in the skin and subcutaneous tissues with a 21 G (orange) needle.

**7** Place the spinal needle on the mark, bevel uppermost, and advance it towards the umbilicus, taking care to keep it parallel to the ground.

**8** The interspinous ligament gives some resistance, and you should notice increased resistance as you go through the tough ligamentum flavum. There is usually an obvious 'give' when the needle is through this. The dura is now only 1–2 mm away. Advance in small steps, withdrawing the stylet after each step.

**9** Cerebrospinal fluid (CSF) should flow freely once you enter the dura. If the flow is poor, rotate the needle in case a nerve root is lying against it.

### Measuring the opening pressure and collecting CSF
**10** Connect the manometer and measure the height of the CSF column (the opening pressure). The patient should uncurl slightly and try to relax at this stage.
**11** Cap the top of the manometer with your finger, disconnect it from the needle and put the CSF in the glucose tube. Collect three samples (about 2 ml each) in the plain sterile bottles.
**12** Remove the needle and place a small dressing over the puncture site.

### Final points
**13** Clear up and dispose of sharps safely. Ensure that the CSF samples are sent promptly to the microbiology laboratory (for red/white cell count, Gram stain, and other tests as indicated: Ziehl–Neelsen stain if suspected tuberculous meningitis, India ink preparation if suspected cryptococcal meningitis, or polymerase chain reaction testing for viral DNA if suspected viral meningitis/encephalitis) and biochemistry laboratory (for protein and glucose concentrations). Write a note of the procedure in the patient's record, documenting: indications/lumbar interspace used/needle size/opening pressure/appearance of CSF/samples sent/any complications.

## Troubleshooting
### You hit bone
- Withdraw the needle. Recheck the patient's position and the bony landmarks. Try again, taking particular care to keep the needle parallel to the ground. If this fails, modify the angle of the needle in the sagittal plane.
- If you are still unsuccessful, try another space or ask a colleague for assistance.

### You obtain heavily blood-stained fluid
- The possibilities are subarachnoid hemorrhage, traumatic tap or puncture of the venous plexus. If the fluid appears to be venous blood (slow ooze) try again in another space, after flushing the needle.

Lumbar puncture

- Subarachnoid hemorrhage results in uniformly blood-stained CSF (as shown by the red cell count in successive samples). Xanthochromia of the supernatant is always found from 12 h to 2 weeks after the bleed; centrifuge the CSF and examine the supernatant by spectrophotometry if available. Otherwise compare against a white background with a 'control' bottle filled with water.

### Deteriorating conscious level after lumbar puncture
- Seek urgent advice from a neurologist or neurosurgeon.
- Give mannitol 20% 100–200 ml (0.5 g/kg) IV over 10 min. Check plasma osmolality: further mannitol may be given until plasma osmolality is 320 mosmol/kg.
- Arrange transfer to the intensive therapy unit in case intubation and ventilation are needed. If intubated, hyperventilate to an arterial $PCO_2$ of 4.0 kPa (30 mmHg).

## Interpreting the results
See Tables 97.2, 97.3.

**TABLE 97.2** Cerebrospinal fluid (CSF): normal values and correction for traumatic tap

| | |
|---|---|
| • Opening pressure: | 7–18 cm CSF |
| • Cell count: | 0–5/mm$^3$, all lymphocytes |
| • Protein concentration: | 0.15–0.45 g/L (15–45 mg/dl) |
| • Glucose concentration: | 2.8–4.2 mmol/L |
| • CSF: blood glucose ratio | >50% |
| • Correction of cell count and protein concentration in traumatic tap: for every 1000 RBC/mm$^3$, subtract 1 WBC/mm$^3$ and 0.015 g/L (15 mg/dl) protein | |

RBC, red blood cells; WBC, white blood cells.
From Normal reference values. *N Engl J Med* 1986; **314**: 39–49.
Gottlieb, A.J. et al. *The whole internist catalog*. Philadelphia: W.B. Saunders, 1980: 127–8.

**TABLE 97.3** Cerebrospinal fluid (CSF) formulae in meningitis and encephalitis

| Element | Pyogenic meningitis | Viral meningitis | Tuberculous meningitis | Cryptococcal meningitis | Viral encephalitis |
|---|---|---|---|---|---|
| White cell count/mm³ | >1000 | <500 | <500 | <150 | <250 |
| Predominant cell type | Polymorphs | Lymphocytes | Lymphocytes | Lymphocytes | Lymphocytes |
| Protein concentration (g/L) | >1.5 | 0.5–1.0 | 1.0–5.0 | 0.5–1.0 | 0.5–1.0 |
| CSF: blood glucose | <50% | >50% | <50% | <50% | >50% |

- The values given are typical, but many exceptions occur
- Red cells may be seen in the CSF in herpes encephalitis, reflecting cerebral necrosis
- Antibiotic therapy substantially changes the CSF formula in pyogenic bacterial meningitis, leading to a fall in cell count, increased proportion of lymphocytes and fall in protein level. However, the low CSF glucose level usually persists

Lumbar puncture

## Further reading

Armon C, Evans RW. Addendum to assessment: prevention of post-lumbar puncture headaches. *Neurology* 2005; 65: 510–12.

Deisenhammer F, et al. Guidelines on routine cerebrospinal fluid analysis. Report from a European Federation of Neurological Societies task force. *Eur J Neurol* 2006; 13: 913–22.

Ellenby MS, et al. Lumbar puncture. *N Engl J Med* 2006; 355: e12.

Lawrence RH. The role of lumbar puncture as a diagnostic tool in 2005. *Crit Care Resusc* 2005; 7: 213–20.

# 98 Aspiration of a knee joint

> **ALERT**
> If you are not familiar with joint aspiration, ask the help of a rheumatologist or orthopedic surgeon.

**TABLE 98.1** Aspiration of a knee joint: indications, contraindications and potential complications

**Indications**
- To confirm or exclude septic arthritis
- To establish the diagnosis in acute mono- or polyarthritis (p. 473)
- To relieve symptoms from a tense effusion

**Contraindications**
- Cellulitis of overlying skin
- Bleeding disorder (including platelet count $<50 \times 10^9$/L, INR >1.5, or receiving anticoagulant-dose heparin): discuss management with a hematologist

**Potential complications**
- Introduction of infection: rarely occurs (<1/10,000) with appropriate sterile technique
- Bleeding into the joint in patients with bleeding disorder
- Cartilage injury

INR, international normalized ratio.

## Technique

**1** Confirm the indications for joint aspiration. Explain the procedure to the patient and obtain consent.

**2** The patient should lie down with the knee slightly flexed. The knee joint can be aspirated from the medial or lateral side. The needle should pass from a skin entry point 1 cm medial or lateral to the superior third of the patella towards the intracondylar notch. Check the bony landmarks and mark the skin entry point with a ballpoint pen.

**3** Put on gloves. Prepare the skin with chlorhexidine or povidone-iodine and apply drapes. Anesthetize the skin with 2 ml of lidocaine 1% using a 25 G (orange) needle. Then infiltrate a further 5 ml of lidocaine along the planned needle path.

**4** Give the local anesthetic time to work. Mount a 21 G (green) needle on a 20 ml syringe and then advance along the anesthetized path, directing the needle behind the patella and towards the intracondylar notch. Aspirate as you advance.

**5** When you enter the effusion, hold the needle steady and aspirate to dryness (two syringes may be needed if the effusion is large). Remove the needle and place a small dressing over the puncture site. Send samples of the effusion for analysis: ethylene diaminetetra-acetic acid (EDTA) tube for white cell count; plain sterile container for Gram stain and culture; plain sterile container for microscopy for crystals.

**6** Clear up and dispose of sharps safely. Write a note of the procedure in the patient's record: approach/appearance of synovial fluid/volume aspirated/samples sent. Ensure the samples are sent promptly for analysis.

## Troubleshooting

### Dry tap

- This may be due to misdiagnosis of effusion, or obesity with resulting difficulty in accurately identifying the bony landmarks.
- Try again from the lateral approach if the medial approach was used, and vice versa.
- If you still cannot obtain fluid, and septic arthritis needs to be excluded, use ultrasound to confirm the presence of the effusion and identify the appropriate puncture site and depth of needle insertion.

## Interpreting the results

See Table 98.2.

## Further reading

Thomsen TW. Arthrocentesis of the knee. *N Engl J Med* 2006; 354: e19.

Aspiration of a knee joint

**TABLE 98.2** Classification of joint effusions

| Classification of effusion | Features | White cell count | Causes |
|---|---|---|---|
| Normal synovial fluid | Clear, colorless, viscous | $<200/mm^3$<br><25% polymorphs | |
| Non-inflammatory | Clear, yellow, viscous | $200-2000/mm^3$<br><25% polymorphs | Common: osteoarthritis, trauma<br>Uncommon: osteochondritis dissecans, neuropathic arthropathy, subsiding or early inflammation, hypertrophic osteoarthropathy, pigmented villonodular synovitis |
| Inflammatory | Cloudy, yellow, watery | $2000-100,000/mm^3$<br>>50% polymorphs | Common: rheumatoid arthritis, acute crystal-induced synovitis<br>Uncommon: Reiter syndrome, ankylosing spondylitis, psoriatic arthritis, arthritis associated with inflammatory bowel disease, rheumatic fever, systemic lupus erythematosus, hypertrophic osteoarthropathy, scleroderma |
| Septic | Purulent | $>80,000/mm^3$<br>>75% polymorphs | Common: bacterial, myobacterial and fungal infection |
| Hemorrhagic | Blood-stained | | Common: hemophilia or other bleeding disorder, trauma with or without fracture<br>Uncommon: neuropathic arthropathy, pigmented villonodular synovitis, synovioma, hemangioma, other benign neoplasms |

Aspiration of a knee joint

# 99 Insertion of a Sengstaken–Blakemore tube

**ALERT**

A Sengstaken–Blakemore tube should only be used to control life-threatening variceal bleeding. If you have not had experience with its placement and use, it is better to manage the patient conservatively because of the risks of complications.

---

**TABLE 99.1** Insertion of a Sengstaken–Blakemore tube: indications, contraindications and potential complications

**Indications**
- Failure to control variceal bleeding despite pharmacological therapy (p. 370)

**Contraindications**
- If the patient has a reduced conscious level (grade 2 encephalopathy or more), endotracheal intubation should be done by an anesthetist before insertion of the tube to prevent misplacement of the tube in the trachea or inhalation of blood

**Potential complications**
- Inhalation of blood and secretions causing respiratory failure/ pneumonia
- Placement of tube in trachea causing respiratory failure
- Esophageal rupture due to inflation of gastric balloon in the esophagus
- Mucosal ulceration after placement of balloon

## Assistance/equipment

- Two assistants: one to manage the patient, including suction of the oropharynx, the other to help with equipment.
- Sengstaken–Blakemore tube (Fig. 99.1). If this has only three lumens, tape a standard medium-bore nasogastric tube with the perforations just above the esophageal balloon to allow aspiration of the esophagus. The lumens of the tube are not always labeled; if not, label them now with tape.
- Sphygmomanometer (for inflation of the esophageal balloon).
- Water (300 ml) for inflation of gastric balloon (with 10 ml of contrast medium (e.g. Gastrografin) added so you can see where it is). The balloon is less likely to deflate (with consequent displacement) if water is used rather than air (400 ml).
- Bladder syringe for aspirating the esophageal drainage tube.
- Suction equipment.

## Technique
### Preparation

1 If the patient has a reduced conscious level (grade 2 encephalopathy or more), endotracheal intubation should be done by an anesthetist before insertion of the tube to prevent misplacement of the tube in the trachea or inhalation of blood.

2 If the patient has a normal conscious level, explain the procedure and obtain consent. Give supplemental oxygen via nasal cannulae, with monitoring of oxygen saturation by oximetry. Attach an ECG monitor. Sedation with midazolam can be given 2 mg (1 mg in the elderly) IV over 30 s, followed after 2 min by increments of 0.5–1 mg if needed (usual range 2.5–7.5 mg) but only if an anesthetist is available in case endotracheal intubation becomes necessary.

3 Put on apron, mask and gloves. Check the suction equipment works. Anesthetize the patient's throat with lidocaine spray.

### Placement of the tube

4 Lubricate the end of the tube with KY jelly and pass it through the gap between your index and middle fingers placed on the tongue: this reduces the chance of the tube curling. Ask the patient to breathe quietly through his or her mouth throughout the procedure. Steadily advance the tube until it is inserted to the hilt. An assistant should aspirate blood from the mouth and from all lumens while you insert the tube.

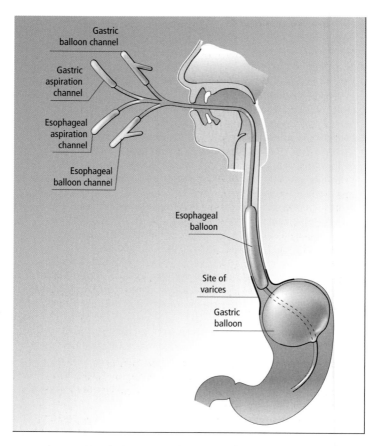

**FIGURE 99.1** Four-lumen Sengstaken–Blakemore tube in place to compress bleeding varices. (From Thompson, R. *Lecture Notes on the Liver*. Oxford: Blackwell Scientific Publications 1985; 37.)

5 If at any stage of the procedure the patient becomes dyspneic, withdraw the tube immediately and start again after endotracheal intubation.

6 Inflate the gastric balloon with the water/contrast mixture (310 ml). Insert a bung or clamp the tube. If there is resistance to inflation,

deflate the balloon and check the position of the tube with X-ray screening. Pull the tube back gently until resistance is felt.

**7** Firm traction on the gastric balloon is usually sufficient to stop the bleeding since this occurs at the filling point of the varices in the lower few centimeters of the esophagus. If not, inflate the esophageal balloon:

- Connect the lumen of the esophageal balloon to a sphygmomanometer via a three-way tap (Fig. 99.2).
- Inflate to 40 mmHg and clamp the tube.
- The esophageal balloon tends to deflate easily so the pressure must be checked every 2 h or so.

**8** Place a sponge pad (as used to support endotracheal tubes in ventilated patients) over the side of the patient's mouth to prevent the tube rubbing. Strap the tube to the cheek. Fixation with weights over the end of the bed is less effective, and may lead to displacement, especially in agitated patients. Mark the tube in relation to the teeth so that movement can be detected more easily.

**9** Obtain a chest X-ray to check the position of the tube. Write a note of the procedure in the patient's record, documenting: monitoring/sedation if given/any complications/postprocedure chest X-ray findings/plan of management.

### Aftercare

**10** It is not necessary to deflate the esophageal balloon every hour as sometimes recommended. Aspirate the esophageal channel every 30 min or more frequently if needed to prevent the accumulation of secretions and to reduce the risk of inhalation.

**11** Continue terlipressin infusion and other supportive therapy (p. 370). If facilities for variceal injection/banding are available, the tube should be removed in the endoscopy suite immediately before this, which can be done as soon as the patient is hemodynamically stable (and usually within 12 h). If endoscopic therapy is not possible, discuss the case with the regional liver unit and arrange transfer if appropriate. Alternatively, start planning for esophageal transection within 24 h if bleeding recurs when the balloon is deflated.

**12** Do not leave the tube in for longer than 24 h because of the risk of mucosal ulceration. Changing the side of the attachment to the cheek every 2 h reduces the risk of skin ulceration, but should be done carefully because of the risk of displacement.

Insertion of a Sengstaken–Blakemore tube

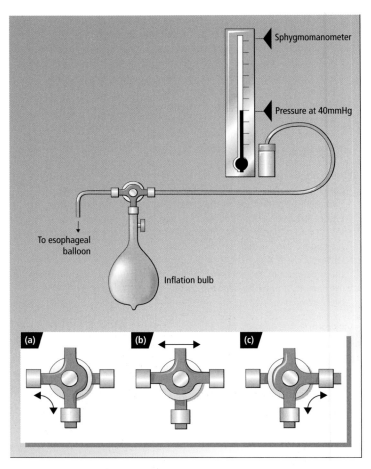

**FIGURE 99.2** Method of filling the esophageal balloon and measuring its pressure. Position of three-way tap: (a) to fill the esophageal balloon; (b) to read the pressure; and (c) maintenance position.

## Further reading

Dearden JC, et al. Does cooling Sengstaken–Blakemore tubes aid insertion? An evidence based approach. *Eur J Gastroenterol Hepatol* 2004; 16: 1229–32. *(The answer is no.)*

# Index